Functional Imaging

Guest Editors

ALEXANDRA J. GOLBY, MD
PETER MCLAREN BLACK, MD, PhD

NEUROSURGERY CLINICS OF NORTH AMERICA

www.neurosurgery.theclinics.com

Consulting Editors

ANDREW T. PARSA, MD, PhD
PAUL C. McCORMICK, MD, MPH

April 2011 • Volume 22 • Number 2

SAUNDERS an imprint of ELSEVIER, Inc.

W.B. SAUNDERS COMPANY

A Division of Elsevier Inc.

1600 John F. Kennedy Blvd. • Suite 1800 • Philadelphia, PA 19103-2899

http://www.theclinics.com

NEUROSURGERY CLINICS OF NORTH AMERICA Volume 22, Number 2
April 2011 ISSN 1042-3680, ISBN-13: 978-1-4557-0472-9

Editor: Jessica Demetriou
Developmental Editor: Donald Mumford

Neurosurgery Clinics of North America (ISSN 1042-3680) is published quarterly by Elsevier Inc., 360 Park Avenue South, New York, NY 10010-1710. Months of issue are January, April, July, and October. Business and Editorial Offices: 1600 John F. Kennedy Blvd., Suite 1800, Philadelphia, PA 19103-2899. Customer Service Office: 11830 Westline Industrial Drive, St. Louis, MO 63146. Periodicals postage paid at New York, NY, and additional mailing offices. Subscription prices are $317.00 per year (US individuals), $492.00 per year (US institutions), $347.00 per year (Canadian individuals), $601.00 per year (Canadian institutions), $443.00 per year (international individuals), $601.00 per year (international institutions), $156.00 per year (US students), and $214.00 per year (international students). International air speed delivery is included in all *Clinics* subscription prices. All prices are subject to change without notice. **POSTMASTER:** Send address changes to *Neurosurgery Clinics of North America*, Elsevier Periodicals Customer Service, 11830 Westline Industrial Drive, St. Louis, MO 63146. **Customer Service: 1-800-654-2452 (US and Canada). From outside the US and Canada, call: 1-314-453-7041. Fax: 1-314-453-5170. E-mail: JournalsCustomerService-usa@elsevier.com (for print support) and journalsonlinesupport-usa@elsevier.com (for online support).**

Reprints. For copies of 100 or more, of articles in this publication, please contact the Commercial Reprints Department, Elsevier Inc., 360 Park Avenue South, New York, NY 10010-1710. Tel. (212) 633-3812; Fax: (212) 462-1935; E-mail: reprints@elsevier.com.

Neurosurgery Clinics of North America is covered in *MEDLINE/PubMed (Index Medicus), EMBASE/Excerpta Medica,* and *Current Contents/Clinical Medicine (CC/CM).*

Printed in the United States of America.

Printed and bound by CPI Group (UK) Ltd, Croydon, CR0 4YY

Transferred to Digital Print 2011

Contributors

CONSULTING EDITORS

ANDREW T. PARSA, MD, PhD
Associate Professor; Principal Investigator,
Brain Tumor Research Center; Reza and
Georgianna Khatib Endowed Chair in Skull
Base Tumor Surgery, Department of
Neurological Surgery, University of California,
San Francisco, San Francisco, California

PAUL C. MCCORMICK, MD, MPH, FACS
Herbert & Linda Gallen Professor of
Neurological Surgery, Department of
Neurological Surgery, Columbia University
Medical Center, New York, New York

GUEST EDITORS

ALEXANDRA J. GOLBY, MD
Associate Professor of Surgery and Radiology,
Harvard Medical School, Departments of
Neurosurgery and Radiology, Brigham and
Women's Hospital, Boston, Massachusetts

PETER MCLAREN BLACK, MD, PhD
Franc D Ingraham Professor of Neurosurgery,
Harvard Medical School, Boston,
Massachusetts

AUTHORS

LINDA S. AGLIO, MD
Associate Professor, Department of
Anesthesia, Harvard Medical School;
Director of Neurophysiologic Monitoring,
Brigham and Women's Hospital, Boston,
Massachusetts

SHAHID BASHIR, PhD
Department of Neurology, Berenson-Allen
Center for Noninvasive Brain Stimulation,
Beth Israel Deaconess Medical Center,
Harvard Medical School, Boston,
Massachusetts

JEFFREY R. BINDER, MD
Professor, Department of Neurology and
Biophysics, Medical College of Wisconsin,
Milwaukee, Wisconsin

NICOLE BRENNAN, BA
Researcher, Functional MRI Laboratory,
Department of Radiology, Memorial
Sloan-Kettering Cancer Center,
New York, New York

EVA CATENACCIO, BA
Research Assistant, Department of Psychiatry,
Functional Neuroimaging Laboratory, Brigham
and Women's Hospital, Harvard Medical
School, Boston, Massachusetts

JACQUES CHIRAS, MD
Department of Neuroradiology, Groupe
Hospitalier Pitié-Salpêtrière, Paris, France

PAMELA DEAVER, MD
Department of Radiology, Brigham and
Women's Hospital, Harvard Medical School,
Boston, Massachusetts

CHRISTINE DELMAIRE, MD, PhD
Centre de NeuroImagerie de
Recherche—CENIR, Groupe Hospitalier
Pitié-Salpêtrière, Paris; Department of
Neuroradiology, CHRU, Lille, France

DYLAN EDWARDS, PhD
Department of Neurology, Berenson-Allen
Center for Noninvasive Brain Stimulation, Beth
Israel Deaconess Medical Center, Harvard
Medical School, Boston, Massachusetts;
Non-Invasive Brain Stimulation and the Human
Motor Control Laboratory, Burke Medical
Research Institute, Inc, New York, New York

JANE EPSTEIN, MD
Lecturer in Psychiatry, Department of
Psychiatry, Functional Neuroimaging
Laboratory, Brigham and Women's
Hospital, Harvard Medical School,
Chestnut Hill, Massachusetts

GARY H. GLOVER, PhD
Professor, Department of Radiology,
Stanford University, Lucas MRI Center,
Stanford, California

ALEXANDRA J. GOLBY, MD
Associate Professor of Surgery and
Radiology, Harvard Medical School,
Departments of Neurosurgery and
Radiology, Brigham and Women's Hospital,
Boston, Massachusetts

LAVERNE D. GUGINO, MD, PhD
Associate Professor, Department of
Anesthesia, Harvard Medical School;
Director of Intraoperative Neurophysiologic
Monitoring, Brigham and Women's
Hospital, Boston, Massachusetts

ANDREI I. HOLODNY, MD
Chief of the Neuroradiology Service, Director,
Functional MRI Laboratory, Department
of Radiology, Memorial Sloan-Kettering
Cancer Center; Professor of Radiology,
Weill Medical College of Cornell University,
New York, New York

LAURA L. HORKY, MD, PhD
Instructor in Radiology, Division of
Nuclear Medicine and Molecular Imaging,
Department of Radiology, Brigham and
Women's Hospital, Harvard Medical School,
Boston, Massachusetts

HUSSEIN KEKHIA, MD
Departments of Neurosurgery and
Radiology, Brigham and Women's
Hospital, Harvard Medical School,
Boston, Massachusetts

DELPHINE LECLERCQ, MD
Centre de NeuroImagerie de
Recherche—CENIR, Groupe Hospitalier
Pitié-Salpêtrière; Department of
Neuroradiology, Groupe Hospitalier
Pitié-Salpêtrière; Centre de Recherche de
l'Institut du Cerveau et de la Moelle épinière
CR-ICM, CNRS, UMR, Paris, France

STÉPHANE LEHÉRICY, MD, PhD
Centre de NeuroImagerie de
Recherche—CENIR, Groupe Hospitalier
Pitié-Salpêtrière; Department of
Neuroradiology, Groupe Hospitalier
Pitié-Salpêtrière; Centre de Recherche de
l'Institut du Cerveau et de la Moelle épinière
CR-ICM, CNRS, UMR, Paris, France

NICOLAS MENJOT DE CHAMPFLEUR, MD
Centre de NeuroImagerie de Recherche—CENIR,
Groupe Hospitalier Pitié-Salpêtrière, Paris;
Department of Neuroradiology, Gui de
Chauliac Hospital, CHU Montpellier,
Montpellier, France

SRINIVASAN MUKUNDAN Jr, PhD, MD
Section Head of Neuroradiology,
Department of Radiology, Brigham and
Women's Hospital; Associate Professor of
Radiology, Harvard Medical School,
Boston, Massachusetts

UMER NAJIB, MD
Department of Neurology, Berenson-Allen
Center for Noninvasive Brain Stimulation,
Beth Israel Deaconess Medical Center,
Harvard Medical School, Boston,
Massachusetts

CHRISTOPHER NIMSKY, MD, PhD
Department of Neurosurgery, University
Marburg, Marburg, Germany

ISAIAH NORTON, BS
Departments of Neurosurgery and Radiology,
Brigham and Women's Hospital, Harvard
Medical School, Boston, Massachusetts

LAUREN J. O'DONNELL, PhD
Laboratory of Mathematics in Imaging (LMI), Department of Radiology; Golby Neurosurgical Brain Mapping Laboratory, Department of Neurosurgery, Brigham and Women's Hospital, Harvard Medical School, Boston, Massachusetts

ALVARO PASCUAL-LEONE, MD, PhD
Department of Neurology, Berenson-Allen Center for Noninvasive Brain Stimulation, Beth Israel Deaconess Medical Center, Harvard Medical School, Boston, Massachusetts; Institut Guttman de Neurorehabilitació, Institut Universitari, Universitat Autonoma de Barcelona, Badalona, Spain

KYUNG K. PECK, PhD
Chief Physicist, Functional MRI Laboratory, Department of Radiology, Memorial Sloan-Kettering Cancer Center, New York, New York

DEISY MARCELA RAMIREZ, MD
Assistant Professor, Department of Psychiatry, Boston University School of Medicine, Boston, Massachusetts

LAURA RIGOLO, MS
Departments of Neurosurgery and Radiology, Brigham and Women's Hospital, Harvard Medical School, Boston, Massachusetts

PETTER RISHOLM, MSc
Department of Radiology, Brigham and Women's Hospital, Harvard Medical School, Boston, Massachusetts

JOSÉ RAFAEL ROMERO, MD
Assistant Professor, Department of Neurology, Boston University School of Medicine, Boston, Massachusetts

ALEXANDER ROTENBERG, MD, PhD
Department of Neurology, Berenson-Allen Center for Noninvasive Brain Stimulation, Beth Israel Deaconess Medical Center, Harvard Medical School; Division of Epilepsy and Clinical Neurophysiology, Department of Neurology, Children's Hospital, Harvard Medical School, Boston, Massachusetts

NINA SHEVZOV-ZEBRUN
Researcher, Functional MRI Laboratory, Department of Radiology, Memorial Sloan-Kettering Cancer Center, New York, New York

EMILY STERN, MD
Director, fMRI Service; Co-Director, Functional and Molecular Neuroimaging, Department of Radiology, Brigham and Women's Hospital, Harvard Medical School, Chestnut Hill, Massachusetts

STEVEN M. STUFFLEBEAM, MD
Athinoula A. Martinos Center for Biomedical Imaging, Department of Radiology, Massachusetts General Hospital, Charlestown; Division of Health Sciences and Technology, Massachusetts Institute of Technology-Harvard University, Cambridge; Department of Radiology, Massachusetts General Hospital, Harvard Medical School, Boston, Massachusetts

S. TED TREVES, MD
Professor of Radiology, Division of Nuclear Medicine and Molecular Imaging, Department of Radiology, Children's Hospital Boston, Boston, Massachusetts

DAVID R. VAGO, PhD
Instructor of Psychology in Psychiatry, Department of Psychiatry, Functional Neuroimaging Laboratory, Brigham and Women's Hospital, Harvard Medical School, Boston, Massachusetts

WILLIAM WELLS III, PhD
Department of Radiology, Brigham and Women's Hospital, Harvard Medical School, Boston, Massachusetts

CARL-FREDRIK WESTIN, PhD
Laboratory of Mathematics in Imaging (LMI), Department of Radiology, Brigham and Women's Hospital, Harvard Medical School, Boston, Massachusetts

Contents

common types of surgical planning that the neurosurgeon faces, including localization of epileptic discharges, determination of the hemispheric dominance of verbal processing, and the ability to locate eloquent cortex. MEG is most useful when it is combined with structural imaging, most commonly with structural magnetic resonance (MR) imaging and MR diffusion imaging. This article reviews the history of clinical MEG, introduces the basic concepts about the biophysics of MEG, and outlines the basic neurosurgical applications of MEG.

Molecular imaging with positron emission tomography (PET) plays an important role in the diagnosis and management of patients with brain tumors and epilepsy. The clinical uses of FDG are discussed, as well as the research applications of novel PET tracers. Where applicable, single-photon emission computed tomography (SPECT) is also discussed.

Diffusion tensor magnetic resonance imaging (DTI) is a relatively new technology that is popular for imaging the white matter of the brain. This article provides a basic and broad overview of DTI to enable the reader to develop an intuitive understanding of these types of data, and an awareness of their strengths and weaknesses.

Image registration is the process of transforming images acquired at different time points, or with different imaging modalities, into the same coordinate system. It is an essential part of any neurosurgical planning and navigation system because it facilitates combining images with important complementary, structural, and functional information to improve the information based on which a surgeon makes critical decisions. Brigham and Women's Hospital (BWH) has been one of the pioneers in developing intraoperative registration methods for aligning preoperative and intraoperative images of the brain. This article presents an overview of intraoperative registration and highlights some recent developments at BWH.

Part II: Applications

Functional magnetic resonance imaging (fMRI) enhances the understanding of neuroanatomy and functions of the brain and is becoming an accepted brain-mapping tool for clinicians, researchers, and basic scientists alike. A noninvasive procedure with no known risks, fMRI has an ever-growing list of clinical applications, including presurgical mapping of motor, language, and memory functions. fMRI benefits patients and allows neurosurgeons to be aware of, and to navigate, the precise location of patient-specific eloquent cortices and structural anomalies from a tumor. Optimizing preoperative fMRI requires tailoring the fMRI paradigm to the patient's clinical situation and understanding the pitfalls of fMRI interpretation.

This article focuses on an important neurosurgical problem for which functional imaging may have a role. Temporal lobe epilepsy surgery typically involves removal of much of the anterior medial temporal lobe, which is critical for encoding and retrieval of long-term episodic memories. Verbal episodic memory decline after left anterior temporal lobe resection occurs in 30% to 60% of such patients. Recent studies show that preoperative fMRI can predict the degree of verbal memory change that will occur, and that fMRI improves prediction accuracy when combined with other routine tests. The predictive power of fMRI appears to be at least as good as the Wada memory test, making fMRI a viable noninvasive alternative to the Wada for preoperative assessment.

Noninvasive brain stimulation is a valuable investigative tool and has potential therapeutic applications in cognitive neuroscience, neurophysiology, psychiatry, and neurology. Transcranial magnetic stimulation (TMS) is particularly useful to establish and map causal brain-behavior relations in motor and nonmotor cortical areas. Neuronavigated TMS is able to provide precise information related to the individual's functional anatomy that can be visualized and used during surgical interventions and critically aid in presurgical planning, reducing the need for riskier and more cumbersome intraoperative or invasive mapping procedures. This article reviews methodological aspects, clinical applications, and future directions of TMS-based mapping.

Diffusion tensor imaging (DTI) tractography is increasingly used in presurgical mapping in tumors located in eloquent areas since it is the only non invasive technique that permits in vivo dissection of white matter tracts. Concordance between the DTI tracts and subcortical electrical intraoperative mapping is high, and DTI tractography has proven useful to guide surgery. However, it presents limitations due to the technique and the tumor, which must be known before using the images in the operative room. This review focuses on the possibilities and limits of DTI imaging in intraoperative tumoral mapping and presents an overview of current knowledge.

Multimodal functional navigation enables removing a tumor close to eloquent brain areas with low postoperative deficits, whereas additional intraoperative imaging ensures that the maximum extent of the resection can be achieved and updates the image data compensating for the effects of brain shift. Intraoperative imaging beyond standard anatomic imaging, that is, intraoperative functional magnetic resonance imaging (fMRI) and especially intraoperative diffusion tensor imaging (DTI), add further safety for complex tumor resections. This article discusses the acquisition of intraoperative fMRI, DTI, and imaging.

Identification of Neural Targets for the Treatment of Psychiatric Disorders: The Role of Functional Neuroimaging   279

David R. Vago, Jane Epstein, Eva Catenaccio, and Emily Stern

Neurosurgical treatment of psychiatric disorders has been influenced by evolving neurobiological models of symptom generation. The advent of functional neuro-imaging and advances in the neurosciences have revolutionized understanding of the functional neuroanatomy of psychiatric disorders. This article reviews neuro-imaging studies of depression from the last 3 decades and describes an emerging neurocircuitry model of mood disorders, focusing on critical circuits of cognition and emotion, particularly those networks involved in the regulation of evaluative, expressive and experiential aspects of emotion. The relevance of this model for neuro-therapeutics is discussed, as well as the role of functional neuroimaging of psychiatric disorders.

Development of a Clinical Functional Magnetic Resonance Imaging Service   307

Laura Rigolo, Emily Stern, Pamela Deaver, Alexandra J. Golby, and Srinivasan Mukundan Jr

One of the limitations of anatomy-based imaging approaches is its relative inability to identify whether specific brain functions may be compromised by the location of brain lesions or contemplated brain surgeries. Of the many techniques available to the surgeon, functional magnetic resonance imaging (fMRI) has become the primary modality of choice because of the ability of MRI to serve as a "one-stop shop" for assessing both anatomy and functionality of the brain. This article discusses the specific requirements for establishing an fMRI program, including specific software and hardware requirements. In addition, the nature of the fMRI CPT codes is discussed.

Neurosurgery Clinics of North America

VISIT THE CLINICS ONLINE!

Access your subscription at:
www.theclinics.com

Preface

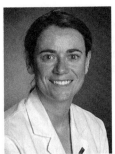

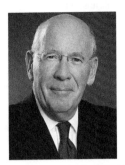

Alexandra J. Golby, MD   Peter McLaren Black, MD, PhD
Guest Editors

The history of neurosurgical progress parallels the development of improved visualization of the brain. From early ventriculography and angiography, to the introduction of the operating microscope, the development of CT and MR imaging, and the increasing adoption of neuronavigation, neurosurgeons have dramatically improved the precision, safety, and effectiveness of brain surgery. Today neurosurgical treatment is increasingly taking advantage of rapid developments in imaging and postprocessing to decrease invasiveness and improve outcomes.

In the last two decades a variety of functional imaging and mapping techniques have been developed which are increasingly able to give surgeons an understanding not only of the complex anatomical relationships of brain lesions, but also of the functional relationship of the lesion to surrounding key cortical areas and white matter structures. Clinical "gold standard" functional studies such as direct electrocortical stimulation testing (ECS) and intracarotid amytal (Wada) testing are now complemented by newer, less invasive techniques, such as functional magnetic resonance imaging (fMRI), transcranial magnetic stimulation (TMS), and others, which are used to map motor, sensory, language, and memory areas. Moreover, it is now possible to map the tracts leading from functional areas through diffusion tensor imaging (DTI).

These techniques are already improving the surgical treatment of patients with brain lesions, including brain tumors, vascular malformations, and epileptic foci. In the future advanced brain mapping techniques will aid the development of more minimally invasive approaches to treating pathology of the CNS by creating a "road map" depicting critical areas noninvasively. Advanced brain mapping may even be able to define new targets for brain modulation, gene therapy, or other treatments. Finally, there are efforts to use techniques such as TMS and real-time fMRI to "rewire" the brain prior to surgery or to help in recovery from neurologic insults.

In this issue of *Neurosurgery Clinics* we are pleased to have brought together experts across a wide range of disciplines related to brain mapping. By their nature, the development of these highly technological brain mapping methods has emerged from cross-disciplinary collaboration. The clinical development of functional brain mapping will further benefit from input by neurophysiologists, radiologists, physicists, and computer scientists. The volume includes in the first section articles on magnetoencephalograpy (MEG), positron emission tomography (PET), fMRI, TMS, and DTI as techniques for brain mapping as well as an article on the important issue of image registration. In the second section it presents the application of these techniques to motor and sensory mapping, memory, intraoperative imaging, and neurosurgical planning. In ordering and interpreting these studies it is essential to understand the physical, physiological, and

Neurosurg Clin N Am 22 (2011) xiii–xiv
doi:10.1016/j.nec.2011.01.005
1042-3680/11/$ – see front matter © 2011 Elsevier Inc. All rights reserved.

psychological underpinnings of the techniques, including, particularly, areas of relative weakness. Differences between the use of brain mapping for neuroscience versus for surgical guidance need also to be borne in mind. Neurosurgeons and other clinicians will have to play a critical role as we move forward in applying the existing techniques, individually and in combination, as well as forthcoming advances, to the particular challenges of neurosurgical patients.

We hope that the articles assembled in this issue of *Neurosurgery Clinics* will serve as a broad overview of, and ready reference to, the rapidly advancing techniques and applications of brain mapping. We look forward to the development of novel therapeutic approaches based on these techniques, which will allow increasing help for many patients suffering from neurologic illnesses.

Alexandra J. Golby, MD
Departments of Neurosurgery and Radiology
Harvard Medical School
Brigham and Women's Hospital
75 Francis Street
Boston, MA 02115, USA

Peter McLaren Black, MD, PhD
Harvard Medical School
25 Shattuck Street
Boston, MA 02115, USA

E-mail addresses:
agolby@partners.org (A.J. Golby)
peter_black@hms.harvard.edu (P. McLaren Black)

Special Surgical Considerations for Functional Brain Mapping

Hussein Kekhia, MD[a,b], Laura Rigolo, MS[a,b],
Isaiah Norton, BS[a,b], Alexandra J. Golby, MD[a,b],*

KEYWORDS

- Surgery • Functional brain mapping • Imaging
- Presurgical planning

To carry out effective and safe neurosurgical interventions for patients with brain lesions, precise information about the unique structural and functional anatomy of that patient is essential. Eloquent cortical areas cannot be recognized solely by identifying known anatomic landmarks even in nonlesional brains.[1–3] In patients with mass lesions or longstanding epilepsy, physical distortion or compensatory reorganization can further alter normal relationships.[4–6] To select patients for surgery, plan the operative approach, and successfully execute the surgical goal, detailed information regarding the individual structural and functional anatomy and the relationship to the lesion is potentially useful. Thus several brain mapping methods that have been developed for neuroscientific brain mapping efforts have been adapted to serve neurosurgical considerations. There are fundamental differences in how these methods are applied to neurosurgical patients and problems. Unlike group studies for neuroscience in which inferences are made about a population based on a sample, neurosurgical planning requires single-subject–specific information, spatial precision, adequate accommodation for impaired task performance, prioritization of sensitivity more than specificity, and robustness in the face of mass lesions. In the last decade, much progress has been made toward fulfilling these needs using several techniques.

This article discusses the particular opportunities and challenges associated with brain mapping as it applies to patient selection, presurgical planning, and intraoperative guidance. The principal methods and their relative strengths and weaknesses are discussed. Approaches for mapping cortical motor, sensory, and language areas are reviewed, as well as the associated white matter connections. Some practical and technical considerations are also discussed, including patient-specific concerns; issues related to data acquisition, analysis, and interpretation; and visualization considerations for planning and intraoperative use. In addition, the specific role of brain mapping in patients with specific pathologic processes including brain tumors, vascular malformations, and medically refractory epilepsy is considered.

This work was supported by the National Institutes of Health (1P41RR019703 and P01-CA67165), the Brain Science Foundation, and the Klarman Family Foundation.
[a] Department of Neurosurgery, Brigham and Women's Hospital, Harvard Medical School, 75 Francis Street, Boston, MA 02115, USA
[b] Department of Radiology, Brigham and Women's Hospital, Harvard Medical School, 75 Francis Street, Boston, MA 02115, USA
* Corresponding author. Department of Neurosurgery, CA 138, Brigham and Women's Hospital, Harvard Medical School, 75 Francis Street, Boston, MA 02115.
E-mail address: AGOLBY@PARTNERS.ORG

Neurosurg Clin N Am 22 (2011) 111–132
doi:10.1016/j.nec.2011.01.004

BRAIN MAPPING TECHNIQUES

Direct cortical stimulation (DCS) and the intracarotid amytal test (IAT) or Wada test are often considered the gold standard procedures for functional mapping and language lateralization, respectively.[7] Their status as gold standard is based on long experience with these procedures as well as the way in which these procedures localize eloquent brain. Both procedures involve deactivation, in which a brain region, either localized in the case of DCS, or nearly hemispheric in the case of IAT, is taken off line, and the patient's neurologic function tested. In this way, the procedures mimic what deficits might be expected after resection. Although these procedures have proved to be effective, they are highly invasive mapping techniques that carry significant risk of morbidity, and which necessitate active patient cooperation during testing. Functionally impaired patients, or those with an altered level of consciousness, may find it difficult to perform the tasks, thus decreasing the value and broad applicability of these procedures. DCS of the gray matter within the depth of the sulci is also usually not readily accessible. Furthermore, DCS is conducted either within the surgical procedure or a short time before it, leaving little time for effective surgical planning or for the contemplation of alternative therapeutic strategies.[8]

Thus, the recent development of less invasive mapping techniques has provided an appealing alternative or adjunct for many neurosurgeons. Most of these techniques map the brain by recruiting the functionality of a particular brain region through a behavioral task (paradigm) and measuring consequent brain changes. For instance, during functional magnetic resonance imaging (fMRI) or magnetoencephalography (MEG), patients are asked to perform a task, such as a language, visual, or movement paradigm, while changes in blood flow, metabolism, or electric activity in activated brain regions is measured. Although this general approach can show all functional brain regions that are involved in the execution of a particular task, it cannot differentiate between brain regions that are essential for execution of the task and those that are merely playing a supportive role. However, inhibition (blocking) methods, like DCS or IAT, temporarily disrupt a specific brain region from functioning, thereby testing for an inducible neurologic deficit. Transcranial magnetic stimulation (TMS) may act as an inhibition method (eg, for language mapping), but more commonly is used for neurosurgical mapping as a direct activator (eg, for motor mapping). This method stimulates a given brain region directly, rather than by engaging the subject in a behavioral paradigm, and can thus depict the causal relationship of the brain tissue in question to the task execution. However, this approach also has limitations. Even direct mapping of the primary motor cortex with TMS may not show all of the areas involved in motor performance. Inhibition methods may fail to show sufficiency. For instance, the disruption of face motor pathways, or even of the temporalis muscle, by TMS could cause speech arrest without interfering with language function per se. In addition, diffusion tensor imaging (DTI) although not a functional mapping study, is able to provide information on the location and trajectory of white matter tracts that may inform interpretation of functional brain areas. Thus, it is critical that the neurosurgeon understands the strengths and weaknesses of each approach to maximize the benefit from presurgical mapping.

Whether the mapping technique is observational, such as positron emission tomography (PET), MEG, or fMRI, an inhibition technique such as TMS, or an advanced structural map such as DTI, these brain mapping modalities are rapidly acquiring an expanded clinical role in the surgical planning phase. Each technique is based on different physiologic properties, thus providing different types of functional maps. Furthermore, each imaging modality is characterized by a specific set of advantages and disadvantages related to spatial and temporal resolution, to the degree of invasiveness, and to the costs of implementation. Combining different functional mapping methods, although resource and time intensive, may provide optimal information by offsetting the strengths of one technique against the weaknesses of another or by integrating functional and structural information. With all of these methods, when used for surgical planning, consideration must be given to sensitivity and specificity: to not miss an eloquent brain region, it is particularly important to avoid false negatives, thus maximizing sensitivity, sometimes at the expense of specificity.

Understanding the physiologic and technical underpinnings of each mapping method is particularly important to use them most effectively for clinical decision making. For example, PET detects the relative position of radioactively labeled compounds within the patient's body, and can thus provide a wide range of functional and physiologic data. PET is emerging as a tool to guide the location of biopsies to avoid sampling error leading to undergrading of tumors that may have heterogeneous histologic characteristics. PET is also frequently used to show areas of interictal hypometabolism associated with epileptogenic foci. Areas being developed include radiotracers targeted to specific receptors, which may eventually guide functional neurosurgery. However, the signal-to-noise ratio (SNR) and temporal resolution of PET are both poor, and the spatial resolution in best-case scenarios is considered to be only moderate. DTI can quantify the magnitude and direction of water diffusion in brain tissue, and is thus able to show the location and trajectory of white matter tracts. However, DTI is vulnerable to signal loss artifacts from air spaces, and provides little information about the functional status of the depicted white matter tract. As routinely deployed, DTI cannot reliably resolve crossing white bundles and can also have difficulty showing tracts with high curvature. However, by combining DTI with fMRI, it may be possible to make inferences about which tracts are important to preserve, based on their physical continuity with cortical areas of interest. MEG non-invasively maps brain activity by measuring changes in the local magnetic fields that accompany neuronal activity. MEG is most commonly used in the presurgical evaluation of epileptic patients. In contrast with PET scanning and DTI, the temporal resolution of MEG is excellent: on the order of 1 millisecond. However, the spatial resolution is variable and dependent on the model used to approximate the source of the signal, and is susceptible to environmental magnetic noise. TMS is an emerging mapping technique that induces neuronal changes by delivering magnetic fields at the scalp that pass unimpeded through the scalp and skull and are able to stimulate the cortex in a manner analogous to DCS. In TMS, electrical activity in a functional brain region may be either stimulated or inhibited depending on the mode of stimulus delivery via a magnetic field change delivered to the scalp. This technique could provide a substantial advantage to the neurosurgeon because it is the only noninvasive modality that can block neuronal function.[8] However, TMS requires dedicated equipment and personnel, has not yet been reliably able to map language function, and may be contraindicated in patients with seizures.[9]

fMRI AS A NONINVASIVE PRESURGICAL MAPPING TECHNIQUE

Presently, the most commonly used functional mapping procedure for surgical planning is fMRI, a functional mapping technique that measures the relative changes in oxygenated and deoxygenated hemoglobin, and thus blood flow, as a surrogate for neuronal activity. Being completely noninvasive and able to be deployed on many clinical magnetic

resonance imaging (MRI) scanners, its clinical role has rapidly expanded. The physiologic information shown by fMRI can be acquired with, and coregistered to, corresponding structural images in a straightforward way. The safety and relative ease with which fMRI can be acquired allows its use not only for planning optimal surgical strategy but also to guide the decision whether to perform surgery and for patient counseling regarding risk. Furthermore, the registration of preoperatively acquired fMRI data into a neuronavigational guidance system can help guide the deployment of intraoperative electrocortical stimulation.[10–14]

WHAT CAN BE EXPECTED FROM FUNCTIONAL MAPPING IN PRESURGICAL PLANNING?

The indications for the use of functional brain mapping continue to evolve as technology develops and becomes more broadly applied. In 1999, Lee and colleagues[15] retrospectively evaluated the effect of fMRI on the treatment plans of 46 patients scheduled for neurosurgical resection of either a tumor or epileptogenic foci. The group determined that fMRI contributed substantially in 3 key areas: (1) allowing the neurosurgeons to assess the risk of inducing a neurologic deficit, allowing them to evaluate the feasibility of the resection; (2) providing substantial neurosurgical guidance by directing the placement of the bone flap or of subdural grids for mapping or electroencephalogram (EEG) recording; and (3) helping to identify patients who required further evaluation through invasive mapping techniques. Overall, the study concluded that fMRI studies were used in at least 1 of the 3 clinical steps in 89% of patients with tumors and 91% of patients with epilepsy. Petrella and colleagues[16] conducted a similar prospective study, analyzing the role of sensorimotor fMRI localization on 39 neuro-oncological patients being evaluated for potential neurosurgical resection. The investigators reported that fMRI altered patient treatment approaches in 49% of patients and allowed the neurosurgeons to further maximize the extent of tumor resection in 45%.

The effect of PET scanning on the neurosurgical treatment of pediatric patients with brain gliomas has also been investigated.[17] The study group concluded that the addition of PET scans into the neuronavigational guidance system substantially improved the diagnostic yield of glioma biopsies, and optimized designated surgical trajectories. In addition, the number of trials needed to reach gliomas situated in remote locations, such as those near the pineal gland, was significantly less when PET scanning was used. The ability of MEG scanning to predict the epileptogenic foci in patients with refractory seizures has been examined and found to be nearly as helpful as intracranial EEG in correctly predicting the epileptogenic foci (MEG, 57%, intracranial video-EEG, 62%).[18]

HOW VALID IS FUNCTIONAL MAPPING FOR SURGICAL PLANNING?

Given the relative newness of the functional mapping methods, there remain numerous issues related to the validity and reliability of the methods in different conditions. One area of note is that several of these methods evolved out of neuroscience efforts, and most publications are related to group results. Functional mapping for neurosurgical planning must inform about individual subjects, and the cost for erroneous results may lead to significant morbidity or, at the other extreme, to undertreatment of a lesion that might be surgically addressed. Thus, ongoing validation of the brain mapping approaches against each other and against the gold standard methods of Wada testing and intraoperative DCS mapping is particularly important. A lot of work has been done examining agreement between mapping approaches and, increasingly, examining effects on patient care.[19–25]

Although fMRI offers substantial advantages to the neurosurgeon, its use in clinical decision making should allow for several technical difficulties. Functional MRI does not assess neural activation directly, but measures the associated variations in the cerebral blood flow using blood oxygen level–dependent (BOLD) contrast on T2*-weighted images. Thus, an intact autoregulatory response is required for proper signal interpretation. Pathologic processes in the brain that disrupt the neural hemodynamic coupling may alter the concordance between neural activity and the cerebral blood flow. For example, the signal can be disrupted by the mass effect of a lesion, or large cerebral veins can induce susceptibilities that can also distort the BOLD signal interpretation. These issues can diminish the sensitivity and specificity of functional brain mapping. Furthermore, fMRI acquisition and analysis as yet have no accepted standard procedure. There is no standardized battery of behavioral paradigms, and determination of the significant threshold of activation is a subjective process. The statistical analysis of the data is diverse; different statistical approaches can be followed in the data interpretation. Furthermore, fMRI only depicts the topography of the functional cortical areas; it does not provide information about the white matter connections, which are equally important in maintaining the proper neuronal functionality of the patient. Because of these limitations,

data interpretation and clinical decisions need to be made with caution.

Several studies have shown a higher incidence of neurologic deficits in patients who underwent resections that were within 0.5 to 2 cm of functional cortex when fMRI alone was used to map functional regions, as opposed to using DCS.[5,26–28] For instance, Mueller and colleagues[29] used fMRI to map the functional cortex and showed that postoperative neurologic deficits occurred in 0%, 33%, and 50% of cases in which the resection margins were beyond 2 cm of the eloquent cortex, within 1 to 2 cm of the eloquent cortex, and less than 1 cm from the eloquent cortex, respectively. Although these studies advocated intraoperative DCS to map functional cortex, when the spatial distance between the lesion and the functional cortex was less than or equal to 2 cm; it should also be emphasized that these early studies concluded that fMRI was a safe and reliable mapping tool that carried great promise for the future.

STATISTICAL ANALYSIS IN CLINICAL IMPLEMENTATIONS OF fMRI

Activation in fMRI is dependent on the statistical threshold and a multitude of other factors. When the statistical threshold is lowered, the area of activation increases, and when the statistical threshold is raised, the area of activation decreases (**Fig. 1**). Thus, fMRI does not measure absolute values, and therefore cannot be used to infer absolute spatial distances. Although a specific description of the statistical methods implemented to analyze fMRI data is beyond the scope of this article, the color-coded maps presented for fMRI studies depict statistical likelihoods, usually as T or Z scores. In addition, variation exists in the magnitude, shape, and location of a signal across different individuals performing an identical task in controlled conditions.[30] The reason for this varied fluctuation has not been precisely determined. Furthermore, there is also intrasubject variability in the signal generation that could be influenced by numerous physiologic and psychological factors, such as caffeine ingestion,[31,32] sleep deprivation,[33] level of attention,[34] and fatigue.[35] For neuroscience applications, group analysis merges the data across different subjects, and random-effects analysis helps to diminish the effect of individual variability. However, for surgical planning, capturing individual variability is the object of the exercise, but avoiding, or at least being aware of, potential artifacts is critical for accurate inferences.

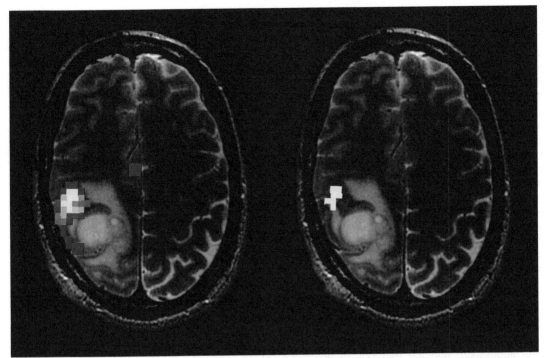

Fig. 1. Axial slices of fMRI hand motor mapping in a patient with a right frontal high-grade glioma. The same data are shown in both panels at 2 different statistical thresholds, illustrating the difference in the relationship of the activation to the lesion.

SPATIAL PRECISION: SMOOTHING AND THE INVERSE SOLUTION

Spatial smoothing is a common step implemented during the analysis of fMRI and PET datasets to improve SNR and because it is a prerequisite for standard statistical analysis using the general linear model. For neuroscientific studies of groups, smoothing is also used to reduce the effect of functional and anatomic variability within and between individual subjects. Smoothing is usually implemented as a convolution of spatial data with a Gaussian kernel. Neighboring voxels within a pre-defined spatial extension are averaged and smoothed into a single voxel value. This processing step optimizes the signal strength and enhances the blob appearance of active brain regions on functional maps. However, this added benefit comes at the undesirable cost (particularly for surgical planning) of decreasing the spatial resolution of the functional maps. The merging of activation centers can blur and shift them distorting their anatomic depiction on the functional maps. In addition, smoothing creates partial volume artifacts along the edge of the brain, because high-intensity brain tissue voxels are averaged with low-intensity voxels outside the brain. Maisog and Chmielowska[36] addressed this issue, and successfully described a method to correct the artifacts along the edges of the brain. Other approaches using data-driven analysis strategies, such as independent component analysis (ICA), have also been proposed that do not require spatial smoothing.[37]

Localization of function (or signal sources) based on the observation of recorded signals at the scalp (ie, MEG and EEG), requires assumptions about a model to which the data are fitted, which is known as the inverse problem of estimating the model parameters based on the data. In the case of MEG and EEG, the inverse solution is ill posed, thus requiring that some assumptions be included to solve the problem. In clinical MEG, a model that is frequently used is the single equivalent current dipole. This model assumes that the generator of the measured signal originates from a single source. In practice, this approximation may result in solutions that do not accurately localize the true source or sources of the signal. Other approaches have been proposed, including distributed solutions, but to date there is no consensus on how best to localize the signals.

In practice, it is important with any mapping method that a measure of the spatial uncertainty be presented with the data. For MEG results, generally only dipoles with goodness of fit of 70% or more are displayed. The written report should also be inspected for a description of how many of the dipoles were discarded, and so forth. For fMRI, the unthresholded or dynamically thresholded statistical maps can provide some information about the location of the boundary of an activation, although there remains no established method of showing the degree of uncertainty. In general, information about acquisition voxel size and the size of the smoothing kernel, if applied, is not given in processed clinical fMRI. Discussion between the individuals acquiring, processing, and interpreting the studies is important in understanding the limits of the data.

SHORTCOMINGS AND CONSIDERATIONS OF PARTICULAR TECHNIQUES

The validity of any functional mapping data interpretation is dependent on numerous preconditions: physiologic assumptions are accurate, adequate SNR, patient cooperation during the data acquisition, and the methods of analysis. Different techniques will be best for different situations and this article describes some technique-specific considerations.

fMRI

Functional MRI indirectly assesses the level of neuronal activation by measuring the relative changes in the concentrations of oxy- and deoxyhemoglobin present in the microvasculature. However, several studies have suggested that signal distortion can also be generated from larger draining veins not directly involved in the activation process (in the so-called vein effect), a phenomenon that can substantially decrease the precision of the spatial localization.[25] Abduljalil and colleagues[38] suggested that the use of spin echo sequences can reduce this distortion from the macrovasculature downstream of the activated area. However, spin echo sequences are less sensitive to magnetic susceptibility effects (which are the basis of the BOLD signal), and thus require longer scanning acquisition times, and cover smaller areas.

Head movement during fMRI acquisition severely degrades data quality. Not only can excessive head motion result in supplemental false activation, it can also decrease or even obscure real activation by altering the signal time course so that the synchronous magnetic resonance (MR) signal from the task paradigm is concealed. This effect can be caused by both abrupt and gradual head movements (**Fig. 2**).[39,40] Krings

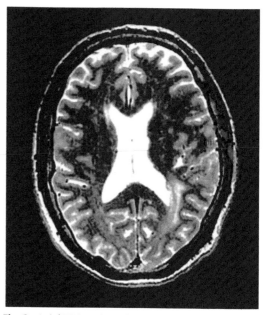

Fig. 2. Axial T2 image with superimposed fMRI activations from a scan with excessive head motion (2.28 mm) resulting in artifactual activation in the skull for a vocalized antonym task.

and colleagues[39] further showed that motion-related signal artifacts in paretic patients occurred in a significantly higher ratio than in patients without a paresis (72% vs 29%). These findings are believed usually to be related to compensatory movement efforts recruiting uninvolved, usually proximal, musculature. We have found that patients have more head motion than healthy controls. In general, if the patient's maximal displacement is more than 2 mm, we repeat the acquisition once to see whether better motion parameters can be achieved. If not, then the data are not deemed interpretable.

Bold fMRI reliance on susceptibility imaging can be problematic. For example, susceptibility artifacts are created at the junction of air and tissue interfaces, such as in the vicinity of the tympano-mastoid air cells of the middle fossa, and from the nasal and sinus airspaces in the orbitofrontal cortex, causing geometric distortions and dropouts in signal intensity.[41] Furthermore, susceptibility artifacts can also be evident in postsurgical patients because of the presence of surgical clips, titanium plates, metal dust from a skull drill, or prior blood products. The presence of these paramagnetic objects can create significant susceptibility that can mask the signal generated from the surrounding neural cortex. Thus constant caution is required in the fMRI data interpretation of postsurgical patients. The customary habit of overlaying the functional brain maps on T1-weighted conventional images can also be troublesome, because the artifacts may no longer be discernible.

MEG

MEG scanners and the shielded room required to house them are expensive, which limits broad clinical applicability outside a few centers. Currently, the cost of installing a MEG scanner can be more than $2 million; MEG scanners also require dedicated personnel. A further drawback of MEG scanners is their extreme susceptibility to surrounding magnetic fields, such as the magnetic noise of the hospital, and even the Earth's own magnetic field.

The clinical applicability of MEG is further hindered by the large spatial distance that separates the source of the signal and the MEG detectors; decreasing both the spatial resolution and the accuracy of signal source localization.[42] Interpreting MEG signals is also problematic whenever multiple sources in the brain become active simultaneously. Then, an infinite number of ways could be used to interpret the signal. For instance Liu and colleagues[43] showed that several signals that were generated from several sources that were 1 to 3 cm apart were erroneously portrayed as a single superimposed signal on MEG scanners.

PET

PET scanners are characterized by a low spatial and temporal resolution. Furthermore, the SNR of PET scanners is weaker than the SNR of other noninvasive mapping techniques such as fMRI. The temporal resolution is especially limited because a substantial temporal delay exists between the imaging phase of the procedure and the visualization phase of the metabolically active foci that discern the neuronal changes. Moreover, PET is a invasive procedure that invokes the administration of a radioactively labeled tracer. Thus, certain patient populations, such as children, are excluded from PET imaging. Similarly to MEG scanning, PET imaging is also expensive, and also requires dedicated personnel. The equipment of PET scanners is also highly priced. Furthermore, a complete PET scanning platform would require a cyclotron to generate radioactive tracers. Similarly to fMRI, PET scanning is also an imaging modality that is hemodynamically based. Thus, it is also a technique that is susceptible to signal distortions from uncoupling issues. PET scanning is also an observational technique and can thus not differentiate functional areas that are essential for the task execution from those

areas that are only supportive to the task execution.

DTI

DTI is presently the only method that can allow the visualization of white matter tracts in vivo. However, several technical limitations still hinder its complete clinical applicability for surgical planning. For instance, three-dimensional (3D) tractography is generally seeded over the whole brain, creating a large mass of fibers that obscure visualization. Several approaches have been developed to aid in the selective visualization of tracts, including seeding from specific anatomic or functional landmarks. Nevertheless, for tracts in close proximity to a brain lesion, it may be difficult to tell whether the tract is running within the lesion or just beyond it. In a recent study, Golby and colleagues[44] addressed these issues by developing an interactive software tool that can show all white bundle tracts within a specific distance from the tumor boundary, and allows the clinician to instantaneously redefine the spatial distance required, enabling the clinician to view all the tract layers around a specific brain lesion. In addition, the software also included the ability to place seedpoints in regions of interests, which also allow the clinician to visualize all the tracts passing through that particular location. Because DTI depends on the fractional anisotropy of white matter to define areas of tightly bundled fibers, anything that lowers the anisotropy, such as tumor infiltration or edema, may falsely obscure the presence of preserved tracts. Also, like some of the functional mapping methods, the visualization of DTI results depends on setting several thresholds such as the fractional anisotropy (FA) and curvature-stopping thresholds. Thus, there is a subjective element to which tracts may be visualized. Furthermore, DTI does not provide any information that relates to the interactions between white bundle tracts and functional cortical regions. Without a priori knowledge acquired from functional mapping such as fMRI, it can be hard to determine the reciprocal interactions between white bundle tracts and the functional cortex. Furthermore, DTI cannot identify eloquent structures within the depicted white bundle tracts, nor can it recognize tracts that are necessary for task execution.

PRACTICAL AND TECHNICAL CONSIDERATIONS
Hardware

All brain mapping techniques require dedicated hardware. For many centers, fMRI will require the least capital investment, because fMRI can be performed on most modern clinical scanners and technical personnel can be trained in additional skills. DTI can also be acquired in addition to any routine clinical studies. In the past 10 years, the most commonly available magnetic field strength was 1.5 T. Today, 3 T field strength is widely being recognized as the optimal strength for most clinical applications.[45] As a notable advantage, the SNR is substantially higher. The signal at 3 T is expected to be 4 times stronger than at 1.5 T, but the noise also increases twofold, and thus only results in a net 2 times factor increase in the SNR. However, this higher resolution in the imaging scans can have important clinical implications, and provides neurosurgeons with a substantial advantage during the surgical planning phase.[46] At 3 T, spatial resolution can be improved, allowing more precise mapping. Advances in coil design have now made multichannel (8- or 16-channel, or even 32-channel) head coils available. The increase in SNR from the multichannel coils can be used to shorten acquisition times or to allow for smaller voxels. Shortening the data acquisition phase can decrease the occurrence of motion artifacts because it is easier for patients to tolerate and makes it more feasible to acquire both structural and functional images in 1 sitting.[47] Overall, designing fMRI scanning paradigms involves making tradeoffs about acquisition time, voxel size, and scan coverage. Although higher field strength and multichannel coils can provide more SNR, the issues of how to effectively maximize acquisitions remain important.

Compared with fMRI, PET and MEG require significant investment. Both methods require expensive scanners, dedicated and specially shielded space, and specially trained personnel. Institutions that already have these suites set up, either for existing clinical applications or research efforts, are likely the sites where these types of studies will be performed in the near future. In addition, functional PET scanning will require the support of nuclear chemists and a cyclotron to maximize the potential. TMS setups are much less expensive to acquire, but have limited penetration in clinical sites to date.

Software

Software plays a critical role in the acquisition and analysis of data from all the brain mapping methods. In addition to the basic processing software, there are frequently issues of separate software systems that need to work together. The most common format for processed images remains Digital Imaging and Communications in Imaging (DICOM; Medical Imaging and Technology Alliance, Arlington, VA, USA), although other formats such as Neuroimaging Informatics Technology Initiative (NIfTI; jointly sponsored by National Institute of Neurological Diseases and Stroke and National Institute of Mental Health) are also being developed. It is particularly important to have personnel with good working knowledge of the software. In going from the acquisition phase on the imaging device to a processing computer and then to a display or navigation system, there are numerous steps in which potential inconsistencies can be introduced. An audit trail of data integrity is particularly important when multiple platforms are used. Some groups have developed fully automated pipelines for data analysis and display that can help to ensure quality control and streamline workflows.

The most commonly used software packages for fMRI and PET have been Brain Voyager[48] and Statistical Parametric Mapping (SPM; Wellcome Department of Neurology, London, United Kingdom). Although these software packages are able to import DICOM images, perform two-dimensional (2D) and 3D statistical data analysis, and analyze single- and multiple-subject data sets, these applications were mainly designed for research use, and they were not tailored for the clinical interpretation of single-subject data or for use by clinicians. With the expanding role of fMRI in the clinical domain, multiple manufactures have begun to develop software tailored for clinical applications. Applications have been designed for use on the major MRI scanner platforms as well as by third-party vendors. Most packages include both stimulus delivery for controlling behavioral paradigms and analysis and visualization software. These software packages, unlike the earlier research packages designed for neuroscience research, do not generally focus on strategies for analyzing multiple-subject data such as normalization and random effects statistics, nor is there the degree of customization generally available in research platforms. Instead, because they have been designed for clinical applications, the focus is on single-subject acquisition, standardization of procedures, ease of use, and regulatory compliance. Several applications have the ability to monitor and display the activation maps with only minimal delay, thus providing direct visualization of statistical maps as the data are being acquired. A substantial advantage of this feature is its ability to monitor the quality of the data at the time of the study. Thus, if poor fMRI maps are being generated, the study can be stopped and any complicating factors, such as stimulus display problems, misunderstanding of task instructions, excessive head motion, and so forth, can be addressed before the patient leaves the suite. The postacquisition packages can perform a semiautomatic in-depth analysis of the datasets that are based in part on the older research software. Thresholding can be performed at the time of acquisition or, ideally, can be dynamically changed by the interpreting clinician. After analysis, data may be represented as contoured or segmented structures on the 2D images or as 3D colored functional maps. In turn, the data can be viewed in any plane, or may be projected onto a reconstruction of the individual's cortical surface, thereby providing a useful surgical planning tool to the neurosurgeon (**Fig. 3**).

DTI visualization has been developed as part of many major research software packages including DTIStudio, FSL, Camino, BrainVisa, MedINRIA, and Slicer. These packages have many features and are highly customizable, but require expert users and are not designed for clinical use. More recently, commercial software designed for clinical use, including BrainLab and Siemens syngo DTI Tractography, has become available. Most clinicians are interested in viewing the tractograms, which show the output of tractography processing. However, reference to the less-processed images, such as the FA maps and the 2D images representing the degree and direction of anisotropy as glyphs, may also be useful.

The software for processing, analysis, and display of MEG data is usually included with the MEG hardware. As such, these FDA-approved software suites are the most commonly used for clinical work. There are also numerous research software platforms developed by both commercial and academic efforts.

Software for TMS has also been developed by both commercial and academic initiatives. The software is used to control the delivery of the magnetic fields as well as to create a digital recording of the events of the session. TMS has also been integrated with frameless navigation for greater spatial accuracy (NexStim, Helsinki, Finland).

INTEGRATING FUNCTIONAL DATA INTO SURGICAL GUIDANCE SYSTEMS

To provide multimodality image guidance to the neurosurgeon during the surgical procedure, navigational systems have developed the capacity to display multiple datasets including functional data, together with any structural data, into a single multimodality platform.[49] The use of such systems for surgical planning before the case is probably underappreciated at present. Using the navigation

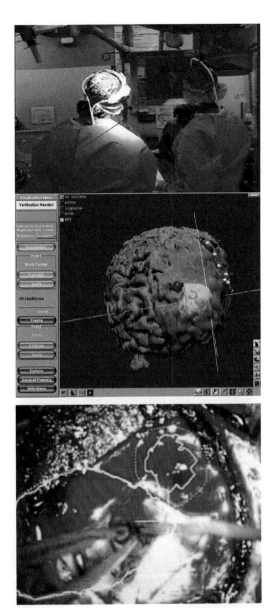

Fig. 3. The screen on which navigational data including fMRI and electrocortical stimulation locations is visible to the surgeon (*top panel*) and navigation system slice view (*middle*). Outlines of segmented structures including the fMRI and tumor may also be visualized through the operating microscope if tracked (*bottom*).

planning system workstation, or research software such as Slicer, the datasets can be merged and viewed. When multiple types of studies acquired at separate sittings on separate platforms are used, accurate coregistration of datasets is critical. Regions, activations, or tracts of interest and the lesion can be highlighted and a surgical plan can be developed. Most commercial neuronavigational guidance systems portray the area of interest as a graphic illustration and both 2D and 3D models (see **Fig. 3; Fig. 4**). In addition, a graphical overlay may be visualized through the surgical microscope provided that the microscope can be tracked by the navigation system. This capacity is available for most modern operating microscopes, though there may be additional components that will need to be purchased. Studies in the literature are beginning to show the added clinical value of integrating multimodal data into neuronavigational guidance systems.[50]

Although a large number of groups have reported success in integrating multimodality data into a single neuronavigational system, several technical challenges still hinder its practical clinical application. For instance, the large amount of functional and structural data that is depicted by each imaging modality can result in incomprehensible data compilations that can make it difficult to identify the precise anatomic and functional features from each imaging technique, particularly within the constraints of the operative setting. This

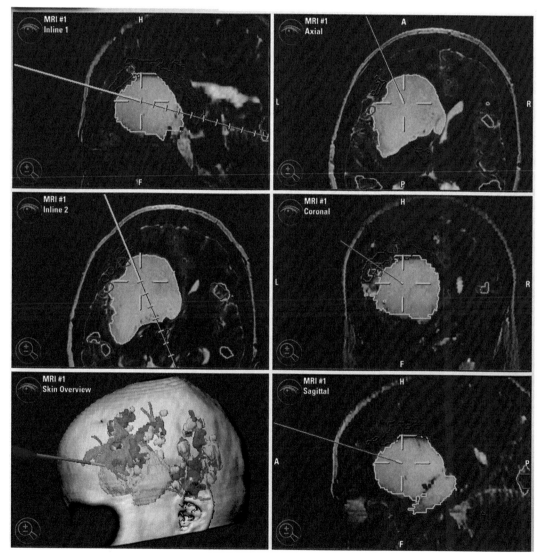

Fig. 4. Intraoperative display of pre- and intraoperatively acquired data coregistered to the patient and displayed by navigation system 3D viewer. Numbered foreground dots indicate intraoperative cortical stimulation locations. Large green model is segmented tumor. Blue model superior to green is tractography. Orange and red models are fMRI activations from language tasks in the patient's first and second language. The surgeon can choose a combination of viewpoints, which is particularly important to appreciate the 3D relations between functional locations and the tumor. Clockwise from top right: standard orthogonal slices, 3D viewer, axial and sagittal in-line views in the plane of the navigation probe.

issue may be exacerbated when the surgical planning phase is not performed by the neurosurgeon conducting the operation or when several different people take part in the creation of the functional maps. Such a large amount of data can frequently slow down the speed with which the navigation system updates the tracking display, meaning that the surgeon must wait a few seconds after pointing the probe in the field. Although this is not a serious downside, it should be noted when many datasets have been loaded into the system.

The integration of functional data such as fMRI, DTI, or MEG into a neuronavigational guidance system is no longer unusual, because of the availability of faster-performing computers, better software/hardware equipment, faster networking, and broader availability of high-field MRI scanners. For instance, Jannin and colleagues[51] successfully integrated MEG, fMRI, and anatomic MR images into a single neuronavigational system to track functional regions in 11 patients with lesions near the central sulcus. In a similar study, Kamada and colleagues[52] also showed that fMRI, MEG, and DTI functional data could also be incorporated into a single integrative platform to provide image guidance during the surgical procedure. In a recent study, Rasmessen and colleagues[53] successfully integrated fMRI and DTI data into a single navigational system, and reported that the incorporation of the functional data into surgical planning provided valuable additional information in a user-friendly way. Even the direct injection of coregistered fMRI images into a surgical microscope with instantaneous portrayal of the functional maps onto the surface of the exposed surgical field is currently available.[54]

However, several technical limitations are still present. For instance, it is challenging for the neurosurgeon to visualize the relationship of the 3D activation maps to the 3D tumor model while the procedure is ongoing (both 2D and 3D views may be helpful). In addition, because viewing the monitor with the structural and functional data cannot be performed simultaneously with surgical action, the neurosurgeon visualizes the neuronavigational data intermittently, thereby limiting his/her ability to comprehend and absorb the data efficiently. In the future, advanced visualization methods, perhaps adopted from military or gaming applications, may help to overcome some visualization challenges.

GUIDANCE OF THE SURGICAL PROCEDURE AND THE PROBLEM OF BRAIN SHIFT

Perhaps, the most important factor that limits the usefulness of preoperative mapping studies is the problem of brain shift. Following the opening of the dural flap, surgical manipulation, CSF drainage, edema, and issues related to gravity and positioning cause the brain to shift, causing an anatomic discrepancy between the preoperatively acquired images and the surgical field. This displacement is exacerbated by the progression of the surgical procedure, during which anatomic displacement greater than 10 mm can occur within an hour of dural opening.[55–59] Reinges and colleagues[60] also showed that the anatomic displacement of superficial cortical structures did not correlate with the displacement of deeper brain structures, further diminishing the usefulness of surgical guidance. Several research groups have addressed these issues by designing algorithms that attempt to correct these anatomic discrepancies.[1] New information may be used to update the images to account for brain shift (eg, ultrasound) (**Fig. 5**).

One solution is the acquisition of intraoperative imaging to allow the neurosurgeon to register the intraoperatively acquired anatomic scans to the preoperatively obtained functional images to further increase the precision and accuracy of the information made intraoperatively available to the neurosurgeon.[1,61] Where available, intraoperative MRI will thus provide a substantial advantage, but, given the amount of time and patient cooperation needed for fMRI, this is unlikely to be possible. Rather, the preoperative functional mapping and tract data may be updated by nonrigidly warping it based on the updated structural image, which uses a segmentation-based model rather than updated imaging.[62,63] Intraoperative DTI has been acquired and has shown that displacements on the order of 1 to 1.5 cm can occur.[64]

CLINICAL CONSIDERATIONS
Selecting the Appropriate Paradigm for Presurgical Motor Mapping

It is critical that the neurosurgeon ordering a brain mapping study for the presurgical evaluation of a patient conveys the clinical aspects of the case to the radiological staff performing the study. Important considerations include the clinical status of the patient, particularly any deficits that may limit the performance of the task or which may influence interpretation of the results. The location of the lesion and the planned trajectory are also important to select the tasks to be tested. The functional architecture of the cerebral cortex involved in voluntary motor movements includes primary motor cortex (M1), the supplementary motor area (SMA), primary somatosensory cortex

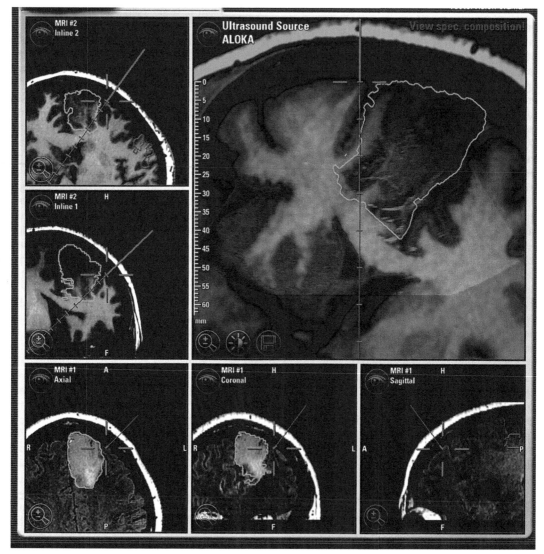

Fig. 5. Neuronavigation screen with coregistered intraoperative ultrasound overlaid on structural MRI images. Ultrasound may be used to perform updated registration to account for some of the brain shift occurring during surgery.

(S1), and the premotor area.[46,65] Within both the M1 and S1 cortex, each body part is disproportionately represented within a distinctive topographic region. The hand region for instance is within the upper portion of the convexity of the motor cortex (the omega region), whereas the leg and tongue regions are respectively on the medial and lateral borders. Thus, the performance of finger tapping paradigms will activate the upper portions of the motor cortex, and will usually not activate the medial and lateral parts. These regions can be mapped using tasks such as toe wiggling or tongue movement, respectively.[29,66] We use toe wiggling rather than movement at the

ankle joint to minimize any transmission of movement to the head, which results in excessive head motion in the z axis. Similarly, lip pursing avoids excessive movement of the jaw or oropharynx, which can cause artifacts.

It is also important to consider the reciprocal neuronal connectivity between the precentral and postcentral gyri for patients who have limited motor function caused by the mass effect or anatomic location of a brain lesion. It may be reasonable to perform passive sensory stimulation tasks on such patients. Brushing or stroking a body part, such as vibrotactile stimulation, can be performed to initiate activity in the S1 cortex.[67] Electrical stimulation of the median and tibial nerves has also been shown to elicit a response from the sensory cortex.[68] Although sensory paradigms are more likely to favor the postcentral sensory gyri, the reciprocal connectivity between the pre- and postcentral gyri can also activate the motor cortex. Such interconnections likely underlie the finding that motor paradigms such as finger tapping can also activate the postcentral sensory cortex. Furthermore, in paralytic patients who have impaired sensation, Stippich and colleagues[69] showed that mere imagination of task execution can elicit a response from the SM1 cortex.

The execution of task paradigms may be problematic for patients who, because of language, attention, or other deficits, are unable to follow the task instructions. For example, it has been shown that the timing of motor performance affects the resultant maps significantly.[70] Although the length of the task block can be extended (eg, from 16 seconds to 30 seconds) to partially compensate for the fluctuating performance, task execution may still prove to be unreliable.[25] Liu and colleagues[71] recently addressed these issues and offered an alternative approach for presurgical motor mapping that relies on measuring spontaneous synchronized changes in brain activation. This approach builds on a finding first described by Biswal and colleagues[72] in which fMRI was used to measure slow, spontaneous brain activity fluctuations to localize distinctive functional brain regions. Participants are asked to close their eyes while fMRI volumes are continuously acquired. Postprocessing then examines the functional connectivity based on temporal correlations between specific functional regions of the brain (such as with the motor network described earlier). This task-free approach, which is known as functional connectivity MR (fcMR), carries great potential for presurgical planning. However, further patient studies will be required to test whether the robustness seen in healthy individuals extends reliably to neurosurgical patients.[73] Another potential advantage of this approach is that multiple brain functions could possibly be probed within a single 20-minute scanning session. Furthermore, the procedure reduces the need for patient compliance. Patients are simply asked to rest or fixate on a crosshair. In certain cases, fcMR has even been conducted on patients who were under the effects of general anesthesia.[71] fcMR imaging has even been performed on human infants, which may allow this approach to be used in children too young to comply with traditional fMRI or other mapping techniques.[74]

Other groups have used TMS for presurgical motor mapping. Although TMS suffers from some disadvantages, by being a technique characterized by poor spatial resolution, and one that can increase seizure risks in patients, it is the only noninvasive mapping technique that is based on direct brain stimulation or inhibition. In 2004, Neggers and colleagues[20] successfully incorporated TMS into a frameless stereotactic navigational system, and showed that the TMS results correlated to within 5 mm of functional mapping by DCS. In 1997, Krings and colleagues[75] also investigated the correlation between DCS and TMS in 2 patients who had tumors infiltrating the functional M1 area, and showed that the correlation was within 1 cm between the 2 techniques.

In addition, DTI can also been used to understand the patient's motor system. The depicted tractography can show the corticospinal tracts, enabling the neurosurgeon to avoid the resection of displaced white bundle tracts that are affected by either the edema or the mass effect of the lesion. DTI can also be helpful during the resection of low-grade gliomas. Some groups have shown that functional white bundle tracts may still be present within the tumor lesion, and tractography can allow the surgeon to plan the resection of the low-grade gliomas while preserving the integrity of the tracts.[76] DTI data have also been combined with fMRI to illustrate motor cortical areas with the associated descending tracts.[52,77–79] Tummala and colleagues[80] successfully used DTI to resect brain tumor lesions in 2 pediatric patients near the optic radiation. No postoperative neurologic deficit was reported in either patient.

Approaches for Language Mapping

Language mapping includes both the determination of the dominant hemisphere (or determination of bilateral support for language) and the localization of language areas. The IAT remains the gold standard for establishing language (and memory) dominance in patients.[7] However, there are significant complications associated with this invasive test, which is also uncomfortable and frightening for patients. A study published in 2008 by Loddenkemper and colleagues[81] included a retrospective evaluation of 677 patients who underwent IAT, and showed that 74 patients (10.9%) developed complications (encephalopathy 7.2%, seizures 1.2%, strokes 0.6%, transient ischemic attacks 0.6%, localized hemorrhage at the catheter insertion site 0.6%, carotid artery dissections 0.4%, or allergic reaction to contrast 0.3%). It can sometimes be difficult to definitively determine language dominance caused by altered cerebrovascular flow: Smith and colleagues[82] evaluated

166 patients undergoing IAT, finding that cross-flow of amobarbital to the contralateral hemisphere occurred to a certain degree in 61 (36.7%) patients. Functional MRI has a reported overall concordance with IAT testing of between 90% and 100%.[21,83–88] Woermann and colleagues[89] compared fMRI data results with IAT in 100 patients with epilepsy and found a 91% concordance rate between the 2 tests. In a different study, Fernandez and colleagues[90] showed that fMRI was as reliable as IAT in its ability to lateralize the regional and global language functions of all investigated patients. Furthermore, Deblaere and colleagues[91] used a low field (1.0 T) MRI scanner to lateralize language functions in 20 patients with epilepsy, showing that fMRI acquired at low magnetic field strength could lateralize language function with a 100% concordance to IAT. Nevertheless, interpretation of the studies is complicated by issues of which regions of interest should be measured and with what metric. Furthermore, several study groups have combined fMRI with DTI data results to further reveal on the anatomic and physiologic causes of asymmetrical language lateralization. Vernooij and colleagues[92] and Powell and colleagues[93] have both proposed that language lateralization is related to structural asymmetry of the white matter tracts in the arcuate fasciculus, which can be measured by DTI, although these findings have not yet led to clinical protocols. Changes in fMRI activation patterns and white matter measures have also been found to reflect handedness.[94] These findings suggest that DTI and measures of white matter structure may one day be useful for predicting structure-function asymmetries in the brain, reflecting language lateralization in patients.

Other groups have also shown that MEG can be used as another noninvasive mapping technique to lateralize language function. MEG is usually used to map the functional cortex that is involved in language reception; in addition to providing the important advantage of enabling the neurosurgeon to track the temporal course of language activation (**Fig. 6**). In 2004, Papinacolaou and colleagues[95] investigated the concordance between MEG and IAT in 100 patients with epilepsy, and found the rate to be 93%. The group concluded that MEG was reliable as a noninvasive mapping technique to replace IAT. In another similar study conducted by Maestu and colleagues,[19] which used a Spanish-based version of the test, the concordance rate between MEG and IAT was found to be 88%. In a recent study conducted by Doss and colleagues,[22] the concordance between MEG and IAT was found to be 86%, whereas the sensitivity and specificity values were reported to be 80% and 100%, respectively.

Language Localization

To date, no single, standardized, robust clinical fMRI language battery has been developed, and no universal paradigm has been defined to plan for the surgical resection of brain lesions near the Broca or Wernicke areas. For instance, different groups have implemented different paradigms such as picture naming,[96] silent word generation,[96,97] rhyme detection,[98] semantic-decision,[96,98,99] word stem completion,[100] and silent reading tasks.[101] Moreover, localization of language function is challenging primarily because of the functional heterogeneity found in perisylvian language areas. The proximity of the brain lesion to the language cortex further complicates interpretation of the functional language localization because of the possibility of lesion-induced plasticity, false negatives related to edema or mass effect, or poor performance because of language impairments. In addition, as with all fMRI, the language-associated region of activation is dependent on the statistical threshold selected, something that remains largely arbitrary. As with all fMRI, lowering the statistical threshold increases the area of activation, and vice versa, when the threshold is increased. Furthermore the extent of activation is also influenced by the baseline task. If a resting baseline is used, then generally more-extensive activations, including sensory and attention areas, will be seen. If a higher-level baseline task (eg, nonword letter strings) is used, then a more restricted activation pattern is likely to be seen. Thus, when implementing fMRI for language mapping, great care must be taken in selecting active and control tasks, and these choices must be incorporated into the review of the final functional maps by the clinician. For these reasons, the validation of fMRI against direct electrocortical stimulation techniques has produced sensitivity and specificity results that have generally been lower than those produced with the motor-sensory brain mapping. Several groups have shown that both the specificity[98] and sensitivity[99] can be increased by having the patients perform multiple linguistic tasks.

DISEASE-SPECIFIC CONSIDERATIONS
Gliomas

The diffuse, infiltrative nature of gliomas can distort the normal anatomy of the brain and induce several pathologic modifications to the cerebral vasculature. High-grade gliomas distort the

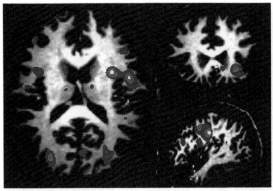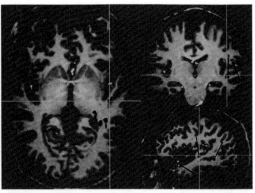

Fig. 6. Functional MRI (*left*) and MEG (*right*) language maps obtained from the same subject performing the same task (vocalized antonym generation with visual stimuli). Although both studies are consistent with left language lateralization, the fMRI shows frontal activations more clearly, whereas the MEG shows more temporal dipole sources.

biochemical environment in the brain and alter the normal composition of ATP, pH, glucose, and lactate levels. High-grade gliomas also induce neovascularization by secreting substances such as vascular endothelial growth factor (VEGF)[102] and rennin,[103] promoting the formation of new blood vessels. However, the architecture of the newly formed blood vessels is weak, disorganized, and immature because of a decreased number of perivascular cells. As a result, focal hemorrhage and fluid transudation leak into the extracellular space, increasing the oxygen availability for activated neural cells.[104–107] The normal oxygen extraction levels of activated neural areas are thus diminished, and the BOLD signal generation is in turn also decreased because of a lower concentration of deoxyhemoglobin causing an uncoupling effect between neural activation and autoregulatory vascular responses. In addition, the mass effect of the rapidly growing tumor can compress the surrounding vasculature, and thus further alter the overall BOLD signal effect. In 2003, Signorelli and colleagues[23] showed that, in postoperative patients, the BOLD signal of activated neural areas that were close to the resection cavity witnessed an increase in the signal intensity compared with the preoperative functional maps. Several reports in the literature have shown that uncoupling can substantially decrease the reliability of fMRI in high-grade glioma, and could be wrongfully interpreted as brain plasticity.

Generally, functional imaging is useful for low-grade gliomas that may contain functional tissue and for which an understanding of the surgical risks often is the key determinant of the surgical plan. The slow-growing nature of low-grade gliomas can allow for a functional adaptation and a cortical topographic reorganization to occur,

which can make interpretation of unusual activation configurations difficult. Russell and colleagues[108] examined the incidence of transient weakness or SMA syndrome in 27 consecutive patients who underwent resection of tumors neighboring or infiltrating the SMA. The incidence of an SMA syndrome was significantly higher among patients with low-grade gliomas, compared with patients with high-grade gliomas, presumably because infiltrated tissue within the SMA retained some functionality. MEG studies in low-grade glioma may be particularly helpful in patients who also have refractory seizures by allowing both functional mapping and a seizure onset localization in a single study.

DTI also may be particularly helpful in low-grade glioma because preserved tracts are seen within lesions (**Fig. 7**). DTI can differentiate infiltration of tracts by the tumor from displacement or destruction of tracts by the tumor. However, edema or tumor infiltration, by lowering FA, may lead to lack of tract visualization when there is a tract present.

Vascular Malformations

Arteriovenous malformations (AVM) are the most common cerebrovascular deformity, and consist of an interconnecting complex of arteries and veins that are devoid of a capillary network. fMRI has proved to be a reliable brain mapping tool that has produced results that closely resemble those of intraoperative brain mapping techniques.[109,110] Functional mapping has also been reported in the preoperative planning of patients undergoing resections of cavernous hemangiomas.[77,111] However, assessing the functional integrity of the brain territories that surround an AVM with fMRI may not always be simple. Because AVM are

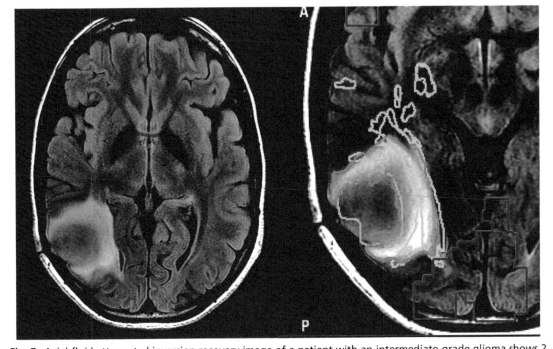

Fig. 7. Axial fluid-attenuated inversion-recovery image of a patient with an intermediate-grade glioma shows 2 distinct regions of abnormality, making the surgical goal unclear.

a direct arteriovenous shunting system, they are characterized by a blood flow that has a high velocity and a low resistance. The blood pressure within the arterial portion of the AVM is characteristically hypotensive, whereas it is hypertensive in the draining venous portion. Because of this irregular pressure difference, the feeding pressure of the artery is lower than normal. This difference can cause a net reduction in the cerebral perfusion pressure in the regions that surround the AVM. Such vascular perturbations do not necessarily decrease the neurologic functionality of the surrounding brain tissues, but can disrupt the BOLD signal and obscure activation in brain regions that are functionally active. Thus, functional mapping with fMRI may erroneously label functionally active brain regions as inactive. This problem is especially important in patients who have AVM with severe flow anomalies (**Fig. 8**). For instance, Juenger and colleagues[112] recently published a case report that showed that MEG and TMS recordings were more reliable than fMRI data in mapping functional regions within the vicinity of an AVM. In this case report, the validity of presurgical mapping techniques was assessed by comparing each of fMRI, MEG, and TMS data results with the results of DCS. However, many patients have AVMs with only moderate, or even inconsiderate, flow irregularities. In such patients, Pouratian and colleagues[113] showed that the correlation between direct electrocortical stimulation and

fMRI can be high, with a 100% and 66.7% sensitivity and specificity, respectively. In a further attempt to minimize the risk of fMRI-based surgical planning for the resection of AVM lesions, Cannestra and colleagues[114] proposed subcategorizing AVM into 3 distinct groups based on the spatial distance between the AVM and the eloquent brain cortex as defined by fMRI. The first group (low risk) included patients who had at least 1 complete gyrus that separated the AVM from the functionally active brain regions. In the second group (high risk), the association between the AVM and the functional brain regions is profound. In the third group (indeterminate risk), the AVM and eloquent cortex were bordering each other. For the patients at low risk, the study group concluded that fMRI alone may be used to plan the surgical resection of the AVM. Patients of the second (high-risk) group are generally considered to be inoperable and are usually referred for radiotherapy, whereas the AVM lesions in the patients of the third group are performed through direct electrocortical stimulation, because the lesion is too close (<1 cm) to the eloquent cortex to rely on fMRI.

Epilepsy

In the presurgical evaluation of epileptic patients, functional brain mapping is particularly important because the target of resection is usually brain tissue

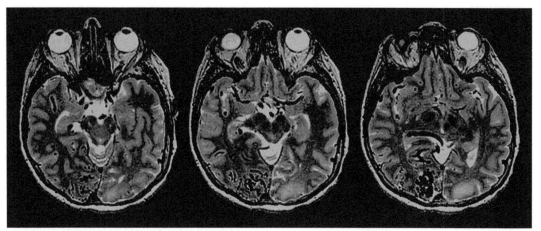

Fig. 8. Visual fMRI scans of a patient with a large occipital AVM. A whole, filed, flashing checkerboard paradigm was delivered. Although the patient had preserved visual perception in the left visual field, the patient did not have any visual activation in the right occipital cortex depicted on fMRI.

rather than tumor or other tissue. Brain mapping can be used to assess numerous functions for preoperative patient selection and procedure planning. The IAT and, more recently, fMRI (including fcMR imaging) have been used to assess memory dominance and risk for postoperative memory loss in patients undergoing temporal lobectomy and amygdalohippocampectomy.[115,116]

IAT, fMRI, and MEG have been used for language lateralization and localization. Compared with a control population, patients with temporal lobe epilepsies have been shown to have more bilateral language activation, during the execution of language paradigms, with less lateralization to either cerebral hemisphere. The degree of activation in the homologous language region of the contralateral hemisphere of these patients was significantly higher than in healthy subjects.[117] Localization of the seizure onset is particularly important in the evaluation of patients with epilepsy. MEG, being a modality that assesses neuronal activity directly, can be used to localize interictal discharges, which may help to localize the seizure focus. Although the correlation is still not perfect, MEG interictal spike recordings are increasingly being used to identify seizure foci. For instance, Mamelak and colleagues[118] used interictal MEG recordings to localize seizure foci to the correct lobe and thereby guide subdural grid placement. In addition, several study groups have used FDG-PET and single-photon emission computed tomography, to identify the seizure foci by analyzing the interictal cellular metabolism and the ictal-interictal metabolism differences, respectively.[119,120] fMRI has acquired a role in the localization of the epileptogenic zone. Krings

and colleagues used fMRI to examine the spatial and temporal course of a patient undergoing a seizure, and were able to successfully identify the location of epileptogenic activation. In a recent promising development, fMRI has been combined with EEG to identify the epileptogenic foci in patients with frequent interictal discharges. So-called spike-triggered fMRI can lateralize medial temporal lobe epilepsies, as well as identify seizure foci by supplementing the spatial resolution of the MRI to the temporal resolution of EEG in the localization of the seizure foci.[121,122]

SUMMARY

The development of numerous functional mapping techniques now gives neurosurgeons many options for preoperative planning. Integrating functional and anatomic data can inform patient selection and surgical planning and makes functional mapping more accessible than when only invasive studies such as IAT and DCS were available. However, the applications of functional mapping to neurosurgical patients are still evolving. Acquisition, processing, interpretation, and visualization of the functional images remain complex and require understanding of the underlying physiologic and imaging characteristics. In particular, the neurosurgeon must be accustomed to interpreting highly processed data. Successful implementation of functional image-guided procedures requires efficient interactions between neurosurgeon, neurologist, radiologist, neuropsychologist, and others, but promises to enhance the care of patients.

REFERENCES

1. Archip N, Clatz O, Whalen S, et al. Non-rigid alignment of pre-operative MRI, fMRI, and DT-MRI with intra-operative MRI for enhanced visualization and navigation in image-guided neurosurgery. Neuroimage 2007;35(2):609–24.
2. Yoo SS, Talos IF, Golby AJ, et al. Evaluating requirements for spatial resolution of fMRI for neurosurgical planning. Hum Brain Mapp 2004; 21(1):34–43.
3. Rolls ET, Grabenhorst F, Franco L. Prediction of subjective affective state from brain activations. J Neurophysiol 2009;101(3):1294–308.
4. Iwasaki S, Nakagawa H, Fukusumi A, et al. Identification of pre- and postcentral gyri on CT and MR images on the basis of the medullary pattern of cerebral white matter. Radiology 1991;179(1):207–13.
5. Ojemann GA. Individual variability in cortical localization of language. J Neurosurg 1979;50(2):164–9.
6. Steinmetz H, Furst G, Freund HJ. Variation of perisylvian and calcarine anatomic landmarks within stereotaxic proportional coordinates. AJNR Am J Neuroradiol 1990;11(6):1123–30.
7. Wada J. A new method for determination of the side of cerebral speech dominance: a preliminary report on the intracarotid injection of sodium amytal in man. Igaku to Seibutsugaki 1949;14:221–2.
8. Tharin S, Golby AJ. Functional brain mapping and its applications to neurosurgery. Neurosurgery 2007;60(4 Suppl 2):185–201 [discussion: 201–2].
9. Sack AT, Linden DE. Combining transcranial magnetic stimulation and functional imaging in cognitive brain research: possibilities and limitations. Brain Res Brain Res Rev 2003;43(1):41–56.
10. Nimsky C, Ganslandt O, Kober H, et al. Integration of functional magnetic resonance imaging supported by magnetoencephalography in functional neuronavigation. Neurosurgery 1999;44(6):1249–55 [discussion: 1255–6].
11. Maldjian JA, Schulder M, Liu WC, et al. Intraoperative functional MRI using a real-time neurosurgical navigation system. J Comput Assist Tomogr 1997; 21(6):910–2.
12. McDonald JD, Chong BW, Lewine JD, et al. Integration of preoperative and intraoperative functional brain mapping in a frameless stereotactic environment for lesions near eloquent cortex. Technical note. J Neurosurg 1999;90(3):591–8.
13. Gumprecht H, Ebel GK, Auer DP, et al. Neuronavigation and functional MRI for surgery in patients with lesion in eloquent brain areas. Minim Invasive Neurosurg 2002;45(3):151–3.
14. Schulder M, Maldjian JA, Liu WC, et al. Functional image-guided surgery of intracranial tumors located in or near the sensorimotor cortex. J Neurosurg 1998;89(3):412–8.
15. Lee CC, Ward HA, Sharbrough FW, et al. Assessment of functional MR imaging in neurosurgical planning. AJNR Am J Neuroradiol 1999;20(8):1511–9.
16. Petrella JR, Shah LM, Harris KM, et al. Preoperative functional MR imaging localization of language and motor areas: effect on therapeutic decision making in patients with potentially resectable brain tumors. Radiology 2006;240(3):793–802.
17. Pirotte B, Acerbi F, Lubansu A, et al. PET imaging in the surgical management of pediatric brain tumors. Childs Nerv Syst 2007;23(7):739–51.
18. Wheless JW, Willmore LJ, Breier JI, et al. A comparison of magnetoencephalography, MRI, and V-EEG in patients evaluated for epilepsy surgery. Epilepsia 1999;40(7):931–41.
19. Maestu F, Ortiz T, Fernandez A, et al. Spanish language mapping using MEG: a validation study. Neuroimage 2002;17(3):1579–86.
20. Neggers SF, Langerak TR, Schutter DJLG, et al. A stereotactic method for image-guided transcranial magnetic stimulation validated with fMRI and motor-evoked potentials. Neuroimage 2004;21(4):1805–17.
21. Arora J, Pugh K, Westerveld M, et al. Language lateralization in epilepsy patients: fMRI validated with the Wada procedure. Epilepsia 2009;50(10):2225–41.
22. Doss RC, Zhang W, Risse GL, et al. Lateralizing language with magnetic source imaging: validation based on the Wada test. Epilepsia 2009;50(10):2242–8.
23. Signorelli F, Guyotat J, Schneider F, et al. Technical refinements for validating functional MRI-based neuronavigation data by electrical stimulation during cortical language mapping. Minim Invasive Neurosurg 2003;46(5):265–8.
24. Giussani C, Roux FE, Ojemann J, et al. Is preoperative functional magnetic resonance imaging reliable for language areas mapping in brain tumor surgery? Review of language functional magnetic resonance imaging and direct cortical stimulation correlation studies. Neurosurgery 2010;66(1):113–20.
25. Tieleman A, Deblaere K, Van Roost D, et al. Preoperative fMRI in tumour surgery. Eur Radiol 2009;19(10):2523–34.
26. FitzGerald DB, Cosgrove GR, Ronner S, et al. Location of language in the cortex: a comparison between functional MR imaging and electrocortical stimulation. AJNR Am J Neuroradiol 1997;18(8):1529–39.
27. Haglund MM, Berger MS, Shamseldin M, et al. Cortical localization of temporal lobe language sites in patients with gliomas. Neurosurgery 1994;34(4):567–76 [discussion: 576].
28. Roux FE, Boulanouar K, Ranjeva JP, et al. Usefulness of motor functional MRI correlated to cortical

mapping in Rolandic low-grade astrocytomas. Acta Neurochir (Wien) 1999;141(1):71–9.

29. Mueller WM, Yetkin FZ, Hammeke TA, et al. Functional magnetic resonance imaging mapping of the motor cortex in patients with cerebral tumors. Neurosurgery 1996;39(3):515–20 [discussion: 520–1].

30. Steinmetz H, Seitz RJ. Functional anatomy of language processing: neuroimaging and the problem of individual variability. Neuropsychologia 1991;29(12):1149–61.

31. Liu TT, Behzadi Y, Restom K, et al. Caffeine alters the temporal dynamics of the visual BOLD response. Neuroimage 2004;23(4):1402–13.

32. Behzadi Y, Liu TT. Caffeine reduces the initial dip in the visual BOLD response at 3 T. Neuroimage 2006;32(1):9–15.

33. Chee MW, Choo WC. Functional imaging of working memory after 24 hr of total sleep deprivation. J Neurosci 2004;24(19):4560–7.

34. Corbetta M, Miezin FM, Dobmeyer S, et al. Selective and divided attention during visual discriminations of shape, color, and speed: functional anatomy by positron emission tomography. J Neurosci 1991;11(8):2383–402.

35. Tartaglia MC, Narayanan S, Arnold DL. Mental fatigue alters the pattern and increases the volume of cerebral activation required for a motor task in multiple sclerosis patients with fatigue. Eur J Neurol 2008;15(4):413–9.

36. Maisog JM, Chmielowska J. An efficient method for correcting the edge artifact due to smoothing. Hum Brain Mapp 1998;6(3):128–36.

37. Tie Y, Whalen S, Suarez RO, et al. Group independent component analysis of language fMRI from word generation tasks. Neuroimage 2008;42(3):1214–25.

38. Abduljalil AM, Robitaille PM. Macroscopic susceptibility in ultra high field MRI. II: acquisition of spin echo images from the human head. J Comput Assist Tomogr 1999;23(6):842–4.

39. Krings T, Reinges MHT, Erberich S, et al. Functional MRI for presurgical planning: problems, artefacts, and solution strategies. J Neurol Neurosurg Psychiatry 2001;70(6):749–60.

40. Hajnal JV, Myers R, Oatridge A, et al. Artifacts due to stimulus correlated motion in functional imaging of the brain. Magn Reson Med 1994;31(3):283–91.

41. Devlin JT, Russell RP, Davis MH, et al. Susceptibility-induced loss of signal: comparing PET and fMRI on a semantic task. Neuroimage 2000;11(6 Pt 1):589–600.

42. Sharon D, Hämäläinen MS, Tootell RBH, et al. The advantage of combining MEG and EEG: comparison to fMRI in focally stimulated visual cortex. Neuroimage 2007;36(4):1225–35.

43. Liu AK, Dale AM, Belliveau JW. Monte Carlo simulation studies of EEG and MEG localization accuracy. Hum Brain Mapp 2002;16(1):47–62.

44. Golby AJ, Kindlmann G, Norton I. Interactive diffusion tensor tractography visualization for neurosurgical planning. Neurosurgery 2011;68(2):496–505.

45. Lin W, An H, Chen Y, et al. Practical consideration for 3T imaging. Magn Reson Imaging Clin N Am 2003;11:615–39.

46. Alkadhi H, Kollias SS, Creilier GR, et al. Plasticity of the human motor cortex in patients with arteriovenous malformations: a functional MR imaging study. AJNR Am J Neuroradiol 2000; 21(8):1423–33.

47. Bellgowan PS, Bandettini PA, van Gelderen P, et al. Improved BOLD detection in the medial temporal region using parallel imaging and voxel volume reduction. Neuroimage 2006;29(4):1244–51.

48. Goebel R. Brainvoyager: a program for analyzing and visualizing functional and structural magnetic resonance data sets. Neuroimage 1996;3(3):S604.

49. O'Donnell LJ, Westin CF, Norton I, et al. The fiber laterality histogram: a new way to measure white matter asymmetry. Med Image Comput Comput Assist Interv 2010;13(Pt 2):225–32.

50. Wu JS, Zhou LF, Tang WJ, et al. Clinical evaluation and follow-up outcome of diffusion tensor imaging-based functional neuronavigation: a prospective, controlled study in patients with gliomas involving pyramidal tracts. Neurosurgery 2007;61(5):935–48 [discussion: 948–9].

51. Jannin P, Morandi X, Fleig OJ, et al. Integration of sulcal and functional information for multimodal neuronavigation. J Neurosurg 2002;96(4):713–23.

52. Kamada K, Houkin K, Takeuchi F, et al. Visualization of the eloquent motor system by integration of MEG, functional, and anisotropic diffusion-weighted MRI in functional neuronavigation. Surg Neurol 2003;59(5):352–61 [discussion: 361–2].

53. Rasmussen IA Jr, Lindseth F, Rygh OM, et al. Functional neuronavigation combined with intraoperative 3D ultrasound: initial experiences during surgical resections close to eloquent brain areas and future directions in automatic brain shift compensation of preoperative data. Acta Neurochir (Wien) 2007;149(4):365–78.

54. Krishnan R, Raabe A, Hattingen E, et al. Functional magnetic resonance imaging-integrated neuronavigation: correlation between lesion-to-motor cortex distance and outcome. Neurosurgery 2004;55(4):904–14 [discussion: 914–5].

55. Nabavi A, Black P, Gering D, et al. Serial intraoperative magnetic resonance imaging of brain shift. Neurosurgery 2001;48(4):787–97 [discussion: 797–8].

56. Nimsky C, Ganslandt O, Cermy S, et al. Quantification of, visualization of, and compensation for brain shift using intraoperative magnetic resonance imaging. Neurosurgery 2000;47(5):1070–9 [discussion: 1079–80].

57. Nimsky C, Ganslandt O, Hastreiter P, et al. Intraoperative compensation for brain shift. Surg Neurol 2001;56(6):357–64 [discussion: 364–5].

58. Hata N, Nabavi A, Wells WM III, et al. Three-dimensional optical flow method for measurement of volumetric brain deformation from intraoperative MR images. J Comput Assist Tomogr 2000;24(4):531–8.

59. Colen RR, Kekhia H, Jolesz FA. Multimodality intraoperative MRI for brain tumor surgery. Expert Rev Neurother 2010;10(10):1545–58.

60. Reinges MH, Nguyen HH, Krings T, et al. Course of brain shift during microsurgical resection of supratentorial cerebral lesions: limits of conventional neuronavigation. Acta Neurochir (Wien) 2004; 146(4):369–77 [discussion: 377].

61. Kekhia H, Colen R, Oguro S, et al. Assessing the significance of intraoperative MRI in glioma surgery: a controlled Volumetric Analysis. Presented at: Spring 2010 Symposium for Research Excellence Awards, Brigham and Women's Hospital. Boston (MA), May 25, 2010.

62. Archip N, Clatz O, Whalen S, et al. Compensation of geometric distortion effects on intraoperative magnetic resonance imaging for enhanced visualization in image-guided neurosurgery. Neurosurgery 2008;62(3 Suppl 1):209–15 [discussion: 215–6].

63. Zhuang DX, Liu YX, Wu JS, et al. A sparse intraoperative data-driven biomechanical model to compensate for brain shift during neuronavigation. AJNR Am J Neuroradiol 2010;32(2):395.

64. Nimsky C, Ganslandt O, Hastreiter P, et al. Preoperative and intraoperative diffusion tensor imaging-based fiber tracking in glioma surgery. Neurosurgery 2005;56(1):130–7 [discussion: 138].

65. Rizzolatti G, Luppino G, Matelli M. The organization of the cortical motor system: new concepts. Electroencephalogr Clin Neurophysiol 1998;106(4):283–96.

66. Hirsch J, Ruge MI, Kim KHS, et al. An integrated functional magnetic resonance imaging procedure for preoperative mapping of cortical areas associated with tactile, motor, language, and visual functions. Neurosurgery 2000;47(3):711–21 [discussion: 721–2].

67. Golaszewski SM, Siedentopf CM, Koppelstaetter F, et al. Human brain structures related to plantar vibrotactile stimulation: a functional magnetic resonance imaging study. Neuroimage 2006;29(3): 923–9.

68. Gasser TG, Sandalcioglu EI, Wiedemayer H, et al. A novel passive functional MRI paradigm for preoperative identification of the somatosensory cortex. Neurosurg Rev 2004;27(2):106–12.

69. Stippich C, Ochmann H, Sartor K. Somatotopic mapping of the human primary sensorimotor cortex during motor imagery and motor execution by functional magnetic resonance imaging. Neurosci Lett 2002;331(1):50–4.

70. Feigl GC, Safavi-Abbass S, Gharabaghi A, et al. Real-time 3T fMRI data of brain tumour patients for intra-operative localization of primary motor areas. Eur J Surg Oncol 2008;34(6):708–15.

71. Liu H, Buckner RL, Talukdar T, et al. Task-free presurgical mapping using functional magnetic resonance imaging intrinsic activity. J Neurosurg 2009;111(4):746–54.

72. Biswal B, Yetkin FZ, Haughton VM, et al. Functional connectivity in the motor cortex of resting human brain using echo-planar MRI. Magn Reson Med 1995;34(4):537–41.

73. Damoiseaux JS, Rombouts S, Barkhif F, et al. Consistent resting-state networks across healthy subjects. Proc Natl Acad Sci U S A 2006;103(37): 13848–53.

74. Fransson P, Skiöld B, Horsch S, et al. Resting-state networks in the infant brain. Proc Natl Acad Sci U S A 2007;104(39):15531–6.

75. Krings T, Buchbinder, Butler WE, et al. Stereotactic transcranial magnetic stimulation: correlation with direct electrical cortical stimulation. Neurosurgery 1997;41(6):1319–25 [discussion: 1325–6].

76. Skirboll SS, Ojemann GA, Berger MS, et al. Functional cortex and subcortical white matter located within gliomas. Neurosurgery 1996;38(4):678–84 [discussion: 684–5].

77. Moller-Hartmann W, Krings T, Coenen VA, et al. Preoperative assessment of motor cortex and pyramidal tracts in central cavernoma employing functional and diffusion-weighted magnetic resonance imaging. Surg Neurol 2002;58(5):302–7 [discussion: 308].

78. Parmar H, Sitoh YY, Yeo TT. Combined magnetic resonance tractography and functional magnetic resonance imaging in evaluation of brain tumors involving the motor system. J Comput Assist Tomogr 2004;28(4):551–6.

79. Witwer BP, Moftakhar R, Hasan KM, et al. Diffusion-tensor imaging of white matter tracts in patients with cerebral neoplasm. J Neurosurg 2002;97(3):568–75.

80. Tummala RP, Chu RM, Liu H, et al. Application of diffusion tensor imaging to magnetic-resonance-guided brain tumor resection. Pediatr Neurosurg 2003;39(1):39–43.

81. Loddenkemper T, Morris HH, Moddel G. Complications during the Wada test. Epilepsy Behav 2008; 13(3):551–3.

82. Smith IM, McGlone J, Fox AJ. Intracarotid amobarbital memory protocol: muteness, dysphasia, and variations in arterial distribution of the drug do not affect recognition results. J Epilepsy 1993;6:75–84.

83. Binder JR, Swanson SJ, Hammeke TA, et al. Determination of language dominance using functional MRI: a comparison with the Wada test. Neurology 1996;46(4):978–84.

84. Bahn MM, Lin W, Silbergeld DL, et al. Localization of language cortices by functional MR imaging compared with intracarotid amobarbital hemispheric sedation. AJR Am J Roentgenol 1997; 169(2):575–9.

85. Hertz-Pannier L, Gaillard WD, Mott SH, et al. Noninvasive assessment of language dominance in children and adolescents with functional MRI: a preliminary study. Neurology 1997;48(4):1003–12.

86. Benson RR, FitzGerald DB, LeSueur LL, et al. Language dominance determined by whole brain functional MRI in patients with brain lesions. Neurology 1999;52(4):798–809.

87. Fernandes MA, Smith ML, Logan W, et al. Comparing language lateralization determined by dichotic listening and fMRI activation in frontal and temporal lobes in children with epilepsy. Brain Lang 2006;96(1):106–14.

88. Sabbah P, Chassoux F, Leveque C, et al. Functional MR imaging in assessment of language dominance in epileptic patients. Neuroimage 2003;18(2):460–7.

89. Woermann FG, Jokeit H, Luerding R, et al. Language lateralization by Wada test and fMRI in 100 patients with epilepsy. Neurology 2003;61(5): 699–701.

90. Fernandez G, Specht K, Weis S, et al. Intrasubject reproducibility of presurgical language lateralization and mapping using fMRI. Neurology 2003; 60(6):969–75.

91. Deblaere K, Boon PA, Vandemaele P, et al. MRI language dominance assessment in epilepsy patients at 1.0 T: region of interest analysis and comparison with intracarotid amytal testing. Neuroradiology 2004;46(6):413–20.

92. Vernooij MW, Smits M, Wielopolski PA, et al. Fiber density asymmetry of the arcuate fasciculus in relation to functional hemispheric language lateralization in both right- and left-handed healthy subjects: a combined fMRI and DTI study. Neuroimage 2007;35(3):1064–76.

93. Powell HW, Parker GJM, Alexander DC, et al. Hemispheric asymmetries in language-related pathways: a combined functional MRI and tractography study. Neuroimage 2006;32(1):388–99.

94. Propper RE, O'Donnell LJ, Whalen S, et al. A combined fMRI and DTI examination of functional language lateralization and arcuate fasciculus structure: effects of degree versus direction of hand preference. Brain Cogn 2010;73(2):85–92.

95. Papanicolaou AC, Simos PG, Castillo EM, et al. Magnetocephalography: a noninvasive alternative to the Wada procedure. J Neurosurg 2004;100(5): 867–76.

96. Deblaere K, Backes W, Hofman P, et al. Developing a comprehensive presurgical functional MRI protocol for patients with intractable temporal lobe epilepsy: a pilot study. Neuroradiology 2002; 44(8):667–73.

97. Vikingstad EM, George KP, Johnson AF, et al. Cortical language lateralization in right handed normal subjects using functional magnetic resonance imaging. J Neurol Sci 2000;175(1):17–27.

98. Seghier ML, Lazeyras F, Pegna AJ, et al. Variability of fMRI activation during a phonological and semantic language task in healthy subjects. Hum Brain Mapp 2004;23(3):140–55.

99. Weber B, Wellmer J, Schür S, et al. Presurgical language fMRI in patients with drug-resistant epilepsy: effects of task performance. Epilepsia 2006;47(5):880–6.

100. Palmer ED, Rosen HJ, Ojemann JG, et al. An event-related fMRI study of overt and covert word stem completion. Neuroimage 2001;14(1 Pt 1):182–93.

101. Gaillard WD, Balsamo L, Xu B, et al. Language dominance in partial epilepsy patients identified with an fMRI reading task. Neurology 2002;59(2): 256–65.

102. Plate KH, Breier G, Weich HA, et al. Vascular endothelial growth factor and glioma angiogenesis: coordinate induction of VEGF receptors, distribution of VEGF protein and possible in vivo regulatory mechanisms. Int J Cancer 1994;59(4):520–9.

103. Ariza A, Fernandez LA, Inagami T, et al. Renin in glioblastoma multiforme and its role in neovascularization. Am J Clin Pathol 1988;90(4):437–41.

104. Jain RK, Munn LL, Fukumura D. Dissecting tumour pathophysiology using intravital microscopy. Nat Rev Cancer 2002;2(4):266–76.

105. Shweiki D, Itin A, Soffer D, et al. Vascular endothelial growth factor induced by hypoxia may mediate hypoxia-initiated angiogenesis. Nature 1992; 359(6398):843–5.

106. Plate KH, Breier G, Weich HA, et al. Vascular endothelial growth factor is a potential tumour angiogenesis factor in human gliomas in vivo. Nature 1992; 359(6398):845–8.

107. Helmlinger G, Yuan F, Dellian M, et al. Interstitial pH and pO_2 gradients in solid tumors in vivo: high-resolution measurements reveal a lack of correlation. Nat Med 1997;3(2):177–82.

108. Russell SM, Kelly PJ. Incidence and clinical evolution of postoperative deficits after volumetric stereotactic resection of glial neoplasms involving the supplementary motor area. Neurosurgery 2007;61(Suppl 1):358–67 [discussion: 367–8].

109. Latchaw RE, Hu X, Ugurbil K, et al. Functional magnetic resonance imaging as a management tool for cerebral arteriovenous malformations. Neurosurgery 1995;37(4):619–25 [discussion: 625–6].

110. Maldjian J, Atlas SW, Howard RS, et al. Functional magnetic resonance imaging of regional brain activity in patients with intracerebral arteriovenous

malformations before surgical or endovascular therapy. J Neurosurg 1996;84(3):477–83.

111. Duffau H, Fontaine D. Successful resection of a left insular cavernous angioma using neuronavigation and intraoperative language mapping. Acta Neurochir (Wien) 2005;147(2):205–8 [discussion: 208].

112. Juenger H, Ressel V, Braun C, et al. Misleading functional magnetic resonance imaging mapping of the cortical hand representation in a 4-year-old boy with an arteriovenous malformation of the central region. J Neurosurg Pediatr 2009;4(4):333–8.

113. Pouratian N, Bookheimer SY, Rex DE, et al. Utility of preoperative functional magnetic resonance imaging for identifying language cortices in patients with vascular malformations. J Neurosurg 2002;97(1):21–32.

114. Cannestra AF, Pouratian N, Forage J, et al. Functional magnetic resonance imaging and optical imaging for dominant-hemisphere perisylvian arteriovenous malformations. Neurosurgery 2004; 55(4):804–12 [discussion: 812–4].

115. Vincent JL, Snyder AZ, Fox MD, et al. Coherent spontaneous activity identifies a hippocampal-parietal memory network. J Neurophysiol 2006; 96(6):3517–31.

116. Yu HY, Shih YH, Su TP, et al. The Wada memory test and prediction of outcome after anterior temporal lobectomy. J Clin Neurosci 2010;17(7):857–61.

117. Adcock JE, Wise RG, Oxbury JM, et al. Quantitative fMRI assessment of the differences in lateralization of language-related brain activation in patients with temporal lobe epilepsy. Neuroimage 2003;18(2):423–38.

118. Mamelak AN, Lopez N, Akhatari M, et al. Magnetoencephalography-directed surgery in patients with neocortical epilepsy. J Neurosurg 2002; 97(4):865–73.

119. Paesschen WV. Ictal SPECT. Epilepsia 2004;45: 35–40.

120. Theodore WH, Sato S, Kufta C, et al. Temporal lobectomy for uncontrolled seizures: the role of positron emission tomography. Ann Neurol 1992; 32(6):789–94.

121. Salek-Haddadi A, Friston KJ, Lemieux L, et al. Studying spontaneous EEG activity with fMRI. Brain Res Brain Res Rev 2003;43(1):110–33.

122. Salek-Haddadi A, Lemieux L, Merschhemke M, et al. Functional magnetic resonance imaging of human absence seizures. Ann Neurol 2003;53(5): 663–7.

Overview of Functional Magnetic Resonance Imaging

Gary H. Glover, PhD

KEYWORDS

- Functional magnetic resonance imaging • BOLD fMRI
- Challenges • Future of fMRI

Functional magnetic resonance imaging (fMRI) is a class of imaging methods developed to demonstrate regional, time-varying changes in brain metabolism.[1–3] These metabolic changes can be consequent to task-induced cognitive state changes or the result of unregulated processes in the resting brain. Since its inception in 1990, fMRI has been used in an exceptionally large number of studies in the cognitive neurosciences, clinical psychiatry/psychology, and presurgical planning (between 100,000 and 250,000 entries in PubMed, depending on keywords). The popularity of fMRI derives from its widespread availability (can be performed on a clinical 1.5 T scanner), noninvasive nature (does not require injection of a radioisotope or other pharmacologic agent), relatively low cost, and good spatial resolution. Increasingly, fMRI is being used as a biomarker for disease,[4,5] to monitor therapy,[6] or for studying pharmacologic efficacy.[7] Thus, it is of interest to review the contrast mechanisms, the strengths and weaknesses, and evolutionary trends of this important tool.

BASIS FOR FMRI

fMRI is of course based on MRI, which in turn uses nuclear magnetic resonance coupled with gradients in magnetic field[8] to create images that can incorporate many different types of contrast such as T1 weighting, T2 weighting, susceptibility, flow, and so forth.[9] To understand the particular contrast mechanism predominantly used in fMRI it is necessary to first discuss brain metabolism.

All the processes of neural signaling in the brain, including formation and propagation of action potentials, binding of vesicles to the presynaptic junction, the release of neurotransmitters across the synaptic gap, their reception and regeneration of action potentials in the postsynaptic structures, scavenging of excess neurotransmitters, and so forth, require energy in the form of adenosine triphosphate (ATP).[10] This nucleotide is produced principally by the mitochondria from glycolytic oxygenation of glucose, and its production results in carbon dioxide as a by-product. When a region of the brain is upregulated (ie, activated) by a cognitive task such as finger tapping, the additional neural firing and other increased signaling processes result in a locally increased energy requirement, in turn resulting in upregulated cerebral metabolic rate of oxygen ($CMRO_2$) in the affected brain region.[11] As the local stores of oxygen in tissues adjacent to capillaries are transiently consumed by glycolysis and waste products build up, various chemical signals (CO_2, NO, H^+) cause a vasomotor reaction in arterial sphincters upstream of the capillary bed, causing dilation of these vessels. The increased blood flow acts to restore the local $[O_2]$ level required to overcome the transient deficit; however, for reasons that are still not fully understood more oxygen is delivered than is needed to offset the increase in $CMRO_2$. As a result, neural upregulation results initially in a buildup of deoxygenated hemoglobin

Supported by NIH Grant P41-RR009784.
The author has no conflicts to declare.
Department of Radiology, Stanford University, Lucas MRI Center, MC 5488, 1201 Welch Road, Stanford, CA 94305–5488, USA
E-mail address: gary.glover@stanford.edu

Neurosurg Clin N Am 22 (2011) 133–139
doi:10.1016/j.nec.2010.11.001

(Hb) and a decrease in oxygenated hemoglobin (HbO$_2$) in the intra- and extravascular spaces, followed within a second or two by a vasodilatory response that reverses the situation to result in an increase in [HbO$_2$] and decrease in [Hb] over that in the resting condition (**Fig. 1**).[12,13] This sequence of processes is described as the hemodynamic response to the neural event.

Thus, there are 2 primary consequences of increased neural activity, and both can be detected by MRI: increased local cerebral blood flow (CBF) and changes in oxygenation concentration (Blood Oxygen Level Dependent, or BOLD, contrast). The change in CBF can be observed using an injected contrast agent and perfusion-weighted MRI, first demonstrated by Belliveau and colleagues,[14] or noninvasively by arterial spin labeling (ASL).[15] However, ASL suffers from reduced sensitivity, increased acquisition time, and increased sensitivity to motion compared with the BOLD contrast method, and its use has therefore centered on obtaining quantitative measurements of baseline CBF for studies modeling the neurobiological mechanisms of activation[11,13] or calibration of vasoreactivity,[16] rather than in routine mapping of brain function.

The second mechanism, termed BOLD contrast, was first demonstrated in rats[17,18] and later in humans,[1–3,19] and is the contrast that is used in virtually all conventional fMRI experiments. BOLD contrast results from the change in magnetic field surrounding the red blood cells depending on the oxygen state of the hemoglobin. When fully oxygenated, HbO$_2$ is diamagnetic and is magnetically indistinguishable from brain tissue.

However, fully deoxygenated Hb has 4 unpaired electrons and is highly paramagnetic.[20] This paramagnetism results in local gradients in magnetic field whose strength depends on the [Hb] concentration. These endogenous gradients in turn modulate the intra- and extravascular blood's T2 and T2* relaxation times through diffusion and intravoxel dephasing, respectively. Using a gradient refocused echo (GRE) MRI pulse sequence,[9] the acquisition is made sensitive to T2* and T2. At 1.5 T and 3 T, the T2* contrast is predominant and is largest in venules,[21] whereas at higher field strength the diffusion-weighted contrast of T2 relaxation becomes more important and, because signals are generated preferentially in capillaries and tissue with spin-echo acquisitions, provides greater spatial specificity.[22,23] Because most fMRI is currently performed at 3 T or below, BOLD fMRI uses primarily GRE methods because of the increased T2* contrast.[24]

Task activation fMRI studies seek to induce different neural states in the brain as the visual, auditory, or other stimulus is manipulated during the scan, and activation maps are obtained by comparing the signals recorded during the different states. Therefore, it is important to collect each image in a snapshot mode to avoid head motion, and prevent physiologic processes of respiration[25] and cardiovascular functions[26,27] from injecting noise signals unrelated to the neural processing being interrogated. In general, most fMRI is performed using an echo planar imaging (EPI) method,[28] which can collect data for a 2-dimensional image in approximately 60 milliseconds at typical resolutions (3.4 × 3.4 × 4 mm^3 voxel size). Whole brain scans with approximately 32 2-dimensional slices typically are acquired with a repetition time (TR) of 2 seconds per volume. Each voxel in the resulting scan produces a time series that is subsequently analyzed in accordance with the task design.

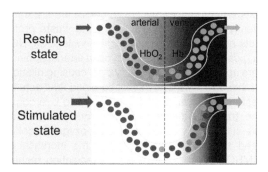

Fig. 1. Sketch of brain tissue containing a capillary during rest (*top*) and activation (*bottom*). Red and blue circles represent red blood cells that are fully oxygenated (HbO$_2$) and fully deoxygenated (Hb), respectively. The MRI signal is depressed in the venous side of the capillary due to the paramagnetic susceptibility of the Hb acting as an endogenous contrast agent (shown darker). In the stimulated condition, increased blood flow causes the Hb to be swept out and replaced by HbO$_2$, causing a BOLD signal increase.

THE FMRI EXPERIMENT

The typical fMRI task activation experiment uses visual, auditory, or other stimuli to alternately induce 2 or more different cognitive states in the subject, while collecting MRI volumes continuously as already described. With a 2-condition design, one state is called the experimental condition and the other is denoted the control condition; the goal is to test the hypothesis that the signals differ between the 2 states. Using a block design, the trials are arranged to alternate between the experimental and control conditions, as shown in **Fig. 2**, with each block typically being a few tens of seconds long. The block design is optimum

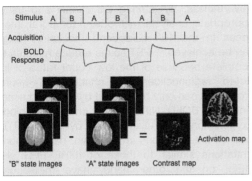

Fig. 2. Block-design fMRI experiment. A neural response to the state change from A to B in the stimulus is accompanied by a hemodynamic response (as shown in **Fig. 1**) that is detected by the rapid and continuous acquisition of MR images sensitized to BOLD signal changes. Using single or multivariate time series analysis methods, the average signal difference between the 2 states is computed for the scan and a contrast map generated. A statistical activation map is finally obtained using a suitable threshold for the difference; the map depicts the probability that a voxel is activated, given the uncertainty due to noise and the small BOLD signal differences.

for detecting activation, but a jittered event-related (ER) design is superior when characterization of the amplitude or timing of the hemodynamic response is desired.[29,30] In the ER design, task events are relatively brief and occur at nonconstant intertrial intervals with longer periods of control condition, which allows the hemodynamic response to return more fully to baseline. Jittering the timing serves to sample the hemodynamic response with higher temporal frequency in the overall time series, but may also be used to induce a desired cognitive strategy, for example, to avoid an anticipatory response or maintain attention.

The degree to which valid inferences can be drawn from the measured time series data depends in large part on careful design of the task. The investigator must take care that only the effect of interest changes between experimental and control conditions, while confounding effects such as attention and valence are maintained constant or irrelevant. In some studies this is straightforward, such as in the use of a sensory task for presurgical mapping, where the goal is only to localize activation so that important brain functions can be maintained after surgery. In this case the signal intensity is of minor interest as long as it is adequate to characterize the functional substrates to be preserved during surgical intervention. In many other cases, however, comparative inferences are desired, such as in parametric studies of the influence of task difficulty on

a cognitive process, and thus control of such factors as learning, adaptation, and salience must be considered.

ANALYSIS METHODS

Once the images have been acquired, the time series data must be processed to obtain maps of brain activation. Because the BOLD contrast is small (<1% in many studies of higher cognitive processes),[31] simply averaging images over the experimental and control conditions and then subtracting (as sketched in **Fig. 2**) is inadequate to reliably determine differences because noise will compete to render false positives and negatives. The noise results from thermal sources in the subject and electronics, bulk motion of the head, cardiac and respiratory-induced noise, and variations in baseline neural metabolism. Because the noise can sometimes be larger than the signal of interest, fMRI analyses compare the signal difference between the states using a statistical test. These tests result in an activation map that is a function of the probability that the brain states differ. The statistical test for activation can use a general linear model,[32,33] cross-correlation with a modeled regressor,[34] or one of several data-driven approaches such as independent components analysis.[35] The models against which the acquired data are tested include the experimental design of interest as well as "nuisance regressors" of no interest such as signal drift, motion, and noise reflected in global or white-matter signals. In all cases, the activation testing is preceded by a series of preprocessing steps.

The steps in preprocessing can include all or some of the following: (1) time-slice correction, to eliminate differences between the time of acquisition of each slice in the volume; (2) motion coregistration, in which affine head motion is detected and the time series of volumes is resampled to register each time frame to a reference frame, such as the first or middle time series point; (3) correction for physiologic noise from breathing and cardiovascular function,[25,26] low pass and/or high pass temporal filtering to improve the statistics while removing spectral components of no interest; (4) spatial smoothing to improve the signal to noise ratio (SNR) and improve the normality of the noise distribution; (5) prewhitening to correct for autocorrelation in the time series.[31] The analysis of fMRI data continues to be a subject of intense research at this time, and is one about which numerous books have been written, to which the reader is referred for further information (eg, Sarty[36]).

COMPARISONS WITH OTHER FUNCTIONAL IMAGING MODALITIES

fMRI can be compared with other imaging methods used to obtained functional assessment of brain metabolism in terms of spatial and temporal resolution and availability. The primary alternatives are positron emission tomography (PET), near-infrared spectroscopy (NIRS), electro-encephalography (EEG), and magnetoencephalography (MEG).[31]

Spatial Resolution

Resolution in fMRI is limited primarily by SNR because of the necessity for rapid acquisition of time series information. For MRI, $SNR \propto p^2 w \sqrt{T_{acq}N}$, where p is the pixel size, w the slice thickness, T_{acq} is the k-space readout time, and N the number of time frames. Thus, as T_{acq} is reduced for single-shot imaging (typically 20–30 milliseconds) the pixel size must be increased over that for conventional anatomic imaging to maintain an acceptable SNR. Accordingly, the typical fMRI pixel size is 3 to 4 mm, although with higher field magnets (7 T) a pixel size of 500 μm or less may be readily achieved.[22] The resolution of PET is limited by the size of the gamma-ray detectors as well as the positron-electron annihilation range, and is typically 5 to 10 mm or more. NIRS resolution is low (10–20 mm) and is limited predominantly by the strong scatter and attenuation of infrared photons (which also limits the depth of cortex that can be imaged within a banana-shaped region connecting optodes), the modest density of optodes, and the ill-conditioned inverse problem of reconstructing 3-dimensional maps of [Hb] from scalp recordings.[37] The resolution in EEG and MEG is similarly limited to greater than 10 to 20 mm by the fact that a unique reconstruction of dipoles is not possible from scalp-based measurements of electrical or magnetic distributions and models, and regularization must be employed for model estimation. Unlike EEG, MEG does not have the confounding factor that scalp recordings may be spatially distorted by heterogeneous electrical conduction paths within the brain/skull.

Temporal Resolution

Temporal resolution of fMRI is limited by hemodynamic response time; typically the BOLD response has a width of ~3 seconds and a peak occurring approximately 5 to 6 seconds after the onset of a brief neural stimulus. This rate is much slower than the underlying neural processes, and temporal information is thereby heavily blurred.

Nevertheless, by jittering ER stimuli and using appropriate analysis methods,[29] temporal inferences in the 100-millisecond resolution range can be achieved.[38] PET scans require minutes to complete because of the low count rates of injected radionuclides, so changes in neural processes can only be studied by repeated scanning. Like BOLD, NIRS reports changes in blood oxygenation and, exacerbated by low SNR of near-infrared photons in the brain, has temporal limitations similar to those of fMRI. EEG and MEG, on the other hand, have millisecond temporal resolution and can easily capture the dynamics of evoked responses that last a few milliseconds to several hundred milliseconds. Multimodal approaches combining fMRI and EEG use fMRI maps as spatial priors to reconstruct high temporal resolution electrophysiology, thereby gaining resolution in both dimensions.[39]

STRENGTHS AND WEAKNESSES OF FMRI

From the foregoing discussion, a primary strength of fMRI is its relatively high spatial resolution and availability. In addition, it is readily available to both clinical and academic researchers, is noninvasive, and can provide high-resolution anatomic scans in the same session to use for localization, vessel identification,[40] or development of maps of white matter connectivity through the use of diffusion tensor imaging.[41]

Because BOLD contrast derives from the sluggish hemodynamic response to metabolic changes, a significant weakness is its low temporal resolution. Another problem is signal dropout and/or spatial distortion in frontal orbital and lateral parietal regions, caused by the difference of approximately 9 ppm in magnetic susceptibility at interfaces between air and brain tissue.[42] This situation can result in erroneous lack of BOLD signal in ventral, temporal, and prefrontal cortex regions important in many cognitive studies. Many methods have been developed to diminish these susceptibility losses, although most involve some trade-off of SNR in magnetically uniform brain regions.[42–48] Other weaknesses include the scanner's loud noise associated with switched magnetic fields, which can cause confounding factors in studies of audition[49,50] and resting state networks[51]; however, methods using interleaved scanning/stimulus delivery epochs can avoid these problems, albeit with some loss of flexibility in experimental design.[49,52] Finally, the high magnetic fields require customized stimulus delivery and subject response systems, again limiting flexibility and complicating multimodal experiments such as concurrent EEG recording.

FUTURE OF FMRI

For the most part, the MRI physics and technology development behind BOLD fMRI acquisitions are mature, and the trade-offs between acquisition speed, resolution, SNR, signal dropout, and contrast are well understood. Over the years, several investigators have attempted to develop alternatives to BOLD contrast using direct neural current detection,[53] although by now it is understood[54] that the weak size of the neural current signal relative to physiologic noise makes a breakthrough unlikely. Another alternative is the use of diffusion-weighted imaging to demonstrate activation-related changes in populations of bound versus free water distributions.[55,56] A potential advantage is that such diffusion-related changes may have more rapid responses than BOLD methods. However, again the signals are weaker than BOLD contrast and their biophysical origin is still unclear.[57] Other experiments have reported the use of spin echo rather than gradient echo acquisitions of BOLD contrast, especially at higher fields where T2* is foreshortened.[22]

While a modest research effort will continue in improving acquisition technology, the bulk of research in the development of fMRI has shifted to its application to answering more complex questions in cognitive neuroscience. One promising area is that of using activation maps as input to classification and state change algorithms to predict or classify cognitive behavior, such as predicting brain states[58,59] (also see, eg, Norman and colleagues[60] for a review). Other emerging uses of fMRI include the development of quantitative measures, that is, biomarkers for disease or monitoring behavioral modification such as reading disorders. A cautionary note, however, is that because of the small BOLD responses typical of cognitive processes, most studies are limited to employing group statistics to make inferences about populations rather than about individuals. Thus the use of fMRI in quantifying individual characteristics may continue to be limited to those tasks for which relatively strong BOLD responses are observed, such as primary sensory systems. Resting state networks and their modification by disease conditions such as Alzheimer disease, depression, and other psychiatric disorders[61] are gaining attention. However, there is growing awareness that these networks may be much more complex in their spatiotemporal dynamics than previously thought,[62] and much more work is indicated to understand their role and utility in predicting individual behavior/physiology. Finally, feedback derived from real-time fMRI has been shown to allow subjects to learn pain-reduction strategies,[63] to enhance sensorimotor control,[64] and to control relevant brain regions in mood disorder experiments.[59] The reader is also referred to Bandettini[65] for additional considerations regarding the future of fMRI.

SUMMARY

Functional MRI has enjoyed an exciting development course with an exponential growth in published studies since its inception in the early 1990s, and it has become commonplace for clinical uses such as presurgical planning, fundamental cognitive neuroscience investigations, behavior modification, and training. Informed by fMRI, more sophisticated modeling of brain networks is certain to lead to new levels of understanding of the human brain.

ACKNOWLEDGMENTS

The author is indebted to C.E. Chang for suggestions on the manuscript.

REFERENCES

1. Bandettini PA, Wong EC, Hinks RS, et al. Time course EPI of human brain function during task activation. Magn Reson Med 1992;25:390.
2. Kwong KK, Belliveau JW, Chesler DA, et al. Dynamic magnetic resonance imaging of human brain activity during primary sensory stimulation. Proc Natl Acad Sci U S A 1992;89:5675.
3. Ogawa S, Lee TM, Kay AR, et al. Brain magnetic resonance imaging with contrast dependent on blood oxygenation. Proc Natl Acad Sci U S A 1990;87:9868.
4. Greicius MD, Srivastava G, Reiss AL, et al. Default-mode network activity distinguishes Alzheimer's disease from healthy aging: evidence from functional MRI. Proc Natl Acad Sci U S A 2004;101:4637.
5. Kim DI, Sui J, Rachakonda S, et al. Identification of imaging biomarkers in schizophrenia: a coefficient-constrainedindependent component analysis of the mind multi-siteschizophrenia study. Neuroinformatics 2010;8(4):213–29.
6. Richards TL, Berninger VW. Abnormal fMRI connectivity in children with dyslexia during a phoneme task: before but not after treatment. J Neurolinguistics 2008;21:294.
7. Wise RG, Preston C. What is the value of human FMRI in CNS drug development? Drug Discov Today 2010;15:973–80.
8. Lauterbur PC. Image formation by induced local interactions. Examples employing nuclear magnetic resonance. Nature 1973;242:190.

9. Bernstein MA, King KF, Zhou XJ. Handbook of MRI pulse sequences. New York: Elsevier Press; 2004.

10. Roland PE. Brain activation. New York: John Wiley & Sons; 1993.

11. Buxton R, Frank L. A model for the coupling between cerebral blood flow and oxygen metabolism during neural stimulation. J Cereb Blood Flow Metab 1997;17:64.

12. Buxton RB, Wong EC, Frank LR. Dynamics of blood flow and oxygenation changes during brain activation: the balloon model. Magn Reson Med 1998;39:855.

13. Davis TL, Kwong KK, Weisskoff RM, et al. Calibrated functional MRI: mapping the dynamics of oxidative metabolism. Proc Natl Acad Sci U S A 1998;95:1834.

14. Belliveau JW, Kennedy DJ, McKinstry RC, et al. Functional mapping of the human visual cortex by magnetic resonance imaging. Science 1991;254:716.

15. Detre JA, Leigh JS, Williams DS, et al. Perfusion imaging. Magn Reson Med 1992;23:37.

16. Bangen KJ, Restom K, Liu TT, et al. Differential age effects on cerebral blood flow and BOLD response to encoding: associations with cognition and stroke risk. Neurobiol Aging 2009;30:1276.

17. Ogawa S, Lee TM. Magnetic resonance imaging of blood vessels at high fields: in vivo and in vitro measurements and image simulation. Magn Reson Med 1990;16:9.

18. Ogawa S, Lee TM, Nayak AS, et al. Oxygenation-sensitive contrast in magnetic resonance image of rodent brain at high magnetic fields. Magn Reson Med 1990;14:68.

19. Ogawa S, Menon RS, Tank DW, et al. Functional brain mapping by blood oxygenation level-dependent contrast magnetic resonance imaging. A comparison of signal characteristics with a biophysical model. Biophys J 1993;64:803.

20. Thulborn KR, Waterton JC, Matthews PM, et al. Oxygenation dependence of the transverse relaxation time of water protons in whole blood at high field. Biochim Biophys Acta 1982;714:265.

21. Weisskoff RM, Zuo CS, Boxerman JL, et al. Microscopic susceptibility variation and transverse relaxation: theory and experiment. Magn Reson Med 1994;31:601.

22. Shmuel A, Yacoub E, Chaimow D, et al. Spatiotemporal point-spread function of fMRI signal in human gray matter at 7 Tesla. Neuroimage 2007;35:539.

23. Yacoub E, Van De Moortele PF, Shmuel A, et al. Signal and noise characteristics of Hahn SE and GE BOLD fMRI at 7 T in humans. Neuroimage 2005;24:738.

24. Boxerman JL, Bandettini PA, Kwong KK, et al. The intravascular contribution to fMRI signal change: Monte Carlo modeling and diffusion-weighted studies in vivo. Magn Reson Med 1995;34:4.

25. Birn RM, Smith MA, Jones TB, et al. The respiration response function: the temporal dynamics of fMRI signal fluctuations related to changes in respiration. Neuroimage 2008;40:644.

26. Chang C, Cunningham JP, Glover GH. Influence of heart rate on the BOLD signal: the cardiac response function. Neuroimage 2009;44:857.

27. Chang C, Glover GH. Relationship between respiration, end-tidal CO(2), and BOLD signals in resting-state fMRI. Neuroimage 2009;47:1381–93.

28. Mansfield P. Multi-planar image formation using NMR spin echoes. J Phys Chem C 1977;10:L55.

29. Buckner RL, Bandettini PA, O'Craven KM, et al. Detection of cortical activation during averaged single trials of a cognitive task using functional magnetic resonance imaging. [see comments]. Proc Natl Acad Sci U S A 1996;93:14878.

30. Liu TT, Frank LR. Efficiency, power, and entropy in event-related FMRI with multiple trial types. Part I: theory. Neuroimage 2004;21:387.

31. Huettel SA, Song AW, McCarthy G. Functional magnetic resonance imaging. Sunderland (MA): Sinauer Associates, Inc; 2004.

32. Friston KJ, Holmes AP, Poline JB, et al. Analysis of fMRI time-series revisited. Neuroimage 1995;2:45.

33. Worsley KJ, Liao CH, Aston J, et al. A general statistical analysis for fMRI data. Neuroimage 2002;15:1.

34. Bandettini PA, Jesmanowicz A, Wong EC, et al. Processing strategies for time-course data sets in functional MRI of the human brain. Magn Reson Med 1993;30:161.

35. Calhoun VD, Adali T, Pearlson GD, et al. A method for making group inferences from functional MRI data using independent component analysis. Hum Brain Mapp 2001;14:140.

36. Sarty GE. Computing brain activity maps from fMRI time series images. Cambridge (UK): Cambridge University Press; 2007.

37. Cui X, Bray S, Bryant DM, et al. A quantitative comparison of NIRS and fMRI across multiple cognitive tasks. Neuroimage 2010. [Epub ahead of print]. PMID: 21047559.

38. Ogawa S, Lee TM, Stepnoski R, et al. An approach to probe some neural systems interaction by functional MRI at neural time scale down to milliseconds. Proc Natl Acad Sci U S A 2000;97:11026.

39. Dale AM, Halgren E. Spatiotemporal mapping of brain activity by integration of multiple imaging modalities. Curr Opin Neurobiol 2001;11:202.

40. Menon RS. Postacquisition suppression of large-vessel BOLD signals in high-resolution fMRI. Magn Reson Med 2002;47:1.

41. Basser PJ, Pajevic S, Pierpaoli C, et al. In vivo fiber tractography using DT-MRI data. Magn Reson Med 2000;44:625.

42. Cho ZH, Ro YM. Reduction of susceptibility artifact in gradient-echo imaging. Magn Reson Med 1992; 23:193.

43. Constable R, Spencer D. Composite image formation in Z-shimmed functional MR imaging. Magn Reson Med 1999;42:110.

44. Glover GH, Law CS. Spiral-in/out BOLD fMRI for increased SNR and reduced susceptibility artifacts. Magn Reson Med 2001;46:515.

45. Hsu JJ, Glover GH. Mitigation of susceptibility-induced signal loss in neuroimaging using localized shim coils. Magn Reson Med 2005;53:243.

46. Stenger VA, Boada FE, Noll DC. Three-dimensional tailored RF pulses for the reduction of susceptibility artifacts in T2*-weighted functional MRI. Magn Reson Med 2000;44:525.

47. Weiger M, Pruessmann KP, Osterbauer R, et al. Sensitivity-encoded single-shot spiral imaging for reduced susceptibility artifacts in BOLD fMRI. Magn Reson Med 2002;48:860.

48. Yang QX, Dardzinski BJ, Li S, et al. Multi-gradient echo with susceptibility inhomogeneity compensation (MGESIC): demonstration of fMRI in the olfactory cortex at 3.0 T. Magn Reson Med 1997;37:331.

49. Gaab N, Gabrieli JD, Glover GH. Assessing the influence of scanner background noise on auditory processing. I. An fMRI study comparing three experimental designs with varying degrees of scanner noise. Hum Brain Mapp 2007;28:703.

50. Gaab N, Gabrieli JD, Glover GH. Assessing the influence of scanner background noise on auditory processing. II. An fMRI study comparing auditory processing in the absence and presence of recorded scanner noise using a sparse design. Hum Brain Mapp 2007;28:721.

51. Gaab N, Gabrieli JD, Glover GH. Resting in peace or noise: scanner background noise suppresses default-mode network. Hum Brain Mapp 2008;29: 858.

52. Edmister WB, Talavage TM, Ledden PJ, et al. Improved auditory cortex imaging using clustered volume acquisitions. Hum Brain Mapp 1999;7:89.

53. Bodurka J, Bandettini PA. Toward direct mapping of neuronal activity: MRI detection of ultraweak, transient magnetic field changes. Magn Reson Med 2002;47:1052.

54. Luo Q, Gao JH. Modeling magnitude and phase neuronal current MRI signal dependence on echo time. Magn Reson Med 2010;64(6):1832–7.

55. Le Bihan D, Urayama S, Aso T, et al. Direct and fast detection of neuronal activation in the human brain with diffusion MRI. Proc Natl Acad Sci U S A 2006; 103:8263.

56. Li T, Song AW. Fast functional brain signal changes detected by diffusion weighted fMRI. Magn Reson Imaging 2003;21:829.

57. Miller KL, Bulte DP, Devlin H, et al. Evidence for a vascular contribution to diffusion FMRI at high b value. Proc Natl Acad Sci U S A 2007;104:20967.

58. Martinez-Ramon M, Koltchinskii V, Heileman GL, et al. fMRI pattern classification using neuroanatomically constrained boosting. Neuroimage 2006;31:1129.

59. Phan KL, Fitzgerald DA, Gao K, et al. Real-time fMRI of cortico-limbic brain activity during emotional processing. Neuroreport 2004;15:527.

60. Norman KA, Polyn SM, Detre GJ, et al. Beyond mind-reading: multi-voxel pattern analysis of fMRI data. Trends Cogn Sci 2006;10:424.

61. Greicius M. Resting-state functional connectivity in neuropsychiatric disorders. Curr Opin Neurol 2008; 21:424.

62. Chang C, Glover GH. Time-frequency dynamics of resting-state brain connectivity measured with fMRI. Neuroimage 2010;50:81.

63. deCharms RC, Maeda F, Glover GH, et al. Control over brain activation and pain learned by using real-time functional MRI. Proc Natl Acad Sci U S A 2005;102:18626.

64. deCharms RC, Christoff K, Glover GH, et al. Learned regulation of spatially localized brain activation using real-time fMRI. Neuroimage 2004;21:436.

65. Bandettini PA. What's new in neuroimaging methods? Ann N Y Acad Sci 2009;1156:260.

Brain Mapping Using Transcranial Magnetic Stimulation

José Rafael Romero, MD[a],*, Deisy Marcela Ramirez, MD[b],
Linda S. Aglio, MD[c], Laverne D. Gugino, MD, PhD[c]

KEYWORDS

- Brain mapping • Transcranial magnetic stimulation
- Cortex • Brain physiology

Localization of eloquent brain regions has evolved in the past few decades with the development of noninvasive techniques for cortical stimulation. Identification of eloquent brain areas such as the motor cortex is highly relevant in various fields ranging from preoperative planning of surgical procedures to studies of functional recovery following stroke, and administration of treatments such as repetitive transcranial magnetic stimulation (TMS) for the treatment of depression. Since its initial description in 1985 by Anthony Barker,[1] TMS has evolved significantly. Initial studies involved blind placement of stimulating coils over the scalp surface. However, the advent of navigation systems using model reconstructions of the brain (mostly based on brain magnetic resonance imaging [MRI]) allowed for more precise positioning of coils during brain stimulation using TMS. Prior studies have shown that this approach reduces significantly the variability of brain regions stimulated,[2] and has significant implications for the diagnostic and therapeutic use of TMS.[3] TMS is considered a safe, noninvasive technique allowing also for assessment of various brain functions. This article reviews the principles underlying the mechanism of action of TMS, and discusses its use to obtain functional maps of the motor and visual cortex, including technical considerations for accuracy and reproducibility of mapping procedures.

PRINCIPLES OF TMS

In the early 1800s, Michael Faraday described the phenomenon of electromagnetic induction, in which an electric current induces a magnetic field, and a magnetic field in turn can induce electrical currents. It was not until 1985 that further use of magnetic stimulation was developed by Barker and colleagues,[1] showing that magnetic pulses applied over the scalp elicit motor responses that can be used for transcranial motor cortex stimulation in a safe and painless fashion.

The magnetic stimulator consists of a component that generates, stores, and releases rapidly a large electrical current pulse through a copper coil, which in turn produces a pulsed magnetic field around the coil windings. The magnetic field then travels in the space underlying the coil, and, if it is impressed on electrically conductive tissue of sufficient volume, a secondary electrical current loop is generated within the tissue, much as in the secondary windings of a transformer. Such current loops are responsible for excitation of neural elements.[4]

TMS stimulates different components of neural tissue, but a predominant descending motor path originating in the motor cortex that is excited by TMS is the corticospinal tract (CST).[5–9] Controversy remains concerning the precise site of action of TMS and its ability to excite CST neurons

[a] Department of Neurology, Boston University School of Medicine, 72 East Concord Street, C-329 Boston, MA 02118, USA
[b] Department of Psychiatry, Boston University School of Medicine, 72 East Concord Street, Boston, MA 02118, USA
[c] Department of Anesthesia, Harvard Medical School, Brigham and Women's Hospital, 75 Francis Street, CWN-L1, Boston, MA 02115, USA
* Corresponding author.
E-mail address: joromero@bmc.org

Neurosurg Clin N Am 22 (2011) 141–152
doi:10.1016/j.nec.2010.11.002
1042-3680/11/$ – see front matter © 2011 Elsevier Inc. All rights reserved.

directly. Some investigators have suggested that CST excitation is mediated by excitation of cortical interneurons.[5,7,10] The latency of motor-evoked potentials (MEP) at all stimulus intensities produced by TMS have a longer latency than those seen using transcranial electrical stimulation (TCES). Day and colleagues,[5] Rothwell[7] and others have reasoned that, because TMS-induced current loops are parallel to the inner cranial surface, they would likewise parallel the surface of the cortical gyral caps. Thus, the current loops would be oriented along the axis of cortical interneurons, an orientation appropriate for cortical interneuron excitation. However, the induced current loops would be orthogonal to CST neurons, which are radially oriented within the cortical gyral caps. This current loop orientation is much less efficient for direct stimulation of CST cortical neurons.

However, other investigators have shown that direct TMS activation of CST neurons was possible with appropriate tilting of the stimulating coil on the scalp.[11] The change in coil orientation on the scalp presumably led to induced current loops that paralleled the orientation of CST neurons (or the neuronal axons) within the cortex. Jalinous[12] showed that large-diameter stimulating coils produce electric fields of greater intensity as a function of cortical depth than smaller coils. A scalp vertex orientation of a large round coil should, theoretically, cause direct excitation of CST cells located within the anterior bank of the central sulcus. At this location, these cells are oriented in a radial direction to both the cortical surface and induced current loops. Amassian and colleagues[13] reasoned that magnetically induced current flowing within the axons tends to exit at the axonal bend, leading to a situation favorable for axonal excitation. Their results were consistent with CST activation deep within the cortex at the junction of the cortex and underlying white matter. They hypothesized that impulse initiation occurred near the axon hillock region or the CST basal dentrites.[13] Rudiak and colleagues,[14] using an analogous approach, found a similar depth for TMS excitation of geniculocalcarine fibers near the primary visual cortex or possibly within the secondary visual cortex.

MOTOR CORTEX MAPPING

TMS applied to restricted areas of the scalp overlying the motor cortex elicits MEPs in contralateral muscles, which may be used to map the location and extent of motor cortical representations for several muscles. Such maps are useful to assess normal motor cortical function as well as brain plasticity as a result of skill acquisition or pathologic lesions.[2,15–17] They may also allow evaluation of brain response to injury (eg, as in stroke recovery), providing a tool to evaluate interventions that enhance recovery, assessment of patients with lesions near eloquent cortex before surgical interventions (eg, presurgical planning for resection of brain tumors near the motor cortex), and evaluation of cortical excitability in diseases affecting the nervous system.

Precision in targeting specific brain regions using TMS is of utmost importance. The functional patterns of the cortical surface are known to vary among individuals.[18,19] Therefore, a cortical mapping technique should relate cortical surface anatomy and function.

Precision of TMS for Brain Mapping

The focality of a coil varies depending on its shape. Cohen and colleagues,[20] using an experimental model, calculated the largest current densities occur under a stimulating coil, showing that a double circular coil produces the greatest focality with respect to magnetically induced stimulating currents. The figure-of-eight coil shows a peak induced electric field under the juxtaposition of the small circular components. The electric field is minimal at the center of each circular coil and has smaller peaks compared with the central contact of the 2 circular coils under the outer wing windings.[21,22] The magnetic field was largest 3 cm from the center of the butterfly coil with a polarity reversal beyond the borders.[20] Epstein and colleagues[23] used 2 different-sized figure-of-eight coils to study the location of TMS-induced direct excitation of CST neurons in humans. A small magnetic coil produces a more intense magnetic field close to the coil surface than is the case with a larger coil. However, the magnetic field attenuates faster with distance from the smaller coil. Because CST neurons have the same threshold for activation, the locus for CST action potential initiation is the same for both types of coil. However, the magnetic coil current intensities are greater for threshold impulse initiation when using the smaller coil. Epstein and colleagues[23] determined the depth within the cortex where CST impulse initiation occurred by knowing the degree of the induced electric field attenuation with distance and the threshold for producing a thumb twitch. Their results were consistent with CST activation deep within cortex located at the junction of the cortex and underlying white matter. They hypothesized that impulse initiation occurred near the axon hillock region or the CST basal dentrites.[23]

Ueno and Matsuda[24] studied the resolution of TMS using a figure-of-eight coil. Single monophasic induced cortical current pulses were used. By optimizing the stimulation technique for focal excitation of the motor cortex distal upper limb foci, he was able to show a resolution of 0.5 cm for discrete TMS muscle activation.

Traditionally, TMS has been delivered using skull/scalp landmarks, in a blind fashion, holding the TMS coil in place while stimulation is delivered. Some have used head frames to immobilize the person's head[25]; others mark the coil contour on a swimming cap worn by the individual being stimulated (**Fig. 1**). However, displacement of the coil may occur, resulting in stimulation of different brain regions from those intended, and potentially affecting the results of the intervention.

We recently described a TMS mapping technique using stereotactic optic guidance.[2,26] The purpose of this technique is to facilitate visualization of the cortical surface, and to guide placement of the TMS coil relative to the cortical surface of an individual. Thus, specific brain regions can be stimulated while controlling for coil movements relative to the person's brain. The mapping procedure is described in the Appendix. In a previous study, we evaluated the precision attained using this optical tracking system[2] using single-pulse TMS in normal volunteers. A blind technique, using markings of the figure-of-eight contour on a swimming cap worn by the volunteer to guide coil placement over the scalp, was compared with a guided technique, using the optical tracking system described. Three levels of TMS stimulation intensity were studied. The accuracy of coil repositioning at the optimal location for the first dorsal interosseus muscle was evaluated using a blind

versus guided approach. Use of the guided technique resulted in smaller cortical regions stimulated (**Fig. 2**). In addition, the distances between the cortical optimal locus and loci stimulated during subsequent stimulation trials were significantly smaller using the guided technique (<2 mm compared with 10–14 mm using a blinded technique). The differences of the three-dimensional (3D) angles achieved during the initial stimulation at the optimal location and subsequent trials attempting to reproduce it were also significantly smaller using the guided technique. These findings were more evident at lower stimulation intensities, as expected, because higher

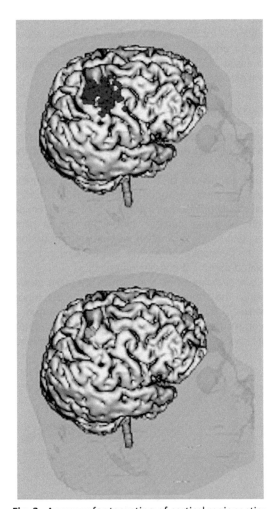

Fig. 2. Accuracy for targeting of cortical regions stimulated using guided (*green*) versus blind (*red*) stimulation techniques. The motor cortical representation for the contralateral first dorsal interosseus muscle is the target region. Note the significantly larger area stimulated using a blind approach, compared with the improved targeted stimulation using a guided technique.

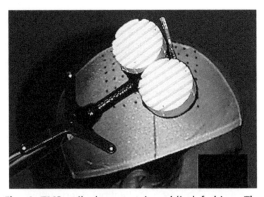

Fig. 1. TMS coil placement in a blind fashion. The subject wears a tight swimming cap on which markings are drawn to guide coil placement. Stimulation is delivered while attempting to maintain coil orientation and positioning.

stimulation intensity is associated with current spread,[27] and responses may be elicited by stimulating a location further from the intended target cortical locus. This study also showed that guided stimulation resulted in higher probability of eliciting MEPs, and that the MEPs obtained were of higher amplitudes and areas, although the coefficients of variation did not decrease significantly. This study also showed significant improvement in the precision to deliver TMS to target cortical regions, and illustrated some of the physiologic consequences.

Other investigators have also found improvement in precision for scalp placement of a coil by using other methods such as a 3D digitizer,[28] or a chin rest and clamping the coil.[29] However, the system developed by our group allows quantification of error in coil placement, real-time optical guidance for stimulation, and is frameless, allowing for greater patient comfort. Optical guidance to assist TMS studies improves the precision for coil placement.

Replication of TMS

A second important consideration when obtaining motor cortical maps is the reproducibility of the maps over time, which is relevant for instances such as the use of TMS in presurgical planning and the study of brain plasticity. Prior studies have investigated this aspect.[15,30–32] Some limitations of these studies include the use of blind techniques,[15,30,32] limiting the mapping procedure to the pericentral cortex in a single session,[31] and limited control of coil placement.[28]

We evaluated this question in a recent study, using the optical tracking system described earlier.[33] In 2 mapping sessions performed 1 month apart, 8 healthy volunteers were stimulated using single-pulse TMS to obtain the functional representation for the first dorsal interosseus (FDI) muscle. After performing a coregistration procedure and calibration of the coil, a grid with intersections every 1 cm was displayed and projected onto the cortical surface (**Fig. 3**). Although the grid was flat, the resulting distance between stimulated cortical loci was less than 1 cm. The coil was placed at each grid intersection visually guided by the tracking system, TMS was delivered, and MEPs recorded for offline analysis until no additional responses were obtained. We used a stimulation intensity set at 85% of stimulator output for mapping, based on prior experience that showed that this intensity is greater than the resting motor threshold for reliably eliciting responses from distal upper limb muscles. In addition, less intracortical current spread is expected than if using 100%. Three TMS stimuli were applied at each intersection point and the coil position was recorded. The MEPs were averaged at each intersection and a 4-point interpolated color cortical surface and scalp topographic map was constructed using the MEP amplitudes as a function of their cortical surface location (**Fig. 4**).

The second mapping session followed the same process (ie, coregistration of the subject's head and calibration of the coil, followed by retrieval of the initial map). The display in the monitor showed the coil orientation achieved during the initial map every time TMS stimuli were delivered. The coil position was shown represented by vectors (**Fig. 5**). Next, the coil was placed on the scalp and, as soon as it was detected by the optical tracking cameras, vectors representing the coil location were displayed. The attempt was then made to match the coil orientation achieved during the first mapping session (by matching the vectors in the display). Once matching of coil placement occurred, TMS was delivered and the MEPs

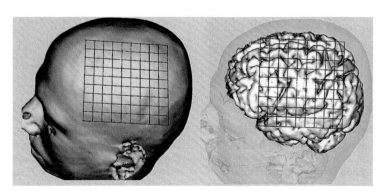

Fig. 3. The virtual grid overlying the scalp and cortical surface. The planar grid intersections are 1 cm apart.

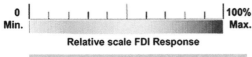

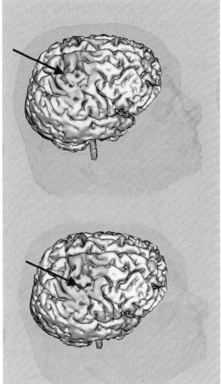

Fig. 4. Interpolated cortical maps of the motor representation for the contralateral FDI muscle. The color scale represents the relative peak-to-peak amplitude of the MEP. The arrow points to the location where the largest averaged peak-to-peak amplitude MEP was elicited (ie, hot spot).

obtained recorded as well as coil position information. This procedure was repeated until all the loci stimulated in the first session were stimulated.

Using this system, accurate coil repositioning could be achieved. Comparison of the coordinates of cortical loci stimulated in the 2 mapping sessions showed excellent prediction of loci stimulated during a second mapping session based on the coordinates achieved in the first session. The system achieved an error of less than 3 mm (distance between cortical loci stimulated in the 2 sessions) in about 95% of the stimulation trials in the study, with a 3D angle difference of less than 3 degrees in about 85% of the trials. Evaluation of the physiologic responses, by comparing the MEPs obtained in the 2 mapping sessions, revealed no significant differences between MEP

latency, amplitude, and area between the 2 sessions. The system again increased the probability of obtaining MEPs. Map response concordance rate was 0.86, reflecting the probability of either eliciting or failing to elicit MEPs in cortical loci stimulated in the 2 mapping sessions. In addition, comparing the motor map parameters revealed no significant differences between map area, volume, and amplitude at the optimal location in the 2 mapping sessions (**Table 1** and **Fig. 6**). The resting motor threshold at the optimal location was not significantly different between mapping sessions. The distance of the amplitude-weighted center of gravity in the 2 maps was 2.6 ($\pm$1.3) mm (mean $\pm$ standard deviation) across subjects. **Table 1** summarizes the map parameters obtained in the 2 mapping sessions.

Other important observations were made. First, some of the subjects showed several cortical loci where large MEPs were obtained, with amplitudes close to that obtained at the optimal location. This finding likely reflects the organization of the motor cortex in neuronal clusters that are closely arranged.[34] This is a relevant consideration because using TMS in a blind fashion may target different brain areas that may elicit similar responses (at least in the motor cortex). Second, there were prominent interindividual differences in the area of motor maps between subjects. This finding is consistent with prior studies,[15,16,30] and is an important consideration further supporting the use of a guided mapping technique.

Guided TMS using an optical tracking system resulted in reliable reproduction of coil placement and motor maps that were stable in the short term in a group of normal volunteers. Other studies support these findings. Mortifee and colleagues[30] reported that motor maps were replicable for a range of 21 to 132 days on 6 normal volunteers. Thus, maps with greater variability might represent abnormalities or plastic changes in the brain as a result of adaptation to underlying disorders or physiologic adaptation, for instance during skill learning.[35,36]

Future applications of the technique described for mapping the motor cortex include use in studies using TMS applied to brain regions other than the motor cortex. In addition, correlation with other mapping methods will provide further clarification of the best method to obtain function cortical maps.

VISUAL CORTEX MAPPING

Previous reports suggest that other brain areas can be mapped using TMS. Although TMS is

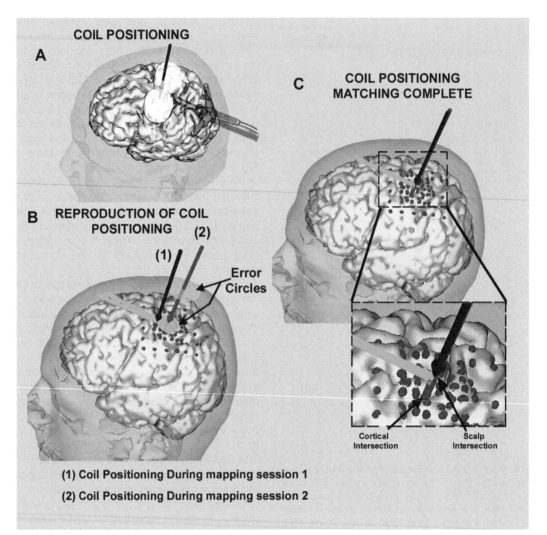

Fig. 5. Live coil positioning guidance by the optical tracking system. (*A*) The vectors representing coil placement. Note the star-shaped probe attached to the figure-of-eight coil containing the 3 light-emitting diodes (LEDs) tracked by infrared cameras. (*B*) Coil positioning achieved during the initial mapping session (represented by the blue vector) and the actual coil position during the second mapping session (represented by the red vector) while the operator is attempting to reproduce coil placement. Note the error circles representing the different 3D angles (ie, tilt and rotation) between the previous and current coil positions. (*C*) Precise coil repositioning, as shown by the disappearance of the error circles and superimposition of the 2 vectors. The insert shows the cortical loci stimulated as represented by the red dots. The pink extension from the vector tip represents the distance from the scalp surface to the cortical surface. (*From* Gugino LD. TMA in the perioperative period. In: Wassermann EM, Epstein CM, Zieman U, et al. The Oxford handbook of transcranial stimulation. New York: Oxford University Press; 2008. p. 320; with permission.)

able to induce cortical responses, as in the case of motor cortex stimulation, it can also suppress cortical activity. This principle is particularly useful to study cognitive phenomena, and obtain functional maps of receptive brain areas such as the visual cortex. In a prior study, our group showed the use of a stereotactic tracking system to map the cortical localization of TMS-induced visual suppression.[37] With a series of experiments, it was first shown that a figure-of-eight coil can effectively suppress visual stimuli contralateral to the site of stimulation at a latency of 80 to 100 milliseconds following presentation of stimulus (**Fig. 7**). This finding reproduced results of previous

Table 1
Motor map characteristics[a]

	Map 1	Map 2
Area (cm²)[a,b]	14.63 ± 8.52	15.75 ± 8.88
Volume[a,c]	384.98 ± 391.06	381.23 ± 330.71
Maximal amplitude (mV)[a,d]	2.23 ± 1.25	2.82 ± 1.59
Resting MT[a,e]	70.2 ± 3.7	69 ± 3.38
Distance between amplitude-weighted CoG (mm)[a,f]	2.6 ± 1.3	
Distance between optimal loci (mm)	10 ± 5.5	

Values are mean of all subjects ± standard deviation.

Abbreviation: CoG, center of gravity.

[a] No statistically significant differences were found across sessions.

[b] Area refers to the number of excitable grid loci.

[c] Volume of the map refers to the sum of the relative MEP amplitudes (%M) across all excitable locations.

[d] Maximal amplitude refers to the highest peak-to-peak amplitude MEP elicited.

[e] The resting MT is expressed as percentage (%) of magnetic stimulator output.

[f] The x, y, and z coordinates for the CoG were recalculated by multiplying the coordinate at each position by its amplitude weight and summing overall positions stimulated.

From Gugino LD. TMA in the perioperative period. In: Wassermann EM, Epstein CM, Zieman U, et al. The Oxford handbook of transcranial stimulation. New York: Oxford University Press; 2008. p. 321; with permission.

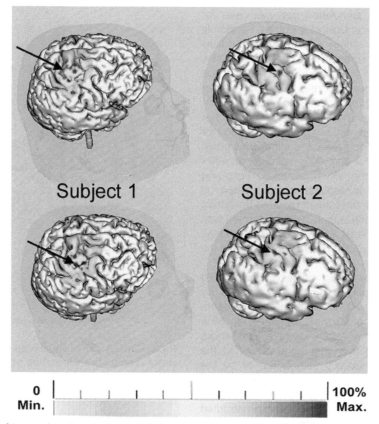

Fig. 6. Example of interpolated cortical maps of the motor representation for the contralateral FDI muscle in 2 separate mapping sessions. The color scale represents the relative peak-to-peak amplitude of the MEP. The arrow points to the location where the largest averaged peak-to-peak amplitude MEP was elicited (ie, hot spot). The 2 subjects shown underwent 2 mapping sessions (initial session top, second session bottom). No significant differences were observed in motor map parameters between the 2 mapping sessions.

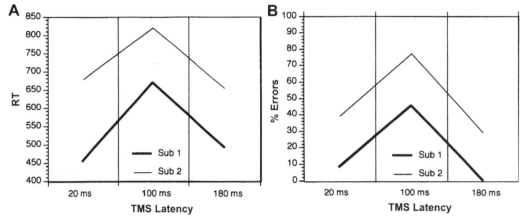

Fig. 7. Visual suppression effect. (*A*) Reaction time versus TMS latency for 2 subjects. Note the slower reaction times for both subjects at the 100-millisecond TMS latency. (*B*) Error rate as a function of TMS latency for the same 2 subjects. Note again the higher error rate at the 100-millisecond TMS latency. (*From* Potts GF, Gugino LD, Leventon ME, et al. Visual hemifield mapping using transcranial magnetic stimulation coregistered with cortical surfaces derived from magnetic resonance images. J Clin Neurophysiol 1998;15:346; with permission.)

studies that used a nonfocal, circular coil.[38] Next, using the visually guided stimulation system, a focal magnetic stimulation coil was used for delivering a stimulus train of 4 pulses. Randomly generated 3-letter strings were presented at fixation on a 35.5-cm screen. At the start of each trial, the subject would focus on a fixation dot at the center of the computer screen. The subject then pushed the computer spacebar to request a stimulus. Five-hundred milliseconds later, a 3-letter string would appear and remain on the screen for 15 milliseconds. Focal magnetic stimulation could occur between 75 and 105 milliseconds after presentation of the visual stimulus. Following TMS stimulation, a response cue appeared on screen. At the cue, the subject reported the letters in the string. Repetitive trials were performed with a separation of at least 30 seconds. For each trial, the coil was moved over different locations on the occiput.

Results from a typical subject showed that disruption of visual processing as indexed by errors in reporting 1 or more of the 3 letters occurred in 40% of 93 trials presented. In 85% of the trials in which errors occurred, the errors were in reporting the letter contralateral to the hemisphere magnetically stimulated, or by the middle and contralateral letter with the ipsilateral letter correctly reported. **Fig. 8** shows the stimulated locations projected onto the reconstructed MRI for 1 subject. Green vectors represent stimulation sites at which all 3 letters were correctly identified (ie, no visual cortex suppression). Violet and red vectors show the stimulated cortical surfaces (ie, involving the primary and secondary

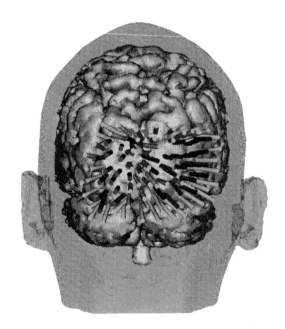

Fig. 8. Cortical map of visual suppression effects. Each vector represents a stimulation site. The color of the vectors represents the effect obtained: green, no effect; red, error reporting right letter or right and center letters but correctly reporting left letter; blue, error reporting left letter or left and center letters but correctly reporting right letter. (*From* Gugino LD. Localization of eloquent cortex using transcranial magnetic stimulation. In: Alexander E, Maciunas R. Advanced Neurosurgical Navigation. New York: Thieme Publications, 1999; with permission.)

visual cortical areas) that produced contralateral right and left visual field suppression, respectively. The cyan vectors represent stimulated cortical surface sites leading to central letter errors only. This study showed that a TMS figure-8 coil can produce a focal effect on visual suppression that can be localized to a specific visual hemifield. In addition, the visually guided tracking system allowed for precise delineation of the neuroanatomical boundaries of the TMS visual suppression effect. In most of the trials, the visual suppression effect localized to secondary visual cortex in area 18 and, to a lesser degree, into area 19 rather than primary visual cortex in area 17 (see **Fig. 8**). This study shows the use of visually guided TMS to improve precision and knowledge of actual cortical regions stimulated using a figure-of-eight TMS coil.

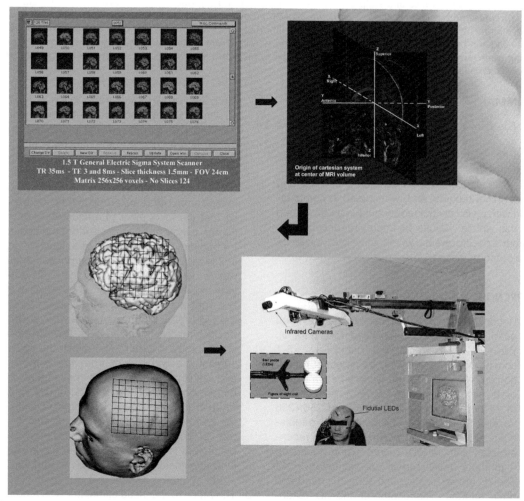

Fig. 9. 3D model reconstruction of the scalp and cortical surface. The left upper insert shows the source MRI images and acquisition parameters. Using customized segmentation algorithms, the 3D model is reconstructed. The center of the MRI volume, as shown in the right upper corner, allows for quantification of distance between cortical loci stimulated and differences in coil position in separate mapping procedures. The stereotactic tracking system is shown in the right lower corner. Note 3 LED detecting cameras mounted on the arm overlying the subject's head. The subject has 5 LEDs taped to his face so that at least 3 of them are detected by the cameras at all times. The insert shows the figure-of-eight coil with a star probe attached, containing 3 LEDs, which allow tracking of the coil under the camera's view and relative to the subject's head. The monitor displays the virtual model of the scalp and cortical surface, as well as the representation of the coil position. The virtual model in the left lower corner displays the scalp and cortical surface with a planar grid superimposed, which is used to guide systematic positioning of the coil.

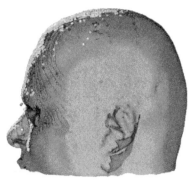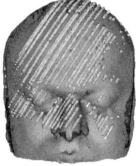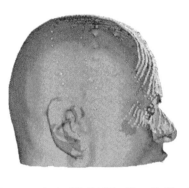

Fig. 10. The subject's face and scalp contours are digitized using a probe mounted with 2 LEDs. The digitized facial representation is then aligned with the 3D MRI model in a 3-step process (manually, interpolated, and fine alignment[39]). After coregistration, the coil is calibrated, making it possible to track its position relative to the head and brain surfaces using the optical tracking system. (*From* Gugino LD. Localization of eloquent cortex using transcranial magnetic stimulation. In: Alexander E, Maciunas R. Advanced Neurosurgical Navigation. New York: Thieme Publications, 1999; with permission.)

SUMMARY

TMS is a novel brain stimulation technique that has advanced the understanding of brain physiology, and has diagnostic value as well as therapeutic potential for several neuropsychiatric disorders. The stimulation involves restricted cortical and subcortical regions, and, when used in combination with a visually guided technique as described in this article, results in improved accuracy to target specific areas, which may also influence the outcome desired.

APPENDIX 1: MAPPING PROCEDURE

1. Reconstruction of a 3D model of the brain and head based on anatomic head MRI (**Fig. 9**). Brain MRI is acquired using a 1.5-T scanner with the following parameters: repetition time 35 milliseconds, echo time 5 milliseconds, slice thickness of 1.5 mm, a field of view of 24 cm, and acquisition matrix of 256×256 voxels. The resulting 124 contiguous double-echo slices are then segmented and reconstructed into a 3D model using multistep algorithms developed in our institution.[2,39–41] The 3D model displays the subject's head and brain surface. The center of the 3D reconstructed model is used as the origin of a Cartesian system that allows precise localization of any coordinate in the scalp or cortical surface.

2. Coregistration procedure to align the subject's head with the virtual 3D model by use of a stereotactic optical tracking system. The tracking procedure depends on the detection of infrared light-emitting diodes (LEDs), taped on the subject's face, by 3 cameras mounted on a mobile arm. LEDs are also secured on

the coil to allow for coil tracking relative to the subject. Using a probe that is a component of the tracking system, several points are then traced and recorded in the subject's face and scalp (**Fig. 10**). The system then coregisters the MRI model with the position of the subjects under the camera's view. Next, the coil position is registered using the probe mentioned earlier, so that the focal point of a figure-of-eight coil (ie, the center point of the bottom surface) can be tracked. The focal point of a figure-of-eight coil is selected for tracking purposes because this is where the peak magnetic field and induced electric field occur. The result is that the optical system tracks the subject's head, the TMS coil under the camera's view, and their position relative to one another. The system has an accuracy of about 1 mm when the coil and subject are within 1 m from the cameras,[39] and detects head and coil movements in 3 dimensions, including detection of coil tilt and rotation (referred to as 3D angle). Details of the geometry premise used for calculation of the 3D angle are available elsewhere.[42] Coil placement is guided in real time; the image is available instantaneously and is updated at a rate of 5 times per second.

3. The MES-10 magnetic stimulator was modified to produce a monophasic current pulse. The pulse is triggered on demand to a figure-of-eight coil (diameter of each coil 4.5 cm) with the 3D pyxis tracking star placed on the center of the upper plane of the coil (see **Fig. 9**). The magnetic stimulus intensity is set constant from 85% to 100% of full power for each mapping session. The coil is then moved in a systematic fashion over the scalp, usually in 1-cm steps (see **Fig. 9**). As each scalp point is

stimulated, recordings of MEPs from all muscle sites are made. The subject is instructed to relax all muscles before stimulation. Interstimulation interval is 30 seconds. The data are stored for offline analysis of MEP parameters. Each response, defined as a peak-to-peak amplitude of greater than 50 μV, is analyzed for take-off latency, area under the response, baseline-to-peak amplitude, and peak-to-trough amplitude. Normalized color maps of each response parameter are superimposed onto the 3D reconstruction of the cortical surface by appropriately color coding each cortical surface point with the value of the myogenic response parameter obtained from stimulation of these points (see **Fig. 4**).

REFERENCES

1. Barker AT, Jalinous R, Freeston IL. Non-invasive magnetic stimulation of human motor cortex. Lancet 1985;1:1106–7.
2. Gugino LD, Romero JR, Aglio L, et al. Transcranial magnetic stimulation coregistered with MRI: a comparison of a guided versus blind stimulation technique and its effect on evoked compound muscle action potentials. Clin Neurophysiol 2001;112:1781–92.
3. Ahdab R, Ayache SS, Brugieres P, et al. Comparison of "standard" and "navigated" procedures of TMS coil positioning over motor, premotor and prefrontal targets in patients with chronic pain and depression. Neurophysiol Clin 2010;40:27–36.
4. Chiappa KH. Transcranial motor evoked potentials. Electromyogr Clin Neurophysiol 1994;34:15–21.
5. Day BL, Dressler D, Maertens de Noordhout A, et al. Electric and magnetic stimulation of human motor cortex: Surface EMG and single motor unit responses. J Physiol 1989;412:449–73.
6. Boyd SG, Rothwell JC, Cowan JM, et al. A method of monitoring function in corticospinal pathways during scoliosis surgery with a note on motor conduction velocities. J Neurol Neurosurg Psychiatr 1986;49:251–7.
7. Rothwell JC. Physiological studies of electric and magnetic stimulation of the human brain. Electroencephalogr Clin Neurophysiol Suppl 1991;43:29–35.
8. Fujiki M, Isono M, Hori S, et al. Corticospinal direct response to transcranial magnetic stimulation in humans. Electroencephalogr Clin Neurophysiol 1996;101:48–57.
9. Edgley SA, Eyre JA, Lemon RN, et al. Excitation of the corticospinal tract by electromagnetic and electrical stimulation of the scalp in the macaque monkey. J Physiol 1990;425:301–20.
10. Brasil-Neto JP, Cammarota A, Valls-Sole J, et al. Role of intracortical mechanisms in the late part of

the silent period to transcranial stimulation of the human motor cortex. Acta Neurol Scand 1995;92:383–6.
11. Amassian VE, Cracco RQ. Human cerebral cortical responses to contralateral transcranial stimulation. Neurosurgery 1987;20:148–55.
12. Jalinous R. Technical and practical aspects of magnetic nerve stimulation. J Clin Neurophysiol 1991;8:10–25.
13. Amassian VE, Eberle L, Maccabee PJ, et al. Modelling magnetic coil excitation of human cerebral cortex with a peripheral nerve immersed in a brain-shaped volume conductor: the significance of fiber bending in excitation. Electroencephalogr Clin Neurophysiol 1992;85:291–301.
14. Rudiak D, Marg E. Finding the depth of magnetic brain stimulation: a re-evaluation. Electroencephalogr Clin Neurophysiol 1994;93:358–71.
15. Levy WJ, Amassian VE, Schmid UD, et al. Mapping of motor cortex gyral sites non-invasively by transcranial magnetic stimulation in normal subjects and patients. Electroencephalogr Clin Neurophysiol Suppl 1991;43:51–75.
16. Wassermann EM, McShane LM, Hallett M, et al. Noninvasive mapping of muscle representations in human motor cortex. Electroencephalogr Clin Neurophysiol 1992;85:1–8.
17. Liepert J, Tegenthoff M, Malin JP. Changes of cortical motor area size during immobilization. Electroencephalogr Clin Neurophysiol 1995;97:382–6.
18. Penfield W, Welch K. Instability of response to stimulation of the sensorimotor cortex of man. J Physiol 1949;109:358–65.
19. Black PM, Ronner SF. Cortical mapping for defining the limits of tumor resection. Neurosurgery 1987;20:914–9.
20. Cohen LG, Roth BJ, Nilsson J, et al. Effects of coil design on delivery of focal magnetic stimulation. Technical considerations. Electroencephalogr Clin Neurophysiol 1990;75:350–7.
21. Brasil-Neto JP, Cohen LG, Panizza M, et al. Optimal focal transcranial magnetic activation of the human motor cortex: effects of coil orientation, shape of the induced current pulse, and stimulus intensity. J Clin Neurophysiol 1992;9:132–6.
22. Cohen D, Cuffin BN. Developing a more focal magnetic stimulator. Part I: some basic principles. J Clin Neurophysiol 1991;8:102–11.
23. Epstein CM, Schwartzberg DG, Davey KR, et al. Localizing the site of magnetic brain stimulation in humans. Neurology 1990;40:666–70.
24. Ueno S, Matsuda T. Magnetic stimulation of the human brain. Ann N Y Acad Sci 1992;649:366–8.
25. Nielsen JF. Logarithmic distribution of amplitudes of compound muscle action potentials evoked by transcranial magnetic stimulation. J Clin Neurophysiol 1996;13:423–34.

26. Ettinger GJ, Leventon ME, Grimson WE, et al. Experimentation with a transcranial magnetic stimulation system for functional brain mapping. Med Image Anal 1998;2:133–42.

27. Pascual-Leone A, Valls-Sole J, Wassermann EM, et al. Responses to rapid-rate transcranial magnetic stimulation of the human motor cortex. Brain 1994; 117(Pt 4):847–58.

28. Miranda PC, de Carvalho M, Conceicao I, et al. A new method for reproducible coil positioning in transcranial magnetic stimulation mapping. Electroencephalogr Clin Neurophysiol 1997;105:116–23.

29. Nielsen JF. Repetitive magnetic stimulation of cerebral cortex in normal subjects. J Clin Neurophysiol 1996;13:69–76.

30. Mortifee P, Stewart H, Schulzer M, et al. Reliability of transcranial magnetic stimulation for mapping the human motor cortex. Electroencephalogr Clin Neurophysiol 1994;93:131–7.

31. Krings T, Buchbinder BR, Butler WE, et al. Stereotactic transcranial magnetic stimulation: Correlation with direct electrical cortical stimulation. Neurosurgery 1997;41:1319–25 [discussion 1325–16].

32. Uy J, Ridding MC, Miles TS. Stability of maps of human motor cortex made with transcranial magnetic stimulation. Brain Topogr 2002;14:293–7.

33. Romero JR, Ramirez M, Aglio L, et al. Benefit of stereotactic optic guidance for reproducibility of motor cortex functional maps using transcranial magnetic stimulation (TMS). 58th Annual Meeting of the American Academy of Neurology. San Diego (CA), April 1–8, 2006.

34. Asanuma H, Babb RS, Mori A, et al. Input-output relationships in cat's motor cortex after pyramidal section. J Neurophysiol 1981;46:694–703.

35. Cohen LG, Brasil-Neto JP, Pascual-Leone A, et al. Plasticity of cortical motor output organization following deafferentation, cerebral lesions, and skill acquisition. Adv Neurol 1993;63:187–200.

36. Pascual-Leone A, Tormos JM, Keenan J, et al. Study and modulation of human cortical excitability with transcranial magnetic stimulation. J Clin Neurophysiol 1998;15:333–43.

37. Potts GF, Gugino LD, Leventon ME, et al. Visual hemifield mapping using transcranial magnetic stimulation coregistered with cortical surfaces derived from magnetic resonance images. J Clin Neurophysiol 1998;15:344–50.

38. Epstein CM, Zangaladze A. Magnetic coil suppression of extrafoveal visual perception using disappearance targets. J Clin Neurophysiol 1996;13: 242–6.

39. Ettinger GJ, Grimson WE, Leventon ME, et al. Non invasive functional brain mapping using registered transcranial magnetic stimulation. IEEE Workshop on mathematical methods in biomedical image analysis. San Francisco (CA), June 21 and 22, 1996.

40. Kapur T, Grimson WEL, Kikinis R. Segmentation of brain tissue from MR images. Proceedings of First International Conference on Computer Vision, Virtual Reality and Robotics in Medicine. Nice (France); 1995. p. 429–33.

41. Shenton ME, Kikinis R, McCarley RW, et al. Harvard brain atlas: a teaching and visualization tool. Proceedings of the '95 Biomedical Visualization. Atlanta (GA), October 30, 1995. p. 10–7.

42. Horn BK. Closed-form solution of absolute orientation using unit quaternions. J Opt Soc Am 1987;4: 629–42.

Clinical Magnetoen-cephalography for Neurosurgery

Steven M. Stufflebeam, MD[a,b,c],*

KEYWORDS

- Epilepsy • Surgery • Brain tumor • Interictal • Localization
- Noninvasive • Connectivity

For presurgical evaluation of resection of a mass or other lesion, noninvasive neuroimaging aids in the surgical planning and in counseling patients about possible risks of the surgery. Magnetoencephalography (MEG) performs the most common types of surgical planning that the neurosurgeon faces, including localization of epileptic discharges, determination of the hemispheric dominance of verbal processing, and the ability to locate eloquent cortex. MEG is most useful when it is combined with structural imaging, most commonly combined with structural magnetic resonance imaging (MRI) and MR diffusion imaging. This article reviews the history of clinical MEG, introduces the basic concepts about the biophysics of MEG, and outlines the basic neurosurgical applications of MEG.

BRIEF HISTORY OF MEG

In 1968, David Cohen (**Fig. 1**) used a room-temperature copper coil as a detector to record the first magnetoencephalogram at the University of Illinois.[1] Later, at the Massachusetts Institute of Technology, he built a more elaborate shielded room. At about the same time, James Zimmerman and colleagues developed the Superconducting Quantum Interference Device (SQUID), which uses the Josephson junction to measure tiny magnetic fields. SQUID requires cooling to liquid

helium temperatures, and has a sensitivity of several hundreds of times that of a copper coil. Zimmerman brought this detector to Cohen's room, and this combination of shielding and detector allowed the first clear measurements of the body's magnetic fields. After they measured the heart, Cohen next recorded the first MEG measured with a SQUID.[2]

For the initial measurements of magnetic brain activity, physicists and neuroscientists used a single or a just few magnetometers. Localizing activity with such a low number of sensors required moving them to maintain sampling from various locations over the head. This process was time consuming and not practical for routine clinical use. Clinical MEG became possible when MEG systems were developed that provided coverage of approximately 7 to 12 cm, enough to produce a field map large enough to visualize the magnetic field lines from a single dipole source; this made it possible to localize the activity in a registered brain MRI.

BIOPHYSICAL PRINCIPLES OF MAGNETOENCEPHALOGRAPHY

Modern MEG systems now provide hundreds of channels that can provide whole-head coverage (**Fig. 2**). This coverage makes it possible to map

a Athinoula A. Martinos Center for Biomedical Imaging, Department of Radiology, Massachusetts General Hospital, 149 13th Street (Mailcode 2301), Charlestown, MA 02129, USA
b Division of Health Sciences and Technology, Massachusetts Institute of Technology-Harvard University, Cambridge, MA, USA
c Department of Radiology, Massachusetts General Hospital, Harvard Medical School, Boston, MA 02115, USA
* Corresponding author. Athinoula A. Martinos Center for Biomedical Imaging, Department of Radiology, Massachusetts General Hospital, 149 13th Street (Mailcode 2301), Charlestown, MA 02129.
E-mail address: sms@nmr.mgh.harvard.edu

Neurosurg Clin N Am 22 (2011) 153–167
doi:10.1016/j.nec.2010.11.006
1042-3680/11/$ – see front matter © 2011 Elsevier Inc. All rights reserved.

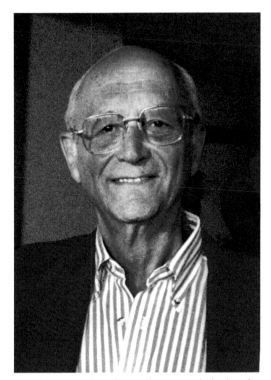

Fig. 1. Dr David Cohen, PhD recorded the first magnetic fields from the brain. His laboratory at Massachusetts Institute of Technology in Boston, Massachusetts pioneered MEG experiments and applications.

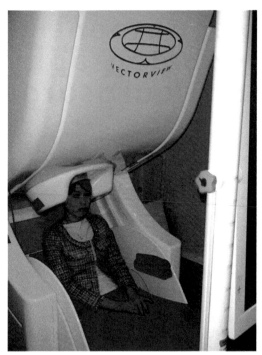

Fig. 2. Typical modern MEG device positioned in the upright position facing a back projection screen.

activity throughout the cerebral cortex and is critical for presurgical mapping of language areas, and for detecting propagating or widespread epileptic activity. Due to interference from extraneous magnetic fields, all MEG measurements must be performed in a magnetically shielded room, which typically consists of 2 to 4 layers of aluminum and multiple layers of ferromagnetic shielding.

Unlike other hemodynamic techniques (functional MRI [fMRI] and positron emission tomography [PET]), both MEG and electroencephalography (EEG) directly measure electric brain activity. The neural generators of the MEG and EEG are identical. There are critical differences that make them both useful and complementary. MEG preferentially detects activity in superficial, nonradial areas of cortex, such as the fissural cortex of the cerebral hemispheres; this is particularly advantageous if the area of interest is also radial, such as the primary somatosensory cortex, which lies in the walls of the sulci.

Much of the neural activity measured by MEG originates as the postsynaptic activity in the pyramidal cells of the cerebral cortex. MEG measures the vector sum of postsynaptic potentials, as contrasted with BOLD (Blood Oxygenation Level Dependent) fMRI and some form of PET imaging that reflects neural activity indirectly through changes in blood flow. MEG localizes neural activity more accurately than EEG because magnetic fields are less perturbed than electrical potentials by overlying brain structures: scalp, skull, cerebrospinal fluid, meninges, and vascular structures. Recently, statistical combination of structural MRI and fMRI with MEG has taken a great stride forward by yielding the maximum benefit from each technique into a single image.[3,4]

The calculation of the magnetic field is more straightforward than that of the electric field because of the symmetries and conductivity distribution of the human head, and because the EEG also is influenced by the extracellular volume current, which is difficult to model accurately. All currents, both intracellular and extracellular, generate magnetic fields, but because of the near spherical shape of the head, one can calculate the resultant magnetic fields caused by primary currents without taking into account the conductivity layers of the head.

INTERPRETATION OF MEG

Intelligent interpretation of MEG requires the examination of the waveforms recorded by the

SQUID sensors, followed by a source estimate that reflects the site of activity in the brain. The raw measurement of MEG is a time-varying magnetic field. For epilepsy discharge mapping, segments of the activity are used for source analysis, often without any signal averaging. To improve the signal-to-noise ratio of measured signals for evoked activity, such as language laterality, it is often necessary to average several (typically around 100 trials) responses from identical or similar stimuli. The signal is typically averaged based on the timing of the presented stimulus, the subject's response, or the peak of activity, such as the peak of an epileptic spike. Averaging lowers the effects of extraneous activity, effectively improving the overall signal-to-noise ratio of the desired activity.

Source Modeling

Source modeling determines the origin of the measured neuromagnetic fields, which is the goal of most MEG measurements. The mathematics behind this analysis is known as the inverse problem. In general, the inverse solution of electromagnetic measurements is nonunique and ill-posed. If proper assumptions are made, however, the solution becomes solvable. Some of most commonly used source analysis methods used clinically are discussed here.

Equivalent current dipole

To make the inverse solution tractable, one can approximate that the activity from primary sensory or motor cortex originates as a single equivalent current dipole (ECD). Physiologically this is plausible, given that a limited patch of cortex is synchronously activated and that the sensors are at least a few centimeters from the source. The ECD provides spatial information, magnitude (current dipole moment), and direction. The ECD is typically computed using a standard iterative least-square algorithm,[5] which can also provide a measure of dipole parameter confidence, as well as the best-fitting parameters such as goodness-of-fit measure.[6]

Thus, by assuming a single source, the inverse problem has a unique solution, which works particularly well for primary sensory areas, focal epilepsies, and higher cognitive areas that have a focal source. Further advances in the ECD approach, for both EEG and MEG, have made it possible to find multiple ECDs with a multidipole approach, such as that developed by Hari and colleagues for somatosensory activation.[7] One approach to investigate temporal changes in different areas of the brain is known as the time-varying dipole model. In this model, a series of dipoles are modeled such that the locations are fixed, but allowing the amplitudes to vary over time (**Fig. 3**). This ECD approach works well for sequentially or simultaneously activated cortical sources, although the fine spatial details are lost because the measurements are obtained at least 3 cm from the brain sources.[6]

Distributed solutions

Minimum norm estimate If a large patch of cortex is activated, or if there are several areas of cortex activity simultaneously, the single ECD solution may be misleading. In practice this may be suspected when a dipole localizes too deep to be physiologically plausible, that is, in the deep white matter. In such cases, distributed solutions such as the minimum norm estimate (MNE), the minimum current estimate, or a beamformer solution may be more accurate. Although numerous other inverse solutions exist,[8,9] this review concentrates on the MNE and beamformer solutions.

Originally pioneered by Hämäläinen and Ilmoniemi,[10] and improved on by Dale and colleagues,[3,4] the MNE is now available in various software packages, from freeware to commercially available software. The MNE does have some important limitations that must be kept in mind especially when used clinically: a depth bias and a difficulty in determining the extent of activation. In its most elementary expression, the source variance is assumed to be equal throughout the volume, and the MNE solution is biased toward the most superficial currents. One approach to lessen this effect is to use a cortical constraint obtained from the anatomic MRIs.[11] In addition to a depth bias, determining the extent of the sources is also problematic. Simulations[11] show that the point-spread function of estimates is a function of location. Further, the spread depends on the assumed source variance.

To compensate for the superficial bias of MNE current sources, Dale and Halgren[4] have suggested producing a dynamic statistical parametric map (dSPM) by normalizing the estimate MNE by the signal noise. Using the dSPM, the point-spread function is more uniform across the brain[12] and removes the superficial bias (see **Fig. 3**). In addition, the dSPM is F-distributed, allowing it to be used for hypothesis testing.[4]

Beamformer Another distributed source solution is commonly termed the beamformer, which is based on the principle of spatial filters. Beamformers typically are applied without a cortical constraint, although they can be modified to do so. Synthetic-aperture magnetometry (SAM)[13] is a beamformer approach that can be applied to

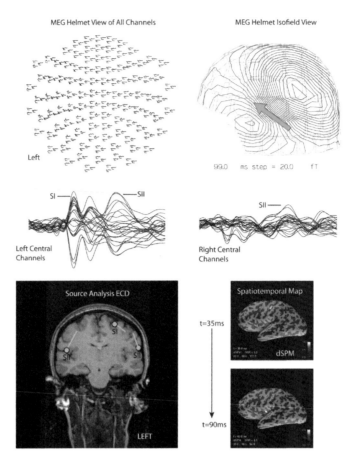

Fig. 3. MEG somatosensory response from median nerve electrical stimulation. (*Upper left*) Equivalent current dipole (ECD) fittings of the primary somatosensory SI (axial T1-wieghted MRI) and secondary SII areas (*lower left*). The 2 locations for SI are for ipsilateral (20 ms latency) and contralateral (35 ms) stimulation. (*Upper right*) The distributed source solution using a noise-normalized minimum norm estimate (MNE) shown at 35 ms and 90 ms after stimulation (*lower right*). dSPM, dynamic statistical parametric map.

both raw data and averaged (evoked) MEG or EEG. More sophisticated methods, such as adaptive spatial filtering[14,15] and dynamic imaging of coherent sources,[16] use a spectral analysis with coherence or other correlations that make it possible to measure functional connectivity in the brain within a particular spectral band. This method makes it possible to localize changes in spectral power or functional connectivity that can be used to make evoked (such as language and motor mapping) or resting state functional connectivity.

ELOQUENT CORTEX EVALUATION
Current Presurgical Methods to Evaluate Eloquent Cortex

In patients with epilepsy or brain masses, lateralization and localization of language functioning may be critical for preserving the quality of life.

At present, there are several methods to evaluate eloquent cortex, including neuropsychological testing, fMRI, MEG, the intracarotid amobarbital procedure (IAP), and invasive electrode mapping.[17–20] Precise localization of the motor cortex and somatosensory cortex (central sulcus) is commonly required for frontal masses or for frontal lobe epilepsy. Verbal memory and language are the most common functions to be affected by a left anterior temporal lobectomy (ATL), a common surgery for medial temporal lobe epilepsy.[21–24] Testing whether a temporal lobe is dominant for verbal function is often referred to as simply determining language lateralization (or verbal memory lateralization). Language cortex, typically the posterior language cortex, also needs to be precisely localized when a lesion is located in the posterior temporal lobe. To better understand how MEG assesses the surgical patient, the author briefly discusses the evaluation of language function.

Neuropsychological testing

Neuropsychological testing assesses the functional status of the hippocampus and predicts the neurocognitive outcome after resection of the hippocampus, but its use as a sole predictor of outcomes is limited. Neuropsychological test performance correlates with mesial temporal lobe epilepsy status and neuropsychological test performance before and after surgery, although the overall specificity is moderate.[23,24] Material-specific memory loss as measured by neuropsychological test performance is observed in 20% to 30% of patients following unilateral ATL.[24–26] Material-specific memory loss is far more common following left- than right-sided ATL, with 25% to 50% of left-sided ATL patients demonstrating verbal memory decline. This outcome is particularly true for patients without significant sclerosis on the surgical side. Declines in visual memory following right-sided ATL are less consistently observed but have been reported on tests that are highly spatial in nature. Accordingly, preoperative scores on material-specific memory tests have demonstrated some utility in the prediction of cognitive morbidity following anterior temporal lobectomy; however, the sensitivity of prediction is modest (56%).

Intracarotid amobarbital procedure

The IAP is used to predict language and memory outcomes following an ATL or for resections near the cortical language area. For an IAP, amobarbital is injected into the internal carotid artery through an arterial catheter, and brief neuropsychological tests are performed. The IAP generally assesses verbal memory and, to a lesser extent, memory for visual items that are not easily encoded verbally, such as scenes or faces **Fig. 4**.[27,28]

Limitations of the IAP Despite its widespread use, some shortcomings to the IAP are widely known and limit its use.[29–31] The IAP is invasive with a small but measurable risk of stroke, vascular damage, and infection.[29,31,32] The results of the IAP have been shown to be unreliable in test-retest studies, which may be due to flow of anesthetic to the opposite hemisphere (transhemispheric cross-flow) and variable penetration of the vasculature to the mesial temporal lobe from the internal carotid artery. Recently there has been a shortage of amobarbital, which has also reduced the use of the procedure, at least temporarily.[33] Pelletier and colleagues[34] suggest 4 requirements are needed before a test could replace the IAP: (1) a high predictive power for the presence or absence of critical functions in specific brain regions; (2) a user-independent statistical

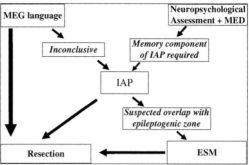

Fig. 4. Current algorithm for presurgical lateralization of language and memory. ESM is the electrical stimulation map with the grid. This diagram depicts language and memory assessment used at many centers, including the author's. In this algorithm, noninvasive language and memory tests are sometimes followed by IAP and, if needed, subdural grid evaluation before resection. (*From* Loddenkemper T. *Quo vadis Wada?* Epilepsy Behav 2008;13(1):1–2; with permission.)

methodology; (3) high spatial resolution; (4) production of reliable activation maps at the individual level. MEG meets these criteria and, in the author's experience, its routine use has led to a reduction in the number of patients who undergo the IAP.

Language evaluation

In part due to advancements in functional neuroimaging, the IAP is being used less and less frequently.[29] Despite the IAP being the consensus gold standard for verbal functional, it has been criticized because of potential cross-flow to the contralateral hemisphere and a typical lack of testing of territory supplied by the posterior circulation. Since the mid 1990s, MEG has been used to determine hemispheric dominance for language as well as regional language mapping of individual language areas.[35–43] MEG of language areas provides an accurate noninvasive method of mapping these areas. In practice, MEG can be used to plan for an IAP and stimulation-based intraoperative mapping techniques.

Determining the location of language processing in a subject requires applying the task that best activates the desired stream of language processing. Specific language processes are complex and often include phonological, lexical, and also semantic processes.[44] Verbal memory encoding and retrieval occurs concurrently in virtually any task, making it difficult to separate "language processing" from "memory." Further supporting language processes are attention, motor planning (speech), and visual or auditory functions. In fMRI, semantic decision and stem completion tasks are popular as they require a response from the patient, which ensures the quality of the patient's responses. For MEG, covert responses are more desirable, as overt (spoken) responses may lead to unacceptable motion artifacts. Nevertheless, some passive sensory paradigms requiring no patient response have been reported in the literature to be successful (see later discussion).

Hemispheric dominance for language Determination of the language-dominant hemisphere is critical in the presurgical evaluation of patients scheduled for temporal or frontal lobe resections. For a left ATL, the determination of language laterality is done routinely with MEG and fMRI. Wada and Rasmussen[20] determined that more than 93% of patients are left-hemisphere dominant for

language, as are more than 96% of right-handed patients, although more recent studies indicate that many patients have more bilateral representation of language than the original studies.[45] In left-handed epilepsy patients, only about 70% of patients demonstrate left hemispheric dominance for language, with about 15% of patients demonstrating bilateral language lateralization.

First proposed by Papanicolaou and colleagues,[46] sequential dipole fitting is a robust method to determine language laterality (**Fig. 5**). The stimuli used by Papanicolaou were both auditory and visual words. The results concur with Wada test results[35] and electrical stimulation mapping.[47] Szymanski and colleagues[42] reported using simple phonetic stimuli, such as the vowel sounds /a/ and /u/, for determining the language-hemispheric dominance

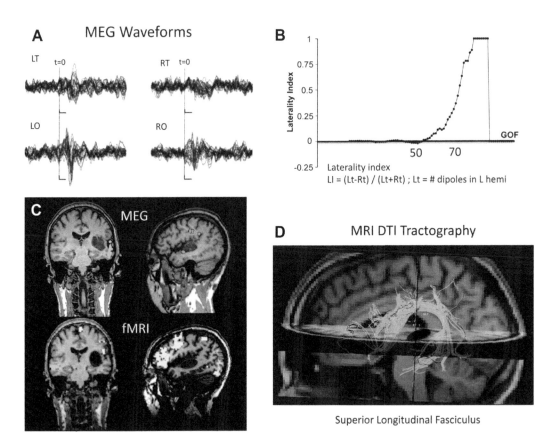

Fig. 5. Multiple imaging modalities for language mapping (MEG, fMRI, and diffusion tensor imaging). (*A*) MEG waveforms for left and right temporal (LT and RT, respectively) and occipital (LO, RO) sensors, showing several peaks related to sensory and language activity. (*B*) Laterality index as a function of the goodness of fit of a sequential equivalent current dipole (ECD) fit to the MEG data, suggesting left-hemisphere dominance. (*C*) Locations of the ECDs for the MEG data (*top*) and fMRI (*bottom*) for a visual reading task, displayed in coronal and sagittal slices of anatomic MRI. Note the cluster of MEG dipoles in the posterior superior temporal gyrus, presumably including Wernicke's area. fMRI shows largest activation in the inferior lateral left frontal cortex. The location of a tumor in the left temporal lobe is highlighted with the red oval. (*D*) MRI tractography showing the superior longitudinal fasciculus (SLF) that connects temporal and frontal language areas. Note that the tumor (*red*) does not interrupt or displace the SLF white matter fiber bundle.

by summing the number of selective dipoles in the late auditory magnetic field on each hemisphere and calculating a lateralization index. Multiple groups report a strong correlation with both intraoperative mapping techniques and the results of the Wada test.[39,42]

Regional language mapping In addition to lateralizing language, MEG also can accurately locate language cortex. MEG localizes, with a high temporal resolution, both receptive and productive brain areas. The spatial resolution can be further increased by combining with fMRI data.[4] For localizing language-specific areas in the cortex, there are several criteria that are important for patient studies as compared with the more frequent use for cognitive neuroscience. First, the neurosurgical application requires precise localization in individual subjects, although for group studies the neuroscientist can average responses over several subjects. Second, presurgical evaluation usually requires mapping the essential language areas, not just participating areas. Removal of essential language areas may result in a language deficit. Participating areas are activated during language paradigms, but do not result in a postoperative language deficit after resection, either because there are areas of redundant processing or because other areas provide the same functions. At present, there is no reliable neuroimaging method to distinguish essential from participating areas with noninvasive imaging, and this remains a major goal of clinical functional imaging. Combining MEG with other technologies such as transcranial magnetic stimulation may make this possible in the near future.

By simply applying a source localization procedure, the same techniques described in determining hemispheric dominance can be used for regional language mapping. The mapping of ECDs of the late auditory evoked fields can be used for both posterior temporal and frontal operculum mapping (see **Fig. 5**).[46,48] Temporal maps of activation have similar profiles to those determined by invasive electrocorticography. On MEG, the latency of Wernicke's area is typically between 210 and 420 milliseconds, and Broca's area 400 to 700 milliseconds, depending on the particular language task and differences in individual subjects. In general, the peak activation of Wernicke's area precedes Broca's area, although occasionally other temporal profiles have been reported.[49] The beamformer technique, such as SAM (**Fig. 6**), maps decreases in specific spontaneous activity power bands, such as beta-band

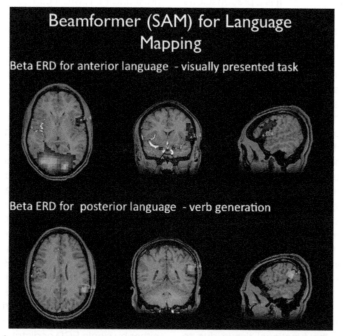

Fig. 6. Beamformer for presurgical mapping. The upper panel shows the map for language using a visually presented word with robust activation of anterior language cortex, comprising Broca's area. A verb generation paradigm was used to map the posterior language areas (Wernicke's area). (*Courtesy of* Dr Erin Simon Schwartz and Dr Timothy Roberts, Children's Hospital, Philadelphia.)

decreases (~20 Hz), known as event-related desynchronization.[50]

A common clinical use of MEG is to aid in the localization of the central sulcus. Even with histologically low-grade tumors, the central sulcus can be distorted by tumor infiltration and/or mass effect, obscuring it on an anatomic MRI. Using a tactile stimulator, the somatosensory cortex homunculus can be easily mapped by successively stimulating finger digits, foot digits, and lip using MEG. Alternatively, an electrical nerve stimulator can be used to map the median, tibial nerve, and lip representative areas. If an electrical nerve stimulator is used, the electrodes are placed and the intensity set such that thumb twitching or toe twitching is elicited. After signal averaging, both the primary (SI) and secondary (SII) somatosensory cortices are detectable with MEG (see **Fig. 3**).

After recording the evoked magnetic fields, the primary somatosensory cortex typically is localized, such as with an ECD method[51–53] or distributed source.[50,54] If an electrical median nerve stimulation technique is used, the N20m—the first identifiable component of the evoked magnetic field—is easily evoked in most patients, including those under deep anesthesia or in a coma.[55,56] The N20m generator is located in the anterior wall of the somatosensory gyrus (Brodmann area 3b), with a nonradial orientation that is ideal for detection with MEG.[7,51,53,55,57] It is a preconscious field that does not synapse in the thalamus and, due to a high signal-to-noise ratio, has a very repeatable localization, with a localization accuracy on the order of millimeters.

MEG identification of the central sulcus has been validated by several groups using intraoperative measurements with a variety of methods including ECDs[45,58–60] and the beamformer approach.[54] Schiffbauer and colleagues,[60] for example, found that regardless of tumor grade, intra-axial brain tumors may border on or invade the somatosensory and auditory cortex. Of importance, low-grade tumors were more likely than high-grade tumors to invade and involve the functionally viable cortex. The investigators concluded that low-grade tumors, due to slow growth, more often demonstrate functional activity within the radiologically abnormal areas than high-grade tumors. High-grade tumors, on the other hand, often show functional activity at the margin of the contrast-enhancing area. The investigators suggested that these findings were caused by physical displacement of the functional tissue due to mass effect of the high-grade tumor. Firsching and colleagues[61] reported that in 30 patients, ECD localization of the tactile neuromagnetic response occurred in the somatosensory cortex, and was in agreement with phase-reversal measurements at the time of surgery, without exception. Further, they concluded that MEG-based functional neuronavigation was practical and reliable. Recent reports of noninvasive multimodal technologies—MEG, fMRI, and others—have noted that when combined they enhance the reliability of identification of the central sulcus. Some have suggested using a functional risk profile, based on MEG findings, to improve surgical decision making.[62] It should be kept in mind that brain tumor patients with known sensory or motor deficits may have diminished evoked fields.[62] Nagarajan and colleagues[54] demonstrated that an adaptive spatial filter, a type of beamformer, can accurately identify the motor cortex and the somatosensory cortex. These investigators further demonstrated that it is more accurate in some circumstances than the ECD approach.

Motor

As already noted, many functional imaging techniques such as fMRI and PET can accurately identify the central sulcus.[63] However, isolating pure motor activity, for example of the precentral gyrus with fMRI, is difficult because of inevitable activation of the adjacent somatosensory cortex. Unlike fMRI and PET, MEG can be used to isolate motor activity due to it's high temporal resolution. In practice, it requires the precise timing of the onset of motor movement to produce an averaged evoked field; this can be achieved by a self-paced button press or by use of a trigger a photo-optic switch. Activity that peaks between 20 and 50 milliseconds before the onset of movement reflects activity in the primary motor cortex.[64]

Alternatively, the motor cortex may be mapped by quantifying the functional connectivity between an electromyogram (EMG) and the MEG sensors, as suggested by Makela and colleagues.[65] Placing bipolar electrodes over the first interosseous muscle and instructing the patient to slowly adduct generates a large signal in both the EMG and MEG. Calculation of the coherence of the MEG-EMG yields a spectrum of a spike centered on or near 20 Hz, strongest over the central sensors. This spectrum represents synchronization of the muscle twitches with the 20-Hz "mu" rhythm, which is known to originate in the motor cortex.[65] By localizing the functional connectivity, either by single ECD or distributed source method, the primary motor cortex is identified. This method isolates the primary motor cortex from the somatomotor network, something that can be difficult with fMRI. Further, MEG identifies the entire neural network activated during the planning and the act of motor movement, including supplementary cortex[66,67] and premotor cortex.[16,68]

Visual Cortex

In patients with lesions lying near visual areas, MEG evaluates the of visual cortex. Mapping of the visual areas is theoretically difficult with MEG because of synchronously active sources that may result in magnetic field cancellation at the scalp. The primary visual cortex can be mapped by a simple ECD of the first visual evoked field from nearly any strong visual stimulus; typically a portion of a visual quadrant is stimulated with a checkerboard. In practice, however, it yields valid results.[69–71] Mapping of the magnetic equivalent of visual evoked potentials N75, P100, and

N145 components is robust, with large visual stimuli with phase-reversal techniques, and can be performed to detect visual field deficits.[69–71]

SPONTANEOUS ACTIVITY: EPILEPTIC SPIKE LOCALIZATION

Localization of epileptic discharges may be performed in the context of a low-grade brain tumor or as part of the workup of surgical epilepsy. Interictal activity is easily captured with MEG. Ictal activity, although more difficult, can also be detected and localized with whole-head MEG systems, particularly if the instrument is located in a hospital where antiepileptic medicines can be tapered. The best MEG measurement of epilepsy is to use a whole-head system with simultaneously recorded EEG. A standard EEG electrode array, manufactured with no magnetic

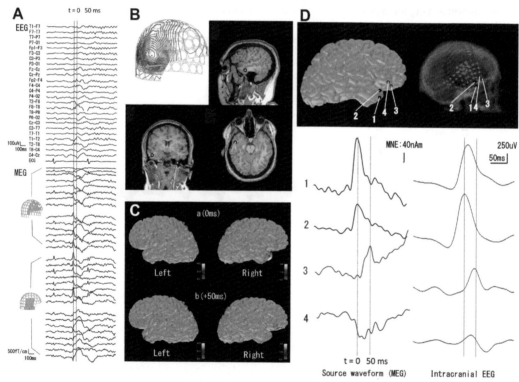

Fig. 7. Localization of epileptic spikes. (A) Simultaneously acquired EEG (top) and MEG (bottom) signals from a patient with epilepsy. An epileptic spike is seen in MEG sensors over the right temporal and frontal regions. (B) An equivalent current dipole (ECD) computed at the peak of the spike ("0 ms"; the corresponding isocontour map of the MEG data, with the ECD as a green arrow, is shown at top left) is localized in the temporal lobe (blue dots superimposed on the anatomic MRI). (C) Distributed source estimates, the noise-normalized minimum-norm estimate (MNE), also known as dynamic statistical parametric map, for the MEG data are displayed on the cortical surface representation reconstructed from anatomic MRI. The source estimates suggest that the activity propagates from a right temporal region ("0 ms") to the right frontal region ("50 ms"). (D) Comparison of MEG data with intracranial EEG. The left panel shows the estimated MEG source waveforms (MNE) at 4 locations ("1" and "2" temporal, "3" and "4" frontal). The right panel shows the intracranial EEG of an epileptic spike at corresponding locations. The MEG and intracranial EEG are consistent in suggesting temporal activity propagating to the frontal lobe over a 50-ms time period. (Figures created by Dr Naoro Tanaka, MD, PhD.)

material, provides a standard EEG classification of ictal or interictal activity. High-density electrode caps are also available if EEG source localization is needed.

Presurgical evaluation of patients with epilepsy typically involves simultaneous whole-head MEG and EEG recording during rest, which records basic rhythmic activity, sleep-related activity, and other spontaneous brain activity, in addition to the epileptic discharges. Localizing the neural source of interictal spikes present in the MEG data (**Fig. 7**) localizes the epileptogenic zone even in the event of propagation.[72–75] The ECD is an important source model for epileptic discharges, typically for localizing the peak of an ictal or interictal epileptic discharge. However, the ECD at times may not match the location of the seizure onset. In particular, source analysis using a distributed source model, such as MNE,[76] and beamformer techniques[77] may be helpful in demonstrating the time course of cortical activation and thereby reveal the generation and propagation of epileptic activity.[78]

MEG Improves Clinical Treatment of Surgical Epilepsy Patients

Several recent studies demonstrate that MEG improves the quality of clinical care in refractory epilepsy patients. Including the MEG in the presurgical evaluation of epilepsy influences clinical decisions and increases the likelihood of surgical success (making a person seizure free).[79–81] MEG also provides nonredundant clinical information in about one-third of the epilepsy cases when performed during the presurgical evaluation.[82]

FUNCTIONAL CONNECTIVITY

Functional connectivity defines correlations of activity across brain regions, whereas effective connectivity measures the influence of brain regions on each other. Corticomuscular coherence is a type of functional connectivity between the motor cortex and the muscle subunits that is used clinically to identify primary motor cortex. Functional connectivity using temporal correlations in

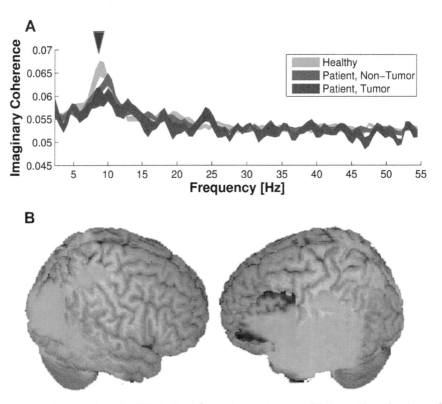

Fig. 8. Frequency spectrum and spatial distribution of imaginary coherence. (*A*) Tumor tissue has lower functional connectivity in the alpha frequency range than nontumor tissue of lesion patients and healthy control subjects. (*B*) The functional connectivity from healthy subjects superimposed on a 3-dimensional brain atlas. High functional connectivity is found in Broca's area and right visual cortex. (*From* Guggisberg AG, Honma SM, Findlay AM, et al. Mapping functional connectivity in patients with brain lesions. Ann Neurol 2008;63:193–203; with permission.)

fMRI has made it possible to map several neural networks, such as the motor system.[83] The high temporal resolution of MEG allows connectivity analysis to be performed at a high temporal resolution. Other abnormalities in functional connectivity include epilepsy. For example, abnormally high functional or effective connectivity across small distances could influence epileptic spike generation. Increased connectivity across brain areas has been hypothesized to be responsible for the propagation and generalization of epilepsy. On the other hand, a failure of integration of perceptions might suggest a failure in "binding" object features within and across brain regions, and may lead to psychiatric diseases such as schizophrenia. Functional connectivity using MEG may help define the epileptogenic cortex, especially in multifocal epilepsy.[84]

Recent work has shown that abnormalities in brain connectivity as measured by MEG have clinical value, such as in patients with brain tumors.[54] Patients with brain tumors have abnormal

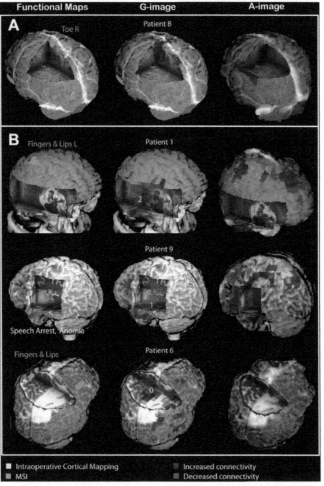

Fig. 9. Functional maps obtained with MEG connectivity and electrical stimulation map (*yellow*) and functional connectivity images of 4 patients with brain tumors are superimposed over their 3-dimensional–rendered individual brain. (*A*) A 25-year-old woman with a right foot with grade III astrocytoma infiltrating the left medial sensorimotor cortex. Functional connectivity in the right foot area of the sensorimotor cortex was decreased. (*B*) MEG functional connectivity in 3 tumor patients without presurgical functional deficits, suggesting functional disconnection (*blue*) of the corresponding tumor tissue (graded 0–2, with 0 indicating smallest proportion of decreased functional connectivity). In agreement with the MEG functional connectivity images and the clinical status, eloquent cortex was mapped outside of decreased connectivity (*blue*) areas by MEG and cortical mapping in all patients. MEG functional connectivity predicts postsurgery function: whereas patient 6 suffered from postsurgical sensible deficits in the left arm and leg, patients 1 and 9 had no postoperative deficits. Red areas indicate increased connectivity. (*From* Guggisberg AG, Honma SM, Findlay AM, et al. Mapping functional connectivity in patients with brain lesions. Ann Neurol 2008;63:193–203; with permission.)

connectivity compared with healthy controls (**Fig. 8**). In patients with brain tumors, eloquent cortex found within abnormal resting-state functional connectivity indicates an increased risk of postoperative deficits (**Fig. 9**). These new clinical applications are potentially useful for MEG in neurosurgical patients.

NEURONAVIGATION AND MEG

Coregistration of MEG and structural images with skin fiducial markers makes it make it possible to delimit the volume containing the lesion and the surgical field.[85–87] Frameless stereotactic systems assist with resection of small, deep-seated tumors during neurosurgery, with a precision approaching 2 mm. Ganslandt and colleagues[88] combined MEG somatosensory mapping with a free-hand stereotactic pointing device in 25 cases of peri-rolandic tumors and masses, and found agreement with intraoperative somatosensory mapping in all cases. Further, they eliminated 11 patients who were not available for open surgery because of tumor infiltration of the motor cortex.[88] Rezai and colleagues[89,90] report the use of a combination of MEG-derived functional mapping and computed tomography scans, MRI, and digital angiography reduces surgical risk. Overcoming the errors associated with shift of brain contents during an operation requires sulcal landmarks on 3-dimensional reconstructions using fMRI, MEG, intracranial EEG, and tractography during surgical planning.

SUMMARY AND FUTURE DIRECTIONS

MEG is now an accepted method of presurgical evaluation in patients with brain tumors and epilepsy. Beyond epileptic discharge mapping and noninvasive mapping of eloquent cortex, clinical research studies suggest that MEG is ready for other neurosurgical applications, including head trauma, Parkinson disease, and other disorders. Combining MEG, EEG, fMRI, and new methods of connectivity are also being evaluated for clinical applications. These studies will continue to change how MEG is applied in neurosurgical evaluations.

REFERENCES

1. Cohen D. Magnetoencephalography: evidence of magnetic fields produced by alpha-rhythm currents. Science 1968;161(843):784–6.
2. Cohen D. Magnetoencephalography: detection of the brain's electrical activity with a superconducting magnetometer. Science 1972;175(22):664–6.
3. Dale AM, Halgren E. Spatiotemporal mapping of brain activity by integration of multiple imaging modalities. Curr Opin Neurobiol 2001;11(2):202–8.
4. Dale AM, Liu AK, Fischl BR, et al. Dynamic statistical parametric mapping: combining fMRI and MEG for high-resolution imaging of cortical activity. Neuron 2000;26:55–67.
5. Marquardt DW. An algorithm for least-squares estimation of nonlinear parameters. SIAM J Appl Math 1963;11(2):431–41.
6. Hamalainen M, Hari R, Ilmoniemi RJ, et al. Magnetoencephalography—theory, instrumentation, and application to noninvasive studies of the working human brain. Rev Mod Phys 1993;65:413–97.
7. Hari R, Karhu J, Hamalainen M, et al. Functional organization of the human first and second somatosensory cortices: a neuromagnetic study. Eur J Neurosci 1993;5(6):724–34.
8. Mosher JC, Leahy RM, Lewis PS. EEG and MEG: forward solutions for inverse methods. IEEE Trans Biomed Eng 1999;46(3):245–59.
9. Mosher JC, Leahy RM. Recursive MUSIC: a framework for EEG and MEG source localization. IEEE Trans Biomed Eng 1998;45(11):1342–54.
10. Hamalainen MS, Ilmoniemi RJ. Interpreting measured magnetic fields of the brain: estimates of current distributions. vol. Report TKK-F-A559. Helsinki (Finland): Helsinki Univ of Technology; 1984.
11. Dale AM, Sereno MI. Improved localization of cortical activity by combining EEG and MEG with MRI cortical surface reconstruction: a linear approach. J Cogn Neurosci 1993;5(2):162–76.
12. Liu AK, Dale AM, Belliveau JW. Monte Carlo simulation studies of EEG and MEG localization accuracy. Hum Brain Mapp 2002;16(1):47–62.
13. Vrba J, Robinson SE. Signal processing in magnetoencephalography. Methods 2001;25(2):249–71.
14. Sekihara K, Sahani M, Nagarajan SS. A simple nonparametric statistical thresholding for MEG spatial-filter source reconstruction images. Neuroimage 2005;27(2):368–76.
15. Sekihara K, Nagarajan SS, Poeppel D, et al. Performance of an MEG adaptive-beamformer technique in the presence of correlated neural activities: effects on signal intensity and time-course estimates. IEEE Trans Biomed Eng 2002;49(12 Pt 2):1534–46.
16. Gross J, Kujala J, Hamalainen M, et al. Dynamic imaging of coherent sources: studying neural interactions in the human brain. Proc Natl Acad Sci U S A 2001;98(2):694–9.
17. Ojemann GA. Individual variability in cortical localization of language. J Neurosurg 1979;50(2):164–9.
18. Bell BD, Davies KG, Haltiner AM, et al. Intracarotid amobarbital procedure and prediction of postoperative memory in patients with left temporal lobe epilepsy and hippocampal sclerosis. Epilepsia 2000;41(8):992–7.

19. Perrine K, Westerveld M, Sass KJ, et al. Wada memory disparities predict seizure laterality and postoperative seizure control. Epilepsia 1995;36(9):851–6.

20. Wada J, Rasmussen T. Intracarotid injection of sodium amytal for the lateralization of cerebral speech dominance. 1960. J Neurosurg 2007;106(6):1117–33.

21. Vaz SA. Nonverbal memory functioning following right anterior temporal lobectomy: a meta-analytic review. Seizure 2004;13(7):446–52.

22. Loring DW. Amobarbital effects and lateralized brain function: the Wada test. New York: Springer-Verlag; 1992. p. 138, xiii.

23. Loring DW, Hermann BP, Meador KJ, et al. Amnesia after unilateral temporal lobectomy: a case report. Epilepsia 1994;35(4):757–63.

24. Loring DW, Meador KJ, Lee GP. Determinants of quality of life in epilepsy. Epilepsy Behav 2004;5(6):976–80.

25. Loring DW, Meador KJ, Lee GP, et al. Structural versus functional prediction of memory change following anterior temporal lobectomy. Epilepsy Behav 2004;5(2):264–8.

26. Loring DW, Murro AM, Meador KJ, et al. Wada memory testing and hippocampal volume measurements in the evaluation for temporal lobectomy. Neurology 1993;43(9):1789–93.

27. Griffith HR, Richardson E, Pyzalski RW, et al. Memory for famous faces and the temporal pole: functional imaging findings in temporal lobe epilepsy. Epilepsy Behav 2006;9(1):173–80.

28. Powell HW, Richardson MP, Symms MR, et al. Preoperative fMRI predicts memory decline following anterior temporal lobe resection. J Neurol Neurosurg Psychiatry 2008;79(6):686–93.

29. Loddenkemper T. Quo vadis Wada? Epilepsy Behav 2008;13(1):1–2.

30. Loddenkemper T, Moddel G, Dinner DS, et al. Language assessment in Wada test: comparison of methohexital and amobarbital. Seizure 2009;18(9):656–9.

31. Loddenkemper T, Morris HH, Moddel G. Complications during the Wada test. Epilepsy Behav 2008;13(3):551–3.

32. Baxendale SA, Thompson PJ, Duncan JS. Evidence-based practice: a reevaluation of the intracarotid amobarbital procedure (Wada test). Arch Neurol 2008;65(6):841–5.

33. Jones-Gotman M, Sziklas V, Djordjevic J, et al. Etomidate speech and memory test (eSAM): a new drug and improved intracarotid procedure. Neurology 2005;65(11):1723–9.

34. Pelletier I, Sauerwein HC, Lepore F, et al. Non-invasive alternatives to the Wada test in the presurgical evaluation of language and memory functions in epilepsy patients. Epileptic Disord 2007;9(2):111–26.

35. Breier JI, Simos PG, Zouridakis G, et al. Lateralization of cerebral activation in auditory verbal and non-verbal memory tasks using magnetoencephalography. Brain Topogr 1999;12(2):89–97.

36. Breier JI, Simos PG, Zouridakis G, et al. Language dominance determined by magnetic source imaging: a comparison with the Wada procedure. Neurology 1999;53(5):938–45.

37. Castillo EM, Simos PG, Venkataraman V, et al. Mapping of expressive language cortex using magnetic source imaging. Neurocase 2001;7(5):419–22.

38. Floel A, Knecht S, Lohmann H, et al. Language and spatial attention can lateralize to the same hemisphere in healthy humans. Neurology 2001;57(6):1018–24.

39. Simos PG, Breier JI, Maggio WW, et al. Atypical temporal lobe language representation: MEG and intraoperative stimulation mapping correlation. Neuroreport 1999;10(1):139–42.

40. Simos PG, Castillo EM, Fletcher JM, et al. Mapping of receptive language cortex in bilingual volunteers by using magnetic source imaging. J Neurosurg 2001;95(1):76–81.

41. Simos PG, Papanicolaou AC, Breier JI, et al. Localization of language-specific cortex by using magnetic source imaging and electrical stimulation mapping. J Neurosurg 1999;91(5):787–96.

42. Szymanski MD, Perry DW, Gage NM, et al. Magnetic source imaging of late evoked field responses to vowels: toward an assessment of hemispheric dominance for language. J Neurosurg 2001;94(3):445–53.

43. Szymanski MD, Rowley HA, Roberts TP. A hemispherically asymmetrical MEG response to vowels. Neuroreport 1999;10(12):2481–6.

44. Poeppel D, Idsardi WJ, van Wassenhove V. Speech perception at the interface of neurobiology and linguistics. Philos Trans R Soc Lond B Biol Sci 2008;363(1493):1071–86.

45. Beisteiner R, Gomiscek G, Erdler M, et al. Comparing localization of conventional functional magnetic resonance imaging and magnetoencephalography. Eur J Neurosci 1995;7(5):1121–4.

46. Papanicolaou AC, Simos PG, Breier JI, et al. Magnetoencephalographic mapping of the language-specific cortex. J Neurosurg 1999;90(1):85–93.

47. Panagiotis B. Grand mal seizures with liver toxicity in a case of clozapine treatment. J Neuropsychiatry Clin Neurosci 1999;11(1):117–8.

48. Breier JI, Simos PG, Wheless JW, et al. Language dominance in children as determined by magnetic source imaging and the intracarotid amobarbital procedure: a comparison. J Child Neurol 2001;16(2):124–30.

49. Kober H, Moller M, Nimsky C, et al. New approach to localize speech relevant brain areas and hemispheric dominance using spatially filtered magnetoencephalography. Hum Brain Mapp 2001;14(4):236–50.

50. Holodny A. Functional neuroimaging: a clinical approach. New York: Informa Healthcare; 2008.

51. Hari R. On brain's magnetic responses to sensory stimuli. J Clin Neurophysiol 1991;8(2):157–69.

52. Hari R. Magnetic evoked fields of the human brain: basic principles and applications. Electroencephalogr Clin Neurophysiol Suppl 1990;41:3–12.

53. Hari R, Forss N. Magnetoencephalography in the study of human somatosensory cortical processing. Philos Trans R Soc Lond B Biol Sci 1999;354(1387): 1145–54.

54. Nagarajan S, Kirsch H, Lin P, et al. Preoperative localization of hand motor cortex by adaptive spatial filtering of magnetoencephalography data. J Neurosurg 2008;109(2):228–37.

55. Hoshiyama M, Kakigi R, Koyama S, et al. Somatosensory evoked magnetic fields following stimulation of the lip in humans. Electroencephalogr Clin Neurophysiol 1996;100(2):96–104.

56. Kakigi R. Somatosensory evoked magnetic fields following median nerve stimulation. Neurosci Res 1994;20(2):165–74.

57. Hari R, Hamalainen H, Hamalainen M, et al. Separate finger representations at the human second somatosensory cortex. Neuroscience 1990;37(1):245–9.

58. Inoue T, Shimizu H, Nakasato N, et al. Accuracy and limitation of functional magnetic resonance imaging for identification of the central sulcus: comparison with magnetoencephalography in patients with brain tumors. Neuroimage 1999;10(6):738–48.

59. Kober H, Nimsky C, Moller M, et al. Correlation of sensorimotor activation with functional magnetic resonance imaging and magnetoencephalography in presurgical functional imaging: a spatial analysis. Neuroimage 2001;14(5):1214–28.

60. Schiffbauer H, Ferrari P, Rowley HA, et al. Functional activity within brain tumors: a magnetic source imaging study. Neurosurgery 2001;49(6):1313–20 [discussion: 1320–1].

61. Firsching R, Bondar I, Heinze HJ, et al. Practicability of magnetoencephalography-guided neuronavigation. Neurosurg Rev 2002;25(1–2):73–8.

62. Hund M, Rezai AR, Kronberg E, et al. Magnetoencephalographic mapping: basic of a new functional risk profile in the selection of patients with cortical brain lesions. Neurosurgery 1997;40(5):936–42 [discussion 942–3].

63. Bittar RG, Olivier A, Sadikot AF, et al. Presurgical motor and somatosensory cortex mapping with functional magnetic resonance imaging and positron emission tomography. J Neurosurg 1999;91(6):915–21.

64. Lewine JD, Orrison WW Jr. Magnetic source imaging: basic principles and applications in neuroradiology. Acad Radiol 1995;2(5):436–40.

65. Makela JP, Kirveskari E, Seppa M, et al. Three-dimensional integration of brain anatomy and function to facilitate intraoperative navigation around the sensorimotor strip. Hum Brain Mapp 2001;12(3): 180–92.

66. Erdler M, Beisteiner R, Mayer D, et al. Supplementary motor area activation preceding voluntary movement is detectable with a whole-scalp magnetoencephalography system. Neuroimage 2000; 11(6 Pt 1):697–707.

67. Erdler M, Windischberger C, Lanzenberger R, et al. Dissociation of supplementary motor area and primary motor cortex in human subjects when comparing index and little finger movements with functional magnetic resonance imaging. Neurosci Lett 2001;313(1–2):5–8.

68. Gross J, Tass PA, Salenius S, et al. Cortico-muscular synchronization during isometric muscle contraction in humans as revealed by magnetoencephalography. J Physiol 2000;527(Pt 3):623–31.

69. Hatanaka K, Nakasato N, Seki K, et al. Striate cortical generators of the N75, P100 and N145 components localized by pattern reversal visual evoked magnetic fields. Tohoku J Exp Med 1997; 182(1):9–14.

70. Nakasato N, Seki K, Fujita S, et al. Clinical application of visual evoked fields using an MRI-linked whole head MEG system. Front Med Biol Eng 1996;7(4):275–83.

71. Nakasato N, Yoshimoto T. Somatosensory, auditory, and visual evoked magnetic fields in patients with brain diseases. J Clin Neurophysiol 2000;17(2): 201–11.

72. Tang L, Mantle M, Ferrari P, et al. Consistency of interictal and ictal onset localization using magnetoencephalography in patients with partial epilepsy. J Neurosurg 2003;98(4):837–45.

73. Tanaka N, Hamalainen MS, Ahlfors SP, et al. Propagation of epileptic spikes reconstructed from spatiotemporal magnetoencephalographic and electroencephalographic source analysis. Neuroimage 2010;50(1):217–22.

74. Shiraishi H, Ahlfors SP, Stufflebeam SM, et al. Application of magnetoencephalography in epilepsy patients with widespread spike or slow-wave activity. Epilepsia 2005;46(8):1264–72.

75. Shiraishi H, Stufflebeam SM, Knake S, et al. Dynamic statistical parametric mapping for analyzing the magnetoencephalographic epileptiform activity in patients with epilepsy. J Child Neurol 2005;20(4):363–9.

76. Shiraishi H, Watanabe Y, Watanabe M, et al. Interictal and ictal magnetoencephalographic study in patients with medial frontal lobe epilepsy. Epilepsia 2001;42(7):875–82.

77. Robinson SE, Nagarajan SS, Mantle M, et al. Localization of interictal spikes using SAM(g2) and dipole fit. Neurol Clin Neurophysiol 2004;2004:74.

78. Shiraishi H, Takano K, Shiga T, et al. Possible involvement of the tip of temporal lobe in Landau-Kleffner syndrome. Brain Dev 2007;29(8):529–33.

79. Knowlton RC. Can magnetoencephalography aid epilepsy surgery? Epilepsy Curr 2008;8(1):1–5.

80. Knowlton RC, Elgavish RA, Bartolucci A, et al. Functional imaging: II. Prediction of epilepsy surgery outcome. Ann Neurol 2008;64(1):35–41.

81. Knowlton RC, Elgavish RA, Limdi N, et al. Functional imaging: I. Relative predictive value of intracranial electroencephalography. Ann Neurol 2008;64(1):25–34.

82. Sutherling WW, Mamelak AN, Thyerlei D, et al. Influence of magnetic source imaging for planning intracranial EEG in epilepsy. Neurology 2008;71(13):990–6.

83. Fox MD, Raichle ME. Spontaneous fluctuations in brain activity observed with functional magnetic resonance imaging. Nat Rev Neurosci 2007;8(9):700–11.

84. Lin FH, Hara K, Solo V, et al. Dynamic Granger-Geweke causality modeling with application to interictal spike propagation. Hum Brain Mapp 2009;30(6):1877–86.

85. Grunert P, Muller-Forell W, Darabi K, et al. Basic principles and clinical applications of neuronavigation and intraoperative computed tomography. Comput Aided Surg 1998;3(4):166–73.

86. Jannin P, Fleig OJ, Seigneuret E, et al. A data fusion environment for multimodal and multi-informational neuronavigation. Comput Aided Surg 2000;5(1):1–10.

87. Jannin P, Morandi X, Fleig OJ, et al. Integration of sulcal and functional information for multimodal neuronavigation. J Neurosurg 2002;96(4):713–23.

88. Ganslandt O, Fahlbusch R, Nimsky C, et al. Functional neuronavigation with magnetoencephalography: outcome in 50 patients with lesions around the motor cortex. J Neurosurg 1999;91(1):73–9.

89. Rezai AR, Hund M, Kronberg E, et al. The interactive use of magnetoencephalography in stereotactic image-guided neurosurgery. Neurosurgery 1996;39(1):92–102.

90. Rezai AR, Mogilner AY, Cappell J, et al. Integration of functional brain mapping in image-guided neurosurgery. Acta Neurochir Suppl 1997;68:85–9.

PET and SPECT in Brain Tumors and Epilepsy

Laura L. Horky, MD, PhD[a],*, S. Ted Treves, MD[b]

KEYWORDS
- Molecular imaging
- Positron emission tomography
- Brain tumor
- Epilepsy

Molecular imaging with positron emission tomography (PET) plays an important role in the diagnosis and management of patients with brain tumors and epilepsy. Where applicable, single-photon emission computed tomography (SPECT) is also discussed.

OVERVIEW OF PET AND SPECT IN NEUROSURGERY: BRAIN TUMORS

Annually in the United States, more than 20,000 people are diagnosed with malignant brain tumors and approximately 13,000 die of primary brain tumors. Another 22,000 are diagnosed with nonmalignant primary brain tumors. Metastatic brain tumors, predominantly from breast, lung, and colon primary cancers are even more common, with approximately 140,000 patients diagnosed each year, and more than 100,000 deaths per year from symptomatic brain metastases.[1–3]

Nuclear molecular imaging can be used for the assessment of treated or untreated primary or metastatic brain tumors. PET is commonly used for assessing and grading brain tumors, assessing aggressiveness and prognosis, distinguishing between recurrence and postradiation necrosis, and guiding biopsy. Brain SPECT is also a useful technique in the assessment of brain tumor activity.

PET Technology

PET was developed in the 1970s by Phelps and Hoffman, as an in vivo imaging application of autoradiography, using radioactively labeled glucose.[4] Briefly, a positron-emitting radiotracer is injected into the patient and taken up selectively by cells possessing certain molecular characteristics, such as the presence of glucose or amino acid transporters. In the target tissue, the radiotracer decays, emitting positrons. The emitted positrons collide with nearby electrons and are annihilated, producing 2 high-energy (511 keV) photons, which are emitted 180° apart. The photons are detected by a PET scanner, which is a ring-shaped, high-energy coincidence detector that surrounds the patient. Registration of millions of coincidence events allows localization of the radiotracer distribution within the patient. The spatial resolution of PET is 4 to 10 mm, depending on the scanner type. It is generally accepted that assessment of lesions smaller than 7 to 8 mm in diameter or 0.5 cm^3 may be limited.

Hybrid PET/computed tomographic (CT) scanners have all but replaced the traditional PET-only scanners. The hybrid scanner uses low-dose multislice helical CT (approximately 10–40 mA and 130 kilovolt [peak]) for the dual purpose of anatomic localization and attenuation correction.[5] Once acquired, PET images may also be fused to a patient's magnetic resonance imaging (MRI). PET/MRI systems are currently under development, in which PET and MRI images are acquired simultaneously.[6]

PET Tracers: FDG

Fluorodeoxyglucose

2-Deoxy-2-(^{18}F)fluoro-D-glucose (^{18}F-FDG or FDG) is the most common clinical nuclear medicine imaging tracer used today to assess brain tumors.

[a] Division of Nuclear Medicine and Molecular Imaging, Department of Radiology, Brigham and Women's Hospital, Harvard Medical School, 75 Francis Street, Boston, MA 02115, USA
[b] Division of Nuclear Medicine and Molecular Imaging, Department of Radiology, Children's Hospital Boston, 300 Longwood Avenue, Boston, MA 02115, USA
* Corresponding author.
E-mail address: lhorky@partners.org

Neurosurg Clin N Am 22 (2011) 169–184
doi:10.1016/j.nec.2010.12.003
1042-3680/11/$ – see front matter © 2011 Elsevier Inc. All rights reserved.

FDG-PET was initially used for functional brain mapping and then became the first PET tracer used for the assessment of brain tumors.[7] An analogue of glucose, FDG uptake correlates with regional glucose metabolism. FDG readily crosses the blood-brain barrier and is transported intracellularly by glucose transporters. Once intracellular, it is phosporylated by glucose 6-hexokinase and trapped in the cell, because it cannot be metabolized. Brain tumors characteristically have a high concentration of glucose transporters and glucose 6-hexokinase and are therefore typically FDG avid.

The brain uses glucose as its main energy source, and glucose is transported by a group of glucose transporters (GLUTs). GLUT1s are expressed in glia, capillary endothelial cells, choroid plexus, and ependymal cells. GLUT3s are expressed in neurons. Gray matter uses 2 to 4 times more glucose than white matter.[8] In brain tumor imaging, the high rate of glucose transport within physiologically active normal brain can obscure the target to background ratio, particularly when the tumor is adjacent to physiologically active gray matter (**Fig. 1**).

TUMOR GRADING WITH FDG

FDG is useful for tumor grading because most high-grade tumors, such as high-grade gliomas, medulloblastoma, and primary central nervous system lymphoma, have high concentrations and activity of GLUTs.[9] Most low-grade tumors have lower concentrations of GLUTs and can be distinguished from high-grade gliomas by the lower FDG uptake on PET. FDG avidity of common benign and malignant primary and metastatic brain tumors is shown in **Box 1**.

As an exception to the rule, some low-grade tumors have a high FDG avidity, which is because of the high concentrations of GLUTs. In pilocytic astrocytomas, for example, the vascular density is high. In this case, glucose uptake does not represent the blood flow but is thought to represent the metabolic activity of the endothelial cells lining the tumor vasculature.[10–12] Endothelial proliferation and metabolism account for the high FDG avidity. Oligoastrocytomas also have variable FDG uptakes, even within the same tumor grade.

Measurements of tumor FDG uptake versus physiologic brain FDG uptake can be used to predict high- versus low-grade brain tumors, both primary and metastatic, with certain exceptions as noted earlier. Semiquantification of glucose uptake is performed using a standardized uptake value (SUV).[13,14] A tumor to gray matter uptake ratio of greater than 0.6 or a tumor to white matter uptake ratio of greater than 1.5 was, in 1 series by Delbeke and colleagues,[15] 100% sensitive and 67% specific for distinguishing high-grade gliomas from low-grade gliomas. Applying the same cutoffs to primary brain tumors and brain metastases yielded 94% sensitivity and 77% specificity. FDG avidity has also been inversely correlated with survival. For example, in a series of 165 patients with highly FDG avid brain tumors, 1-year survival was only 29%, as opposed to 94% in patients with tumors with low FDG avidity.[16]

Recurrence versus Postradiation Necrosis with FDG

In primary or metastatic tumors treated with radiotherapy, tumor growth as seen on contrast MRI

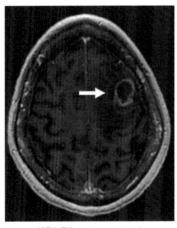
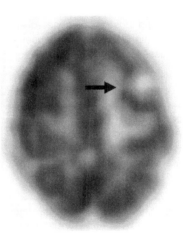

MRI, T1 post-contrast   FDG-PET

Fig. 1. A 62-year-old woman with metastatic lung cancer to the left frontal lobe 18 months after stereotactic radiosurgery. The ring-like contour of FDG avidity corresponding to the rim-enhancing lesion on MRI (*left*) could represent either the tumor or the surrounding gyrus. Biopsy demonstrated that the uptake corresponded to normal gyrus rather than to tumor.

Box 1
FDG avidity in primary and metastatic brain tumors and sources of false-positive uptake

High

   High-grade gliomas (grades III and IV)

   Medulloblastoma

   Primary central nervous system lymphoma

   Pineoblastoma

   Central neurocytoma

   Pilocytic astrocytoma

   Pituitary adenoma

Variable

   Metastases

   Oligodendroglioma

   Meningioma

Low

   Most low-grade gliomas

   Primitive neurectodermal tumor

   Vestibular schwannomas

False positive

   Infection

   Inflammation

   Seizure activity

Malignant tumors are given in italics.

is often indistinguishable from postradiation necrosis, both appearing as enlarging, contrast-enhancing lesions. Approximately 70% of radiation necrosis cases are diagnosed in the first 2 years following radiation treatment, which is similar to the expected time frame for tumor recurrence. The incidence of radiation necrosis increases with the radiation dose and is particularly high in cases in which chemotherapy is concurrently administered.[17–19] FDG-PET is a useful tool in distinguishing postradiation necrosis from tumor progression, both in high-grade gliomas and brain metastases. In general, recurrent tumor is FDG avid (**Fig. 2**), and radiation necrosis is not FDG avid. In the first 3 to 6 months after radiation, FDG-avid radiation-induced inflammatory cells such as macrophages can have the same appearance as a tumor. Inflammatory cells are seen in the setting of edema, neovascularity, demyelination, and necrosis, which begin to occur in the first hours to months after radiation treatment.[17–19] As discussed in later sections, techniques such as dual-phase FDG-PET imaging and PET imaging with investigational radiotracers can help to improve the accuracy of PET imaging by increasing the target to background ratio.

The sensitivity of FDG-PET for distinguishing tumor recurrence (primary and metastatic) ranges from 80% to 86%, with a specificity of 40% to 88%.[18,20–25] In some centers, PET images are fused to MRI and delayed-phase PET images are obtained. Both methods have been shown to improve the accuracy of FDG-PET. Fusion of

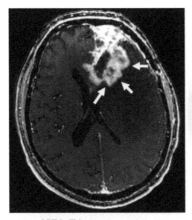 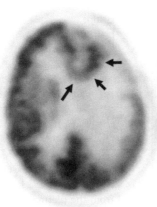 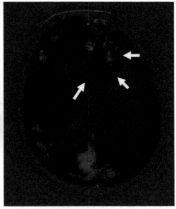

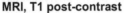

   MRI, T1 post-contrast   **FDG-PET**   **PET/MRI fusion**

Fig. 2. A 54-year-old man with left frontal glioblastoma multiforme presenting with increased enhancement and mass effect on MRI (*left*) 4 months after radiation therapy. He was referred to evaluate for progression versus pseudoprogression (posttreatment necrosis). FDG-PET (*center*) demonstrates intense hypermetabolism (*arrows*) corresponding to the lesion in question. PET/MRI fusion (*right*) helps to confirm that the uptake corresponds to the lesion rather than to the adjacent physiologically active cortex.

FDG-PET images to contrast MRI images is helpful for anatomic correlation and helps to distinguish uptake within a lesion from uptake in an adjacent, functionally active gray matter. This ability may be helpful in cases in which the rounded contour of a rim-enhancing lesion may look similar to the contour of a gyrus, which closely surrounds the lesion, as in **Fig. 1**.

In one series, the sensitivity of FDG-PET in assessing for recurrent brain metastasis versus radiation necrosis without fusion to MRI was 65% and 85%, respectively, and after PET/MRI fusion, sensitivity increased to 86% and specificity to 80%.[25]

Dual-Phase FDG-PET Imaging

Dual-phase FDG-PET imaging has been shown to increase accuracy in distinguishing recurrence from postradiation necrosis in gliomas and brain metastases.[26,27] This method enhances the tumor to background ratio and is based on differences in FDG tracer kinetics between tumor and normal brain parenchyma. When FDG-PET is normally performed at 45 to 60 minutes after tracer injection, FDG tracer kinetics are similar between tumor and gray matter. In other words, transport of the tracer through the blood-brain barrier and into the cells is similar for the tumor and normal brain (**Fig. 3**). Phosphorylation of the tracer by glucose 6-hexokinase, which traps the FDG intracellularly, may be higher in the tumor than in normal gray matter because tumors may have abnormally high levels of glucose 6-hexokinase. Dephosphorylation via glucose 6-phosphatase is higher in normal brain parenchyma than in tumor. Over

time, trapping and retention of the tracer by the tumor is greater than that of normal brain parenchyma. This process is most pronounced at 3 to 6 hours after tracer injection.[26]

In the authors' clinic, dual-phase imaging was performed on a series of 25 patients with treated brain metastases (predominantly breast, lung, and melanoma primary cancer) and enlarging contrast-enhancing lesions on MRI suspicious for recurrence versus radiation necrosis. Of the 25 patients, 22 received radiation, most often stereotactic radiosurgery. The other 3 received chemotherapy without radiation. SUVmax was calculated for the lesion and normal gray matter at 2 imaging sessions, first at 45 to 60 minutes after tracer injection and the second at a mean of 225 minutes after the initial scan. The ratio of SUVmax of the lesion to gray matter was measured at early and late time points, using the following formula: [(L2/GM2−L1/GM1)/(L1/GM1)] where L1 = early SUVmax lesion; L2 = late SUVmax lesion; GM1 = early SUVmax normal contralateral gray matter; GM2 = late SUVmax normal contralateral gray matter. Using receiver operating characteristic (ROC) analysis, the change in this ratio over time was the most accurate parameter for distinguishing recurrence and posttreatment necrosis. When this increase was 19% or more between the early and late imaging sessions, the sensitivity and specificity for detecting tumor were 95% and 100%, respectively. This ROC cutoff is currently being tested prospectively in brain metastases and primary brain tumors.[27] An example of dual-phase imaging is shown in **Fig. 4**.

Several investigational PET tracers provide more specific information about tumor properties

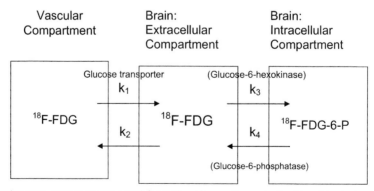

Fig. 3. FDG tracer kinetics. FDG is transported from the plasma through the blood-brain barrier via GLUTs (k_1) and from the extracellular space to the intracellular space within the brain (k_3). Dephosphorylation by glucose 6-phosphatase enables transport of FDG to the extracellular compartment (k_4). Once dephosphorylated, FDG can reenter the plasma (k_2). (*Data from* Sokoloff L, Reivich M, Kennedy C, et al. The [14C]-deoxyglucose method for the measurement of local cerebral glucose utilization: theory, procedure, and normal values in the conscious and anesthetized albino rat. J Neurochem 1977;28:897–916 and Phelps ME, Huang SC, Hoffman EJ, Selin C, Sokoloff L, Kuhl DE, Tomographic measurement of local cerebral glucose metabolic rate in humans with (F-18) 2-fluoro-2-deoxy-D-glucose: validation of method. Ann Neurol 1979;6:371–88.)

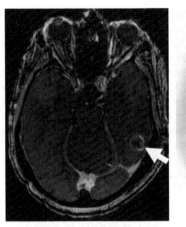 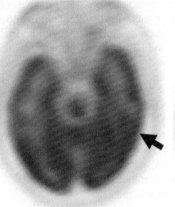 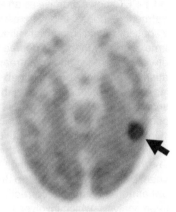

| MRI, T1 post-contrast | Early phase FDG-PET (60 min.) | Late phase FDG-PET (6.5 hrs.) |

Fig. 4. A 69-year-old man with non–small cell lung cancer metastatic to the left temporal lobe 6 months after chemoradiotherapy, with increasing size on MRI (*left*); arrow indicates the lesion. Lesion SUVmax increased from 4.7 to 7.5 between early phase images (*center*) performed 1 hour after FDG tracer injection and delayed-phase images (*right*) performed 5.5 hours later. In contrast, the SUVmax of the surrounding gray matter decreased from 3.9 to 2.9. The change in the lesion to surrounding gray matter ratio over time was 146%, compatible with viable metastasis as opposed to radiation necrosis.

such as cellular proliferation, protein synthesis, and hypoxia.

Proliferation: 3-Deoxy-3-[¹⁸F]Fluorothymidine

3-Deoxy-3-[¹⁸F]fluorothymidine (FLT) is an imaging biomarker of mitotic activity. FLT uptake correlates with the activity of thymidine kinase-1, an enzyme expressed during the S phase (DNA synthesis) of the cell cycle. FLT tracer uptake within normal brain parenchyma is negligible because it does not significantly cross the blood-brain barrier and most normal brain cells do not divide. This scenario allows for an excellent tumor to background ratio. FLT uptake is high in high-grade gliomas because of their high mitotic index and blood-brain barrier permeability. Conversely, FLT uptake is low in low-grade gliomas because of a low mitotic index and an impermeable blood-brain barrier. FLT is more sensitive than FDG in detecting de novo and recurrent high-grade gliomas. Both tracers are useful for glioma grading, as they are generally insensitive in low-grade gliomas (**Fig. 5**).[28]

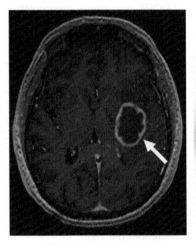 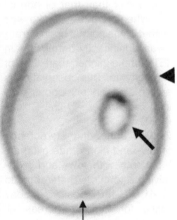

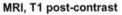

| MRI, T1 post-contrast | FLT-PET |

Fig. 5. A 70-year-old man with left subinsular glioblastoma multiforme. FLT uptake corresponds to the enhancing tumor on MRI (*large arrows*). Central photopenia corresponds to the necrotic portion of the tumor. FLT uptake is also seen in the venous sinuses (*small arrow*) and the bone marrow of the skull (*arrowhead*). Uptake in the normal brain parenchyma is limited.

FLT-PET shows promise as an early predictor of treatment response. In an interesting pilot study of 19 patients with recurrent glioblastoma multiforme, a greater than 25% decrease in FLT uptake between baseline and posttreatment scans in patients receiving bevacizumab and irinotecan was able to predict outcome, with a 3-fold greater survival in metabolic responders than in nonresponders (mean 10.8 vs 3.4 months).[29]

Optimal assessment of FLT uptake in brain tumors (ie, in baseline vs posttreatment scans) may require kinetic modeling with prolonged dynamic imaging times of up to 90 minutes.[30] Furthermore, metabolite correction optimizes FLT image analysis, which involves collection of blood samples for measurement of radioactive metabolites of FLT.[30] FLT imaging is therefore more cumbersome than FDG for both the patient and the image analyst.

Amino Acid Transport and Protein Synthesis

The essential amino acids are transported into the brain by the large neutral amino acid (LNAA) transport system. Amino acid transport via the LNAA transport system is markedly increased in low- and high-grade gliomas. Advantageously, amino acid tracers cross the blood-brain barrier and label both low- and high-grade gliomas, and uptake in the gray matter is low.

[11]C-Methionine (^{11}C-MET) is perhaps the most well-studied amino acid tracer. Increased ^{11}C-MET uptake is not seen in all low-grade gliomas, and uptake levels are a predictor of biologic behavior. In a series of patients with low-grade gliomas, one-third of patients had a MET uptake that was similar to or lower than that of normal brain parenchyma.[31] When ^{11}C-MET uptake was equal to or less than that of the normal brain parenchyma, prognosis was significantly better than in patients with a MET uptake higher than that of the normal brain parenchyma. This observation is similar to the results using an analogous ^{18}F-labeled amino acid radiotracer, O-(2-^{18}F-fluoroethyl)-L-tyrosine (FET).[32]

[11]C-MET is useful in optimizing stereotactic biopsy guidance of low- and high-grade gliomas. In a group of 32 patients with low- and high-grade gliomas receiving a total of 70 stereotactic biopsies, 100% of 61 ^{11}C-MET-positive biopsy sites were diagnostic for tumor, whereas all ^{11}C-MET-negative biopsy sites were negative for tumor or nondiagnostic.[33] Because ^{11}C-MET does not easily discriminate between low- and high-grade tumor, correlation with FDG-PET is helpful in guiding the biopsy to the highest grade portion of the tumor. Amino acid PET also shows promise in optimizing neurosurgical resections of gliomas and radiation planning for gliomas.[33–35]

The short ^{11}C radioactive half-life of 20 minutes limits availability of ^{11}C-MET to hospitals with an on-site cyclotron. ^{18}F-labeled amino acid tracers such as ^{18}F-FDOPA (3,4-dihydroxy-6-[^{18}F]-fluoro-L-phenylalanine) and ^{18}F-FET may be produced off-site because of the longer half-life (110 minutes). These tracers are generally considered to be functionally interchangeable with ^{11}C-MET because their LNAA transport systems are similar and tumor uptake is primarily due to increased transport.[8,36–38]

FDOPA

Before the application of FDOPA to brain tumor imaging, it was primarily used for assessing the striatal dopamine pathway in patients with movement disorders.[39] Applied to gliomas, FDOPA has been shown to be 98% sensitive and 86% specific in distinguishing tumor from radiation necrosis, using a tumor:striatum SUV cutoff ratio of 0.75.[40] Like other amino acid tracers, it is useful in characterizing low-grade gliomas and in distinguishing recurrent tumor from radiation-induced necrosis.

FET

Like other amino acid tracers, FET is useful in distinguishing radiation necrosis from glioma recurrence. FET-PET was used in 45 patients with MRI suspicious for recurrent glioma and was 93% sensitive and 100% specific in making the distinction between recurrence and postradiation necrosis.[41] It has also been shown that analysis of amino acid tracer kinetics using FET and FDOPA accurately distinguishes low- and high-grade gliomas.[42,43]

Hypoxia: ^{18}F-Misonidazole

The most well-studied PET hypoxia tracer is ^{18}F-misonidazole (MISO), a derivative of nitroimidazole. Oxygen consumption of brain tumors is lower than that of the normal brain because of disturbed angiogenesis. MISO is lipophilic, uniformly diffuses throughout the brain, and is trapped only by hypoxic cells. Its uptake is higher in high-grade gliomas because these tumors are typically more hypoxic. Because hypoxia is associated with radioresistance, it is thought that imaging biomarkers of hypoxia may be helpful in treatment planning.[44–46]

The tumor imaging tracers discussed here are summarized in **Table 1**. It should be mentioned that nuclear brain imaging extends beyond PET. SPECT imaging, using a different detector system, is widely clinically available and a valuable

Table 1
Summary of PET radiotracers

Biomarker	Radiotracer	Clinical/ Investigational
Glucose transport and metabolism	^{18}F-FDG	Clinical
DNA synthesis	^{18}F-FLT	Investigational
Protein synthesis and/or transport	^{11}C-MET	Investigational
	^{18}F-FDOPA	Investigational
	^{18}F-FET	Investigational
Hypoxia	^{18}F-FMISO	Investigational

complement and/or alternative to FDG-PET. SPECT radiotracers include thallium 201, ^{99m}Tc-sestamibi and [111]Indium-pentreotide (OctreoScan). Each of these tracers demonstrates low background uptake in the brain, which allows for a high target to background ratio. [111]Indium-pentreotide is a somatostatin analogue and is taken up by neuroendocrine tumors, including meningiomas. [111]Indium-pentreotide is most sensitive in well-differentiated meningiomas, which express high levels of somatostatin receptors, but is less useful in dedifferentiated, atypical meningiomas.[47]

Thallium 201, an analogue of potassium, enters viable cells via the Na[+], K[+]-ATPase pump. Thallium does not cross the blood-brain barrier and is therefore used in assessing MRI contrast-enhancing lesions to differentiate tumor recurrence (primary or metastatic) from radiation necrosis.[48–54] Thallium uptake correlates with the tumor grade and proliferative index and is most sensitive in high-grade lesions.[55] Thallium 201 is reportedly up to 100% sensitive in distinguishing tumor (primary and metastatic) recurrence from postradiation necrosis in as little as 6 to 12 weeks after standard radiation therapy or radiosurgery.[56] Recent hemorrhage, infarct, or the presence of an abscess may give a false positive result.[57]

[99m]Tc-sestamibi is another useful tracer for distinguishing recurrent tumor (high-grade glioma or metastasis) from radiation necrosis. It is a cation that accumulates in negatively charged mitochondria. It does not cross the blood-brain barrier, and background uptake is minimal, aside from the choroid plexus. For distinguishing tumor recurrence from radiation necrosis, its sensitivity ranges from 67% to 100% and specificity from 91% to 100%, with the highest accuracy in the setting of high-grade gliomas.[58–61]

[111]Indium-pentreotide is a somatostatin analogue and is taken up by neuroendocrine tumors, including meningiomas. [111]Indium-pentreotide is

most sensitive in well-differentiated meningiomas that express high levels of somatostatin receptors but is less useful in dedifferentiated, atypical meningiomas.[47]

SPECT imaging is of limited sensitivity for tumors smaller than approximately 10 to 15 mm compared with 7 to 10 mm for FDG-PET. However, if lesions meet this size threshold, SPECT imaging is as sensitive as FDG-PET. SPECT is particularly advantageous in tumors that are not characteristically FDG avid, including some lobular breast cancers and renal cell carcinomas, and in lesions situated near the physiologically active cortex. These tracers are a useful part of the clinical portfolio and will endure as long as PET tracers beyond FDG remain strictly investigational.

Lastly, it should be mentioned that whole-body PET/CT is at times a useful adjunct to brain imaging in patients presenting with a new primary brain tumor versus brain metastasis.[62] Diagnostic biopsy in a more easily accessible site elsewhere in the body may help to preclude a more invasive intracranial biopsy.

OVERVIEW OF PET AND SPECT IN NEUROSURGERY: EPILEPSY

Approximately 150,000 people in the United States are diagnosed with epilepsy annually.[63] Of these, two-thirds suffer from focal or partial epilepsy and one-third have generalized epilepsy.[64] About 70% of patients with epilepsy can be managed medically, but medically refractory patients may benefit from surgical resection of the ictal focus.[65] Surgical treatment is successful in 60% to 90% of patients with unilateral temporal lobe epilepsy (TLE) and 22% to 65% of patients with extratemporal epilepsy.[66,67] Surgical success is defined as resolution of seizures for a period of 2 years after resection.[15]

Accurate localization of the seizure focus is an important prerequisite for successful epilepsy surgery. Noninvasive tools for localization include MRI, SPECT, FDG-PET, and video electroencephalography (EEG) monitoring. Most patients who have epilepsy surgery have structural abnormalities on MRI, such as hippocampal or mesial temporal sclerosis, and these patients statistically are most likely to be seizure-free postsurgically.[68,69] PET and SPECT are useful functional imaging tools for the presurgical assessment of patients with partial epilepsy, particularly in patients without a focal abnormality on MRI that coincides with a localizing epileptogenic focus on EEG. These nuclear imaging modalities can help to guide the placement of long-term intracranial EEG electrodes or, in some cases, can obviate intracranial electrodes, because of accurate locali-zation of a single focus or identification of multiple seizure foci; the latter case would decrease the like-lihood of surgical success.[70] Surgical success is defined as the resolution of seizures for a period of 2 years after resection. Within the criteria for success, patients may continue to take antiepi-leptic medication and may continue to experience auras.[71]

Nuclear imaging studies include ictal SPECT, in-terictal SPECT, and interictal FDG-PET. SPECT defines the seizure focus on the basis of altered cerebral perfusion, and FDG-PET defines the seizure focus on the basis of abnormal glucose metabolism. For defining the epileptic focus, ictal SPECT is considered to be the most sensitive study, followed by interictal PET and then by inter-ictal SPECT. SPECT is performed with perfusion tracers, most commonly technetium Tc 99m ethyl cysteinate dimer (ECD) and technetium Tc 99m hexamethylpropyleneamine oxime (HMPAO). The SPECT scan is routinely performed twice in each patient, with 1 ictal injection and scan (tracer injec-tion given during a seizure) and 1 postictal injection and scan (tracer injection given during the resting state between seizures). These 2 SPECT studies are usually performed 1 or more days apart. The ictal period begins at the time of electroclinical seizure onset. After a seizure, a postictal or recovery period may last for approximately 2 to 6 hours. In the interictal state, the normal resting brain perfusion is imaged. This period begins approximately 2 to 6 hours after the most recent seizure. This recovery period is needed because brain perfusion is altered for several hours postic-tally, with periods of hyperperfusion and rebound hypoperfusion.[72–74]

Ictal SPECT

Ictal SPECT is considered to be the most accurate indicator of the seizure focus, with a sensitivity of 96% reported in 1 meta-analysis.[73] This sensitivity is compared with an interictal SPECT sensitivity of 44% and a postictal (>30 seconds after seizure onset) sensitivity of 75%.[73] Ictal SPECT is labor intensive and requires a tracer injection as soon as possible once a seizure is electroclinically de-tected. It is performed in conjunction with video EEG monitoring in specialized centers. The lipo-philic technetium Tc 99m–labeled SPECT perfu-sion radiopharmaceuticals ECD and HMPAO readily cross the blood-brain barrier and reach the brain by approximately 20 seconds after a peripheral intravenous tracer injection is trapped in the brain parenchyma, with a high first pass extraction of 5% to 7% of the injected dose.[75]

Distribution of the tracer correlates with the cere-bral blood flow. Once within the brain, HMPAO is retained in the brain parenchyma by conversion to a hydrophilic compound. ECD gains a negative charge in the brain and is trapped by this mecha-nism in the brain. The tracers remain fixed in the brain parenchyma for more than 4 hours after injection, and quality images are obtained from 30 minutes to 4 or more hours after tracer injec-tion. After ictal tracer injection, the patient is trans-ported from the video EEG suite to the SPECT scanner in the nuclear medicine clinic. As the tracer is already fixed in the brain, sedatives and antiepileptic medications may be used to ensure that the patient is able to remain still for a 20- to 45-minute imaging session.

Successful ictal SPECT depends on several variables. Most importantly, injection should be performed as soon as possible after seizure onset (**Fig. 6** A, B, D). The following criteria are also crit-ical: seizures should be quickly detected by the staff; nurses or physicians injecting the tracer should be well-trained and experienced and should be familiar with the patient's ictal EEG and clinical characteristics; the aura preceding the seizure is ideally brief, as a prolonged aura can delay the injection; and the injection should be delivered intravenously into a preexisting, well-maintained intravenous line.[75,76]

Subtraction of interictal from ictal SPECT images (**Fig. 6** C, E) helps to increase the accuracy of the diagnosis. This subtraction can be per-formed visually or with the use of postprocessing software. The processed subtraction SPECT image may then be fused to the patient's MRI (known as subtraction ictal SPECT coregistered to MRI or SISCOM), a method that provides improved sensitivity and specificity as compared with visual subtraction.[77]

Devices to automatically inject the radiotracer on detection of EEG changes compatible with the patient's known seizure pattern are under development.[16] Other methods are currently in use, in which the lead-shielded radiotracer dose is mounted to an intravenous pole and can be in-jected quickly once the electroclinical seizure is detected by the EEG technician and the patient's nurse.[78]

FDG-PET

FDG-PET demonstrates regional glucose metabo-lism. It is particularly useful in cases in which ictal SPECT is difficult to obtain or ictal SPECT results are equivocal. Its spatial resolution is approxi-mately 5 mm as opposed to approximately 10 to 12 mm for SPECT, and therefore, interictal PET is more sensitive than interictal SPECT. Once FDG

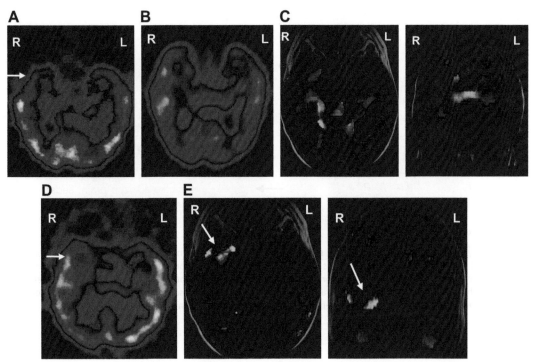

Fig. 6. Example of a case of late ictal injection and a prompt repeat ictal injection in a 12-year-old boy with a seizure disorder. (*A*) Interictal SPECT demonstrates mild relative hypoperfusion in the right temporal lobe (*arrow*). (*B*) Postictal SPECT, in which the perfusion tracer injected more than 30 seconds after the seizure onset fails to demonstrate a definite, single seizure focus, although right temporal activity perfusion is increased. (*C*) Postictal SPECT subtraction images (ictal-interictal scans) fused to MRI (SISCOM) in axial and coronal planes fail to demonstrate a definite, single seizure focus. (*D*) Ictal SPECT (injection 2 seconds after seizure onset) demonstrates right temporal hyperperfusion. (*E*) Ictal subtraction SPECT (ictal minus interictal) fused to MRI, shown in both axial and coronal planes, demonstrates relative hyperperfusion in the right temporal lobe. One month after these images were obtained, the patient underwent a right frontotemporal craniotomy with microsurgical resection of lateral and mesiotemporal structures, including the hippocampus. As of 6 months after surgery, the patient experienced 2 auras but no seizures while remaining on his seizure medication.

is phosphorylated by glucose 6-hexokinase, it remains trapped intracellularly and is not further metabolized. PET is most commonly performed in the interictal state, or between seizures (**Fig. 7**), as it is difficult to time an ictal PET injection. FDG is taken up by the brain over a period of minutes to hours, and if a seizure occurs between the time of tracer injection and imaging, the uptake pattern can reflect both ictal and postictal states, as well as cortical spread. There are some cases of clear seizure identification within ictal PET; however, these cases are rare and often acquired fortuitously, as the tracer in these cases is injected before the seizure occurred (**Fig. 8**). For interictal PET, the patient would ideally be seizure-free for 24 hours before tracer injection; however, in some centers a minimum of 2 to 12 hours is considered acceptable. The postictal recovery period is necessary because glucose metabolic patterns are distorted by seizure activity. If injected with FDG too soon after a seizure, metabolic patterns may be impossible to interpret. In some centers, the patient is monitored with video EEG during the 45- to 60-minute uptake period between injection and scanning so that any seizure activity can be documented. Information about the patient's most recent seizures can aid with image interpretation if a seizure focus is not clearly identifiable.

Interictally, the seizure focus appears as a relatively hypometabolic zone on FDG-PET (case 2). The actual mechanism for this hypometabolism is not understood, but it may be because of neuronal loss or functional disturbance.[70] Interictal PET has been shown to be most helpful in cases of TLE, with sensitivity ranging from 70% to 85%.[79,80] Automated analysis of PET images has shown improved sensitivity of PET to 86% to 90% in 27 patients with TLE and to 67% in a series of 22 patients with extratemporal epilepsy. Automated analysis involves anatomic standardization

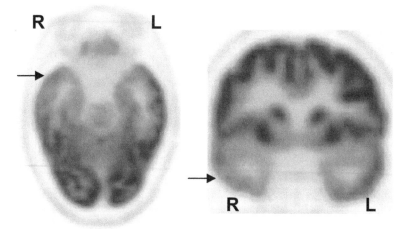

Fig. 7. A 51-year-old man with adult-onset epilepsy characterized predominantly by auras and complex partial seizures. MRI was nonlesional, and EEG was localizing to the right temporal lobe, with right temporal slowing and sharp wave-and-spike discharges, predominantly in the anterior temporal pole. FDG-PET demonstrated asymmetric hypometabolism in the right temporal lobe, quantified as a decrease of 18% relative to the left temporal lobe. A subsequent Wada test demonstrated dominant left-hemispheric language and memory.

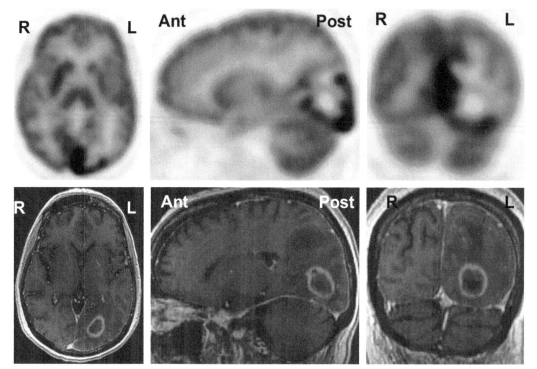

Fig. 8. Occasionally, an unplanned ictal PET scan is obtained. In this case, a 66-year-old man with metastatic lung cancer to the left occipital lobe presented with increased tumor size after stereotactic radiosurgery. The rim-enhancing focus in the left occipital lobe is not FDG avid, compatible with radiation necrosis as opposed to tumor; however, there is markedly increased cortical uptake surrounding the enhancing lesion. This intense, supraphysiologic cortical uptake in the left occipital cortex most likely represents intermittent subclinical seizure activity.

and creation of 3-dimensional stereotactic surface projections and projection onto MRI, followed by comparison to an age-matched database.[81]

Relative temporal lobe hypometabolism of at least 15% has been shown to correlate with seizure-free outcomes after temporal lobe resection, most notably in patients who also underwent preoperative subdural electrode placement.[82] In a different series of 75 patients with TLE, a temporal lobe asymmetry index was calculated for each patient, using statistical parametric mapping, and patients with asymmetry indices of 40% or more were less likely to become seizure-free after surgery.[83] Higher asymmetry indices may indicate a greater degree of dysfunction of the abnormal temporal lobe or a higher degree of asymmetry of bilateral temporal lobe involvement, with asymmetrically lower uptake on the side of the epileptic focus.[83,84]

Interictal FDG-PET is most helpful in patients with normal MRI findings. The pattern of hypometabolism in mesial TLE may involve the mesial and anterolateral temporal cortex and temporal pole, with occasional extension to the basal ganglia and thalamus.[79,85] For extratemporal epilepsy, interictal PET has a much lower sensitivity of approximately 45%.[80,86] Patterns of temporal hypometabolism differ in patients with and without MRI findings of mesial temporal sclerosis. Although MRI-positive mesial temporal sclerosis is associated with anterior inferomesial hypometabolism on PET, focal hypometabolism is more commonly present in the inferolateral temporal neocortex in patients without MRI evidence of hippocampal sclerosis.[87] The pathophysiologic basis for these different patterns of hypometabolism is unclear. In the setting of MRI-positive hippocampal sclerosis, the additional value of PET has been questioned because FDG hypometabolism in the ipsilateral hippocampus is almost always seen.[88] However, the pattern of FDG uptake may differ within this patient population, and it has been hypothesized that because the seizure onset may occur in the temporal pole as well as the hippocampus, the pattern of temporal cortical hypometabolism may help surgeons to decide whether a standard temporal lobectomy or a selective amygdalohippocampectomy would be more appropriate for each individual patient.[70] Likewise, it has been hypothesized that in patients with lateral temporal neocortical hypometabolism in the absence of hippocampal sclerosis on MRI, the surgical approach could possibly be more limited, with sparing of the mesial structures.[87] This fact has yet to be determined. Furthermore, certain regions of hypometabolism may be secondary, such as in the case of frontal hypometabolism associated with temporal hypometabolism in patients with TLE. In this scenario, frontal hypometabolism may represent neuronal inhibition caused by the primary epileptogenic focus in the temporal lobe.[89]

In neocortical epilepsy imaging of cortical dysplasia, a developmental malformation, FDG-PET has been shown to have approximately a 78% concordance with MRI findings (case 4) and may be helpful in delineating the region of functional deficit, which may extend beyond the area of detectable abnormality on MRI.[90,91] FDG-PET may also reveal focal hypometabolism in focal cortical dysplasia that appears normal on MRI (Fig. 9).[92] Decreased FDG-PET uptake of 30% to 50% relative to the contralateral cortex has been shown to be helpful in identifying the cortical

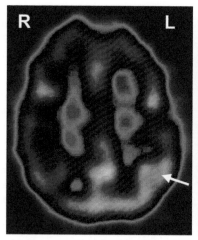
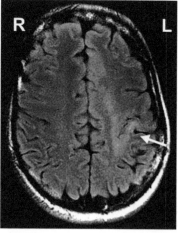

Fig. 9. A 39-year-old woman with daily intractable focal motor seizures localizing to the right arm. Ictal SPECT revealed focal hyperperfusion correlating to left posterior cortical dysplasia on fluid attenuation inversion recovery MRI. Subsequent magnetoencephalography localized a seizure focus to the same region.

tubers that are epileptogenic in patients with tuberous sclerosis complex.[93]

γ-AMINOBUTYRIC ACID RECEPTOR IMAGING WITH [¹¹C]FLUMAZENIL

γ-Aminobutyric acid (GABA) is the most abundant inhibitory neurotransmitter within the forebrain. It is hypothesized that within the epileptic focus, inhibitory neurotransmission is faulty.[94] GABA receptor binding is abnormally low in the seizure focus, suggestive of neuronal loss.[95,96] Since approximately 1988, the experimental PET tracer [¹¹C]flumazenil ([¹¹C]FMZ) has been used as an imaging biomarker of central benzodiazepine receptor (GABA$_A$) binding.[95] Subsequent studies have confirmed that a decreased [¹¹C]FMZ uptake is seen in the medial temporal lobe in patients with or without hippocampal sclerosis.[97–99] The zone of abnormal [¹¹C]FMZ uptake is generally more focal than the zone of hypometabolism seen on FDG-PET in epilepsy patients, and larger regions of ([¹¹C]FMZ) uptake have been shown to directly correlate with the patient's seizure frequency.[89,100]

It has been suggested that [¹¹C]FMZ-PET may be a helpful prognostic indicator of a successful response to surgery in patients with TLE and hippocampal sclerosis. In this patient population, preoperative periventricular uptake of FMZ correlated with poor outcome.[101] [¹¹C]FMZ-PET also shows promise in identifying the seizure focus in extratemporal epilepsy. In a small group of 10 pediatric patients with medically refractory extratemporal epilepsy, [¹¹C]FMZ-PET outperformed FDG-PET in identifying the epileptogenic focus.[102]

As a measure of receptor density, [¹¹C]FMZ-PET images can be variable within the same patient on repeat examination as early as 1 week afterward, indicating short-term plasticity of benzodiazepine receptors after seizures; it has been suggested that the accuracy of [¹¹C]FMZ-PET imaging may be optimized by imaging patients within a few days after a seizure.[103,104]

SEROTONIN RECEPTOR IMAGING WITH A-[¹¹C]METHYL-L-TRYPTOPHAN PET

Similar to [¹¹C]FMZ, the PET tracer A-[¹¹C]methyl-L-tryptophan (AMT) has a half-life of only 20 minutes, as opposed to 110 minutes for [¹⁸F] FDG. This shorter half-life confers a lower radiation dose to patients, which is particularly important in the pediatric population. [¹¹C]AMT-PET has shown promise in identifying the active or epileptogenic tubers in patients with tuberous sclerosis complex.[105] The concentrations of serotonin and its metabolite 5-hydroxyindoleacetic acid are elevated in tissue specimens of human epileptic foci.[106–108] After intravenous injection, the [¹¹C] AMT tracer is taken up by serotoninergic terminals but not metabolized by monoamine oxidase. It accumulates in the nerve terminals, resulting in an increased signal intensity on imaging.[109,110] [¹¹C]AMT is also used in the presurgical assessment of some patients with tuberous sclerosis. In about two-thirds of a series of patients with tuberous sclerosis, uptake of [¹¹C]AMT was 20% to 188% higher in epileptogenic tubers as compared with that in quiescent tubers.[105,110]

SUMMARY

Clinical imaging with perfusion SPECT and FDG-PET, as well as experimental molecular imaging with the research PET tracers [¹¹C]FMZ and [¹¹C] AMT, has been shown to provide useful biomarkers of the epileptogenic focus. In choosing the most appropriate test for each patient, it is helpful to know if the seizures are temporal or extratemporal, if there is a known lesion on MRI, and whether each patient's seizure characteristics would allow for a prompt ictal injection. Interpretation of nuclear images is optimized by correlation with the patient's clinical history and complementary tests, such as EEG and MRI.

ACKNOWLEDGMENTS

The authors thank Jon Hainer for help with PET/MRI image coregistration and BWH Nuclear Medicine technologist James Semer for his help with FLT-PET acquisition.

REFERENCES

1. Central Brain Tumor Registry of the United States (CBTRUS). Statistical report: primary brain tumors in the United States, 1998–2002. North American Brain Tumor Coalition; 2005. Available at: http://www.nabraintumor.org/facts.html. Accessed March 1, 2010.

2. Cancer facts and figures Report 2009. American Cancer Society; 2009. Available at: http://www.cancer.org/research/cancerfactsfigures/cancerfacts figures/cancer-facts-figures-2009. Accessed March 1, 2010.

3. Medical encyclopedia: metastatic brain tumor. Medline plus; 2006. Available at: http://www.nlm.gov/medlineplus/print/ency/article/000769.htm. Accessed March 1, 2010.

4. Phelps ME, Hoffman EJ, Mullani NA, et al. Application of annihilation coincidence detection to transaxial reconstruction tomography. J Nucl Med 1975;16(3):210–24.

5. Czernin J, Dahlbom M, Ratib O, et al. Atlas of PET/CT imaging in oncology. Berlin: Springer-Verlag; 2004.

6. Catana C, Wu Y, Judenhofer MS, et al. Simultaneous acquisition of multislice PET and MR images: initial results with a MR-compatible PET scanner. J Nucl Med 2006;47(12):1968–76.

7. Di Chiro G, DeLaPaz RL, Brooks RA, et al. Glucose utilization of cerebral gliomas measured by [18F] fluorodeoxyglucose and positron emission tomography. Neurology 1982;32(12):1323–9.

8. Herholz K, Herscovitch P, Heiss WD. NeuroPET: PET in neuroscience and clinical neurology. , Berlin: Springer-Verlag; 2004.

9. Warburg O. On the origin of cancer cells. Science 1956;123(3191):309–14.

10. Murovic JA, Nagashima T, Hoshino T, et al. Pediatric central nervous system tumors: a cell kinetic study with bromodeoxyuridine. Neurosurgery 1986;19(6):900–4.

11. Fulham MJ, Radu EW, Hausmann O, et al. Neuroimaging of juvenile pilocytic astrocytomas: an enigma. Radiology 1993;189(1):221–5.

12. Roelcke U, Radu EW, Hausmann O, et al. Tracer transport and metabolism in a patient with juvenile pilocytic astrocytoma. A PET study. J Neurooncol 1998;36(3):279–83.

13. Strauss LG, Conti PS. The applications of PET in clinical oncology. J Nucl Med 1991;32(4):623–48 [discussion 649–50].

14. Huang SC. Anatomy of SUV. Standardized uptake value. Nucl Med Biol 2000;27(7):643–6.

15. Delbeke D, Meyerowitz C, Lapidus RL, et al. Optimal cutoff levels of F-18 fluorodeoxyglucose uptake in the differentiation of low-grade from high-grade brain tumors with PET. Radiology 1995;195(1):47–52.

16. Padma MV, Said S, Jacobs M, et al. Prediction of pathology and survival by FDG PET in gliomas. J Neurooncol 2003;64(3):227–37.

17. Hustinx R, Pourdehnad M, Kaschten B, et al. PET imaging for differentiating recurrent brain tumor from radiation necrosis. Radiol Clin North Am 2005;43(1):35–47.

18. Langleben DD, Segall GM. PET in differentiation of recurrent brain tumor from radiation injury. J Nucl Med 2000;41(11):1861–7.

19. Arnold SM, Patchell RA. Diagnosis and management of brain metastases. Hematol Oncol Clin North Am 2001;15(6):1085–107, vii.

20. Janus TJ, Kim EE, Tilbury R, et al. Use of [18F]fluorodeoxyglucose positron emission tomography in patients with primary malignant brain tumors. Ann Neurol 1993;33(5):540–8.

21. Ricci PE, Karis JP, Heiserman JE, et al. Differentiating recurrent tumor from radiation necrosis: time for re-evaluation of positron emission tomography? AJNR Am J Neuroradiol 1998;19(3):407–13.

22. Valk PE, Budinger TF, Levin VA, et al. PET of malignant cerebral tumors after interstitial brachytherapy. Demonstration of metabolic activity and correlation with clinical outcome. J Neurosurg 1988;69(6):830–8.

23. Kim EE, Chung SK, Haynie TP, et al. Differentiation of residual or recurrent tumors from post-treatment changes with F-18 FDG PET. Radiographics 1992; 12(2):269–79.

24. Kahn D, Follett A, Bushnell DL, et al. Diagnosis of recurrent brain tumor: value of 201Tl SPECT vs 18F-fluorodeoxyglucose PET. AJR Am J Roentgenol 1994;163(6):1459–65.

25. Chao ST, Suh JH, Raja S, et al. The sensitivity and specificity of FDG PET in distinguishing recurrent brain tumor from radionecrosis in patients treated with stereotactic radiosurgery. Int J Cancer 2001; 96(3):191–7.

26. Spence AM, Muzi M, Mankoff DA, et al. 18F-FDG PET of gliomas at delayed intervals: improved distinction between tumor and normal gray matter. J Nucl Med 2004;45(10):1653–9.

27. Horky LL, Hsiao ME, Weiss ES, et al. Dual phase FDG-PET imaging of brain metastases provides superior assessment of recurrence versus post-treatment necrosis. J Neurooncol 2010. [Epub ahead of print].

28. Chen W, Clough esy T, Kamdar N, et al. Imaging proliferation in brain tumors with 18F-FLT PET: comparison with 18F-FDG. J Nucl Med 2005; 46(6):945–52.

29. Chen W, Delaloye S, Silverman DH, et al. Predicting treatment response of malignant gliomas to bevacizumab and irinotecan by imaging proliferation with [18F] fluorothymidine positron emission tomography: a pilot study. J Clin Oncol 2007;25(30): 4714–21.

30. Muzi M, Spence AM, O'Sullivan F, et al. Kinetic analysis of 3'-deoxy-3'-18F-fluorothymidine in patients with gliomas. J Nucl Med 2006;47(10):1612–21.

31. Herholz K, Holzer T, Bauer B, et al. 11C-methionine PET for differential diagnosis of low-grade gliomas. Neurology 1998;50(5):1316–22.

32. Floeth FW, Pauleit D, Sabel M, et al. Prognostic value of O-(2-18F-fluoroethyl)-L-tyrosine PET and MRI in low-grade glioma. J Nucl Med 2007;48(4): 519–27.

33. Pirotte B, Goldman S, Massager N, et al. Comparison of 18F-FDG and 11C-methionine for PET-guided stereotactic brain biopsy of gliomas. J Nucl Med 2004;45(8):1293–8.

34. Levivier M, Wikler D Jr, Massager N, et al. The integration of metabolic imaging in stereotactic procedures including radiosurgery: a review. J Neurosurg 2002; 97(Suppl 5):542–50.

35. Levivier M, Massager N, Wikler D, et al. Use of stereotactic PET images in dosimetry planning of

radiosurgery for brain tumors: clinical experience and proposed classification. J Nucl Med 2004; 45(7):1146–54.

36. Langen KJ, Jarosch M, Muhlensiepen H, et al. Comparison of fluorotyrosines and methionine uptake in F98 rat gliomas. Nucl Med Biol 2003; 30(5):501–8.

37. Weber WA, Wester HJ, Grosu AL, et al. O-(2-[18F] fluoroethyl)-L-tyrosine and L-[methyl-11C]methionine uptake in brain tumours: initial results of a comparative study. Eur J Nucl Med 2000;27(5): 542–9.

38. Grosu AL, Weber WA. PET for radiation treatment planning of brain tumours. Radiother Oncol 2010; 96(3):325–7.

39. Garnett ES, Firnau G, Nahmias C. Dopamine visualized in the basal ganglia of living man. Nature 1983;305(5930):137–8.

40. Chen W, Silverman DH, Delaloye S, et al. 18F-FDOPA PET imaging of brain tumors: comparison study with 18F-FDG PET and evaluation of diagnostic accuracy. J Nucl Med 2006;47(6):904–11.

41. Rachinger W, Goetz C, Popperl G, et al. Positron emission tomography with O-(2-[18F]fluoroethyl)-l-tyrosine versus magnetic resonance imaging in the diagnosis of recurrent gliomas. Neurosurgery 2005;57(3):505–11 [discussion: 505–11].

42. Popperl G, Kreth FW, Mehrkens JH, et al. FET PET for the evaluation of untreated gliomas: correlation of FET uptake and uptake kinetics with tumour grading. Eur J Nucl Med Mol Imaging 2007; 34(12):1933–42.

43. Schiepers C, Chen W, Cloughesy T, et al. 18F-FDOPA kinetics in brain tumors. J Nucl Med 2007; 48(10):1651–61.

44. Bruehlmeier M, Roelcke U, Schubiger PA, et al. Assessment of hypoxia and perfusion in human brain tumors using PET with 18F-fluoromisonidazole and 15O-H2O. J Nucl Med 2004;45(11): 1851–9.

45. Valk PE, Mathis CA, Prados MD, et al. Hypoxia in human gliomas: demonstration by PET with fluorine-18-fluoromisonidazole. J Nucl Med 1992; 33(12):2133–7.

46. Gray LH, Conger AD, Ebert M, et al. The concentration of oxygen dissolved in tissues at the time of irradiation as a factor in radiotherapy. Br J Radiol 1953;26(312):638–48.

47. Di Chiro G, Hatazawa J, Katz DA, et al. Glucose utilization by intracranial meningiomas as an index of tumor aggressivity and probability of recurrence: a PET study. Radiology 1987;164(2):521–6.

48. Ancri D, Basset JY, Lonchampt MF, et al. Diagnosis of cerebral lesions by thallium 201. Radiology 1978;128(2):417–22.

49. Mountz JM, Raymond PA, McKeever PE, et al. Specific localization of thallium 201 in human

high-grade astrocytoma by microautoradiography. Cancer Res 1989;49(14):4053–6.

50. Kaplan WD, Takvorian T, Morris JH, et al. Thallium-201 brain tumor imaging: a comparative study with pathologic correlation. J Nucl Med 1987; 28(1):47–52.

51. Maria BL, Drane WB, Quisling RJ, et al. Correlation between gadolinium-diethylenetriaminepentaacetic acid contrast enhancement and thallium-201 chloride uptake in pediatric brainstem glioma. J Child Neurol 1997;12(6):341–8.

52. Black KL, Hawkins RA, Kim KT, et al. Use of thallium-201 SPECT to quantitate malignancy grade of gliomas. J Neurosurg 1989;71(3):342–6.

53. Rubinstein R, Karger H, Pietrzyk U, et al. Use of 201Thallium brain SPECT, image registration, and semi-quantitative analysis in the follow-up of brain tumors. Eur J Radiol 1996;21(3):188–95.

54. Dierckx RA, Martin JJ, Dobbeleir A, et al. Sensitivity and specificity of thallium-201 single-photon emission tomography in the functional detection and differential diagnosis of brain tumours. Eur J Nucl Med 1994;21(7):621–33.

55. Kline JL, Noto RB, Glantz M. Single-photon emission CT in the evaluation of recurrent brain tumor in patients treated with gamma knife radiosurgery or conventional radiation therapy. AJNR Am J Neuroradiol 1996;17(9):1681–6.

56. Lorberboym M, Mandell LR, Mosesson RE, et alThe role of thallium-201 uptake and retention in intracranial tumors after radiotherapy. J Nucl Med 1997;38(2):223–6.

57. Tomura N, Hirano H, Kato H, et al. Unexpected accumulation of thallium-201 in cerebral infarction. J Comput Assist Tomogr 1998;22(1):126–9.

58. Soler C, Beauchesne P, Maatougui K, et al. Technetium-99 m sestamibi brain single-photon emission tomography for detection of recurrent gliomas after radiation therapy. Eur J Nucl Med 1998;25(12): 1649–57.

59. Maffioli L, Gasparini M, Chiti A, et al. Clinical role of technetium-99 m sestamibi single-photon emission tomography in evaluating pretreated patients with brain tumours. Eur J Nucl Med 1996;23(3): 308–11.

60. Stefanescu C, Meignan M, Rusu V. [The value of scintigraphic imaging with 99mTc-MIBI for the diagnosis of gliomas]. Rev Med Chir Soc Med Nat Iasi 1995;99(3–4):99–107 [in French].

61. O'Tuama LA, Treves ST, Larar JN, et al. Thallium-201 versus technetium-99 m-MIBI SPECT in evaluation of childhood brain tumors: a within-subject comparison. J Nucl Med 1993;34(7):1045–51.

62. Jeong HJ, Chung JK, Kim YK, et al. Usefulness of whole-body (18)F-FDG PET in patients with suspected metastatic brain tumors. J Nucl Med 2002;43(11):1432–7.

63. National Institutes of Health Consensus Conference. Surgery for epilepsy. JAMA 1990;264(6):729–33.

64. Proposal for revised clinical and electroencephalographic classification of epileptic seizures. From the Commission on Classification and Terminology of the International League Against Epilepsy. Epilepsia 1981;22(4):489–501.

65. Goffin K. Neuronuclear assessment of patients with epilepsy. Semin Nucl Med 2008;38(4):227–39.

66. Wiebe S, Blume WT, Girvin JP, et al. A randomized, controlled trial of surgery for temporal-lobe epilepsy. N Engl J Med 2001;345(5):311–8.

67. Elsharkawy AE, Pannek H, Schulz R, et al. Outcome of extratemporal epilepsy surgery experience of a single center. Neurosurgery 2008;63(3):516–25 [discussion 525–6].

68. Berkovic SF, McIntosh AM, Kalnins RM, et al. Preoperative MRI predicts outcome of temporal lobectomy: an actuarial analysis. Neurology 1995;45(7):1358–63.

69. Bien CG, Szinay M, Wagner J, et al. Characteristics and surgical outcomes of patients with refractory magnetic resonance imaging-negative epilepsies. Arch Neurol 2009;66(12):1491–9.

70. Knowlton RC. The role of FDG-PET, ictal SPECT, and MEG in the epilepsy surgery evaluation. Epilepsy Behav 2006;8(1):91–101.

71. Treves ST. Pediatric nuclear medicine/PET. 3rd edition. New York: Springer; 2007. xvii, p. 538.

72. Lee SK, Lee SY, Yun CH, et al. Ictal SPECT in neocortical epilepsies: clinical usefulness and factors affecting the pattern of hyperperfusion. Neuroradiology 2006;48(9):678–84.

73. Devous MD Sr, Thisted RA, Morgan GF, et al. SPECT brain imaging in epilepsy: a meta-analysis. J Nucl Med 1998;39(2):285–93.

74. Newton MR, Berkovic SF, Austin MC, et al. Ictal postictal and interictal single-photon emission tomography in the lateralization of temporal lobe epilepsy. Eur J Nucl Med 1994;21(10):1067–71.

75. Bartolini A. Regional arm-brain mean transit time in the diagnostic evaluation of patients with cerebral vascular disease. Stroke 1981;12(2):241–5.

76. Locharernkul C. Factors influencing successful ictal SPECT injections during epilepsy presurgical evaluation. Neurol Asia 2004;9(Suppl 1):111.

77. O'Brien TJ, So EL, Mullan BP, et al. Subtraction ictal SPECT co-registered to MRI improves clinical usefulness of SPECT in localizing the surgical seizure focus. Neurology 1998;50(2):445–54.

78. Shoeb A, Edwards H, Connolly J, et al. Patient-specific seizure onset detection. Conf Proc IEEE Eng Med Biol Soc 2004;1:419–22.

79. Henry TR, Engel J Jr, Mazziotta JC. Clinical evaluation of interictal fluorine-18-fluorodeoxyglucose PET in partial epilepsy. J Nucl Med 1993;34(11):1892–8.

80. Spencer SS. The relative contributions of MRI, SPECT, and PET imaging in epilepsy. Epilepsia 1994;35(Suppl 6):S72–89.

81. Drzezga A, Arnold S, Minoshima S, et al. 18F-FDG PET studies in patients with extratemporal and temporal epilepsy: evaluation of an observer-independent analysis. J Nucl Med 1999;40(5):737–46.

82. Theodore WH, Sato S, Kufta C, et al. Temporal lobectomy for uncontrolled seizures: the role of positron emission tomography. Ann Neurol 1992;32(6):789–94.

83. Lin TW, de Aburto MA, Dahlbom M, et al. Predicting seizure-free status for temporal lobe epilepsy patients undergoing surgery: prognostic value of quantifying maximal metabolic asymmetry extending over a specified proportion of the temporal lobe. J Nucl Med 2007;48(5):776–82.

84. Engel J, Pedley TA. Epilepsy the comprehensive CD-ROM. Philadelphia: Lippincott Williams & Wilkins; 1999. p. 1.

85. Hajek M, Antonini A, Leenders KL, et al. Mesiobasal versus lateral temporal lobe epilepsy: metabolic differences in the temporal lobe shown by interictal 18F-FDG positron emission tomography. Neurology 1993;43(1):79–86.

86. Ell PJ, Gambhir SS. Nuclear medicine in clinical diagnosis and treatment. New York. 3rd edition. Edinburgh: Churchill Livingstone; 2004. 2 v (xxiv, 1924. p. 150).

87. Carne RP, Cook MJ, MacGregor LR, et al. "Magnetic resonance imaging negative positron emission tomography positive" temporal lobe epilepsy: FDG-PET pattern differs from mesial temporal lobe epilepsy. Mol Imaging Biol 2007;9(1):32–42.

88. Theodore WH, Holmes MD, Dorwart RH, et al. Complex partial seizures: cerebral structure and cerebral function. Epilepsia 1986;27(5):576–82.

89. la Fougere C, Rominger A, Forster S, et al. PET and SPECT in epilepsy: a critical review. Epilepsy Behav 2009;15(1):50–5.

90. Lee N, Radtke RA, Gray L, et al. Neuronal migration disorders: positron emission tomography correlations. Ann Neurol 1994;35(3):290–7.

91. Cohen-Gadol AA, Ozduman K, Bronen RA, et al. Long-term outcome after epilepsy surgery for focal cortical dysplasia. J Neurosurg 2004;101(1):55–65.

92. Kim SK, Na DG, Byun HS, et al. Focal cortical dysplasia: comparison of MRI and FDG-PET. J Comput Assist Tomogr 2000;24(2):296–302.

93. Szelies B, Herholz K, Heiss WD, et al. Hypometabolic cortical lesions in tuberous sclerosis with epilepsy: demonstration by positron emission tomography. J Comput Assist Tomogr 1983;7(6):946–53.

94. Savic I, Svanborg E, Thorell JO. Cortical benzodiazepine receptor changes are related to frequency of partial seizures: a positron emission tomography study. Epilepsia 1996;37(3):236–44.

95. Savic I, Persson A, Roland P, et al. In-vivo demonstration of reduced benzodiazepine receptor binding in human epileptic foci. Lancet 1988;2(8616):863–6.

96. Henry TR, Frey KA, Sackellares JC, et al. In vivo cerebral metabolism and central benzodiazepine-receptor binding in temporal lobe epilepsy. Neurology 1993;43(10):1998–2006.

97. Szelies B, Weber-Luxenburger G, Mielke R, et al. Interictal hippocampal benzodiazepine receptors in temporal lobe epilepsy: comparison with coregistered hippocampal metabolism and volumetry. Eur J Neurol 2000;7(4):393–400.

98. Debets RM, Sadzot B, van Isselt JW, et al. Is 11C-flumazenil PET superior to 18FDG PET and 123I-iomazenil SPECT in presurgical evaluation of temporal lobe epilepsy? J Neurol Neurosurg Psychiatry 1997;62(2):141–50.

99. Hammers A, Koepp MJ, Hurlemann R, et al. Abnormalities of grey and white matter [11C]flumazenil binding in temporal lobe epilepsy with normal MRI. Brain 2002;125(Pt 10):2257–71.

100. Savic I, Thorell JO, Roland P. [11C]flumazenil positron emission tomography visualizes frontal epileptogenic regions. Epilepsia 1995;36(12):1225–32.

101. Hammers A, Koepp MJ, Brooks DJ, et al. Periventricular white matter flumazenil binding and postoperative outcome in hippocampal sclerosis. Epilepsia 2005;46(6):944–8.

102. Muzik O, da Silva EA, Juhasz C, et al. Intracranial EEG versus flumazenil and glucose PET in children with extratemporal lobe epilepsy. Neurology 2000; 54(1):171–9.

103. Ryvlin P, Bouvard S, Le Bars D, et al. Transient and falsely lateralizing flumazenil-PET asymmetries in temporal lobe epilepsy. Neurology 1999;53(8): 1882–5.

104. Bouvard S, Costes N, Bonnefoi F, et al. Seizure-related short-term plasticity of benzodiazepine receptors in partial epilepsy: a [11C]flumazenil-PET study. Brain 2005;128(Pt 6):1330–43.

105. Chugani DC, Chugani HT, Muzik O, et al. Imaging epileptogenic tubers in children with tuberous sclerosis complex using alpha-[11C]methyl-L-tryptophan positron emission tomography. Ann Neurol 1998;44(6):858–66.

106. Louw D, Sutherland GR, Glavin GB, et al. A study of monoamine metabolism in human epilepsy. Can J Neurol Sci 1989;16(4):394–7.

107. Pintor M, Mefford IN, Hutter I, et al. Levels of biogenic amines, their metabolites, and tyrosine hydroxylase activity in the human epileptic temporal cortex. Synapse 1990;5(2):152–6.

108. Trottier S, Evrard B, Vignal JP, et al. The serotonergic innervation of the cerebral cortex in man and its changes in focal cortical dysplasia. Epilepsy Res 1996;25(2):79–106.

109. Missala K, Sourkes TL. Functional cerebral activity of an analogue of serotonin formed in situ. Neurochem Int 1988;12(2):209–14.

110. Kagawa K, Chugani DC, Asano E, et al. Epilepsy surgery outcome in children with tuberous sclerosis complex evaluated with alpha-[11C]methyl-L-tryptophan positron emission tomography (PET). J Child Neurol 2005;20(5):429–38.

An Introduction to Diffusion Tensor Image Analysis

Lauren J. O'Donnell, PhD[a,b,*], Carl-Fredrik Westin, PhD[a]

KEYWORDS

- Diffusion Tensor MRI • DTI • Brain imaging
- Tractography • Review

Diffusion tensor magnetic resonance imaging (DTI) is a relatively new technology that is popular for imaging the white matter of the brain. This article provides a basic and broad overview of DTI to enable the reader to develop an intuitive understanding of these types of data, and an awareness of their strengths and weaknesses. The authors have tried to include equations for completeness, but these are not necessary for understanding the content. Wherever possible, more in-depth technical articles or books are suggested for further reading. The authors especially recommend the new diffusion MRI textbook,[1] the introductory paper on fiber tracts and tumors,[2] the white matter atlas book,[3] and the review of potential pitfalls in DTI analysis.[4] The remainder of this article addresses basic questions about DTI (the what, why, and how of DTI), followed by a discussion of issues in interpretation of DTI, and finally an overview of more advanced diffusion imaging methods and future directions.

WHY DTI? A BRIEF HISTORY OF DTI AND ITS IMPACT ON CLINICAL RESEARCH

The diffusion tensor was originally proposed for use in MRI by Peter Basser in 1994.[5,6] Before DTI, diffusion MRI[7,8] had developed from research in diffusion nuclear magnetic resonance.[9] Before the diffusion tensor model was introduced, the orientation of the axons in a tissue sample had to be known to measure anisotropic diffusion, and therefore only fixed samples could be scanned, such as the axon of the giant squid.[10] The introduction of the diffusion tensor model allowed, for the first time, a rotationally invariant description of the shape of water diffusion. The invariance to rotation was crucial because it enabled application of the DTI method to the complex anatomy of the fiber tracts in the human brain.[11] However, the diffusion tensor is not able to fully describe crossing of the fiber tracts.[12,13]

The popularity of DTI has been enormous. It has been applied to a tremendous variety of neuroscientific studies,[14–16] including schizophrenia,[17] traumatic brain injury,[18] multiple sclerosis,[19,20] autism,[21] and aging.[22] Anatomic investigations have been undertaken regarding the structure of the language network,[23,24] the asymmetry of the white matter in twins and siblings,[25] and the location, asymmetry, and variability of the fiber tracts.[26] Recent investigations have attempted to model the human "connectome" by analyzing structural versus functional brain connectivity as measured with DTI and functional MRI.[27,28] DTI has also been applied for neurosurgical planning and navigation.[29–32] A large prospective study showed that addition of preoperative DTI to

The authors acknowledge the following support: R25CA089017 (LJO), NIH R01MH074794, and NIH P41RR013218 (CFW). Thanks to Gordon Kindlmann for the eigenvalue-based formula for mode.

[a] Laboratory of Mathematics in Imaging (LMI), Department of Radiology, Brigham and Women's Hospital, Harvard Medical School, 75 Francis Street, Boston, MA 02115, USA

[b] Golby Neurosurgical Brain Mapping Laboratory, Department of Neurosurgery, Brigham and Women's Hospital, Harvard Medical School, 75 Francis Street, Boston, MA 02115, USA

* Corresponding author. Laboratory of Mathematics in Imaging (LMI), Department of Radiology, Brigham and Women's Hospital, Harvard Medical School, 75 Francis Street, Boston, MA 02115.

E-mail address: odonnell@bwh.harvard.edu

neuronavigation increased tumor resection and survival and decreased neurologic morbidity.[33]

WHAT IS DTI?

DTI is a sensitive probe of cellular structure that measures the diffusion of water molecules. The measured quantity is the diffusivity or diffusion coefficient, a proportionality constant that relates diffusive flux to a concentration gradient[8] and has units of $\frac{mm^2}{s}$. Unlike the diffusion in a glass of pure water, which would be the same in all directions (isotropic), the diffusion measured in tissue varies with direction (is anisotropic). The measured macroscopic diffusion anisotropy is the result of microscopic tissue heterogeneity.[6] In the white matter of the brain, diffusion anisotropy is primarily caused by cellular membranes, with some contribution from myelination and the packing of the axons.[11,34,35] Anisotropic diffusion can indicate the underlying tissue orientation (**Fig. 1**).

The diffusion tensor describes the diffusion of water molecules using a Gaussian model. Technically, it is proportional to the covariance matrix of a three-dimensional Gaussian distribution that models the displacements of the molecules. The tensor is a 3 × 3 symmetric, positive-definite matrix, and these matrix properties mean that it has three orthogonal (mutually perpendicular) eigenvectors and three positive eigenvalues. The major eigenvector of the diffusion tensor points in the principal diffusion direction (the direction of the fastest diffusion). In anisotropic fibrous tissues, the major eigenvector also defines the fiber tract axis of the tissue,[6] and thus the three orthogonal eigenvectors can be considered a local fiber coordinate system. (This interpretation is only strictly true in regions where fiber tracts do not cross, fan, or branch.) The three positive eigenvalues of the tensor $(\lambda_1, \lambda_2, \lambda_3)$ give the diffusivity in the direction of each eigenvector. Together, the eigenvectors and eigenvalues define an ellipsoid that represents an isosurface of (Gaussian) diffusion probability: the axes of the ellipsoid are aligned with the eigenvectors and their lengths are $\sqrt{2\tau\lambda_i}$.[6] **Fig. 2** shows three diffusion tensors chosen from different regions of the human brain to illustrate possible shapes of the ellipsoid.

HOW IS DTI MEASURED?

To measure diffusion using MRI, magnetic field gradients are used to create an image that is sensitized to diffusion in a particular direction. Through repeating this process of diffusion weighting in multiple directions, a three-dimensional diffusion model (the tensor) can be estimated. In simplified terms, diffusion imaging introduces extra gradient pulses whose effect "cancels out" for stationary water molecules, and causes a random phase shift for molecules that diffuse. Because of their random phase, signal from diffusing molecules is lost. This loss of signal creates darker voxels (volumetric pixels), meaning that white matter fiber tracts parallel to the gradient direction will appear dark in the diffusion-weighted image for that direction (**Fig. 3**).

Next, the decreased signal (S_k) is compared with the original signal (S_0) to calculate the diffusion tensor (D) by solving the Stejskal-Tanner Equation (1).[36] This equation describes how the signal intensity at each voxel decreases in the presence of Gaussian diffusion:

$$S_k = S_0 e^{-b\hat{g}_k^T D \hat{g}_k} \tag{1}$$

In this equation, S_0 is the original image intensity at the voxel (measured with no diffusion-sensitizing gradient) and S_k is the intensity measured after the application of the kth diffusion-sensitizing gradient in the (unit) direction $\hat{g}_k$. The product $\hat{g}_k^T D \hat{g}_k$ represents the diffusion coefficient (diffusivity) in direction $\hat{g}_k$. Because the entire set of diffusion-weighted images is used (giving many

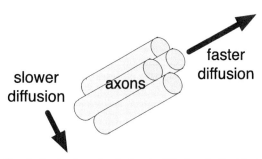

Fig. 1. Illustration of anisotropic diffusion, in the ideal case of a coherently oriented tissue. This example compares the diffusion measured parallel and perpendicular to the axons in a white matter fiber tract.

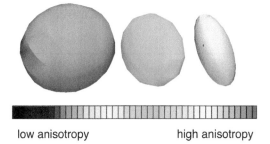

low anisotropy   high anisotropy

Fig. 2. Three example diffusion tensors, selected from a diffusion tensor magnetic resonance imaging scan of the human brain to illustrate differences in tensor anisotropy and orientation.

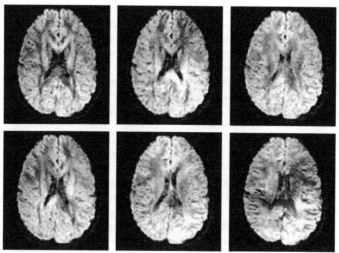

Fig. 3. Six diffusion-weighted images (the minimum number required for tensor calculation). In diffusion MRI, magnetic field gradients are used to sensitize the image to diffusion in a particular direction. The direction is different for each image, resulting in a different pattern of signal loss (*dark areas*) from anisotropic diffusion.

values for S_k and $\hat{g}_k$), this is actually a system of equations that is solved for D, the diffusion tensor. To calculate the six independent numbers in the 3×3 symmetric matrix D, at least seven images are needed: six diffusion-weighted images from six gradient directions (giving six values for S_k) plus one baseline image (giving S_0). However, in clinical research today, a higher number of images are almost always used. The above system of equations can be solved via the least squares method at each voxel.

Equation (1) also contains b, LeBihan's[9] factor describing the pulse sequence, gradient strength, and physical constants. The b-factor is near $0 \frac{s}{mm^2}$ for the image S_0, which is T2-weighted, and the b-factor is near $1000 \frac{s}{mm^2}$ for the diffusion-weighted images S_k in DTI. For rectangular gradient pulses, the b-factor is defined by $b = \gamma^2 \delta^2 (\Delta - \frac{\delta}{3})|g|^2$, where γ is the proton gyromagnetic ratio (42 MHz/Tesla), $|g|$ is the strength of the diffusion sensitizing gradient pulses, δ is the duration of the diffusion gradient pulses, and

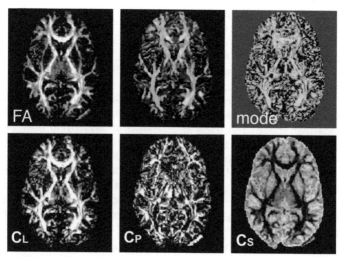

Fig. 4. Scalar measures derived from DTI include FA, mode, C_L, C_P, and C_S. Also shown (*top row, middle*) is a mapping of the major eigenvector orientation to colors. See the text for more information about the definition of these measures.

Δ is the time between diffusion gradient RF pulses.[37]

Information on the MR physics of DTI[8] and more information on the tensor calculation process[5,37] are provided elsewhere. Goodlett and colleagues[38] provide a comparison of tensor calculation methods (including least squares and weighted least squares) in the presence of noise.

HOW IS DTI DISPLAYED?

DTI is usually displayed through condensing the information contained in the tensor (**Fig. 4**) into either one number (a scalar), or four (to give an RGB color and a brightness value). The diffusion tensor can also be viewed using glyphs, which are small three-dimensional representations of the major eigenvector or whole tensor. Finally, DTI is often viewed through estimating the course of white matter tracts through the brain using a process called *tractography*.

Scalars Derived from DTI

This section describes commonly used scalar quantities, which can be divided into two categories: diffusion magnitude measures and anisotropy measures. The eigenvalues of the symmetric, positive-definite diffusion tensor D are referred to using $\lambda_1 \geq \lambda_2 \geq \lambda_3 \geq 0$. Pierpaoli and colleagues[11] originally measured and compared several scalar measures, and the eigenvalues, in different regions of the human brain.

Measures of diffusion magnitude

The simplest and possibly most useful scalar is the average of the tensor's eigenvalues. This average may be referred to as the *mean diffusivity* (MD)[39]; the bulk mean diffusivity ($\langle D \rangle$)[40]; or the apparent diffusion coefficient (ADC) map. In clinical imaging, ADC maps may be measured using fewer diffusion gradients than needed for the tensor. A similar quantity to the MD is the sum of the eigenvalues, called the *trace* of the tensor.

The trace and MD relate to the total amount of diffusion in a voxel, which is related to the amount of water in the extracellular space. The trace is clinically useful in early stroke detection because it is sensitive to the initial cellular swelling (cytotoxic edema) that restricts diffusion.[41] In the normal human brain, the trace is high in cerebrospinal fluid, around $9.6 \times 10^{-3}\frac{mm^2}{s}$, and relatively constant in normal brain parenchyma (white and gray matter), between $1.95 \times 10^{-3}\frac{mm^2}{s}$ and $2.2 \times 10^{-3}\frac{mm^2}{s}$.[11] For comparison, the self-diffusion coefficient of water (the diffusivity measured in pure water without any tissue) at a body temperature of 37°C is $3 \times 10^{-3}\frac{mm^2}{s}$,[42]

which would give a trace of $9 \times 10^{-3}\frac{mm^2}{s}$. The MD and trace measured in ventricles or in edema can be higher than in water because of fluid flow or enhanced perfusion, respectively.[7]

Measures of diffusion anisotropy

Tensor anisotropy measures are ratios of the eigenvalues that are used to quantify the shape of the diffusion. These measures are useful for describing the amount of tissue organization and for locating voxels likely to contain a single white matter tract (without crossing or fanning). The following measures are normalized and all range from 0 to 1, except for the mode, which ranges from –1 to +1.

The fractional anisotropy (FA)[43] is the most widely used anisotropy measure. Its name comes from the fact that it measures the fraction of the diffusion that is anisotropic. This measure can be considered the difference of the tensor ellipsoid's shape from that of a perfect sphere. FA is basically a normalized variance of the eigenvalues:

$$FA = \frac{1}{\sqrt{2}} \frac{\sqrt{(\lambda_1 - \hat{\lambda})^2 + (\lambda_2 - \hat{\lambda})^2 + (\lambda_1 - \hat{\lambda})^2}}{\sqrt{\lambda_1^2 + \lambda_2^2 + \lambda_3^2}} \quad (2)$$

where $\hat{\lambda}$ is the mean diffusivity. FA is often considered a measure of white matter integrity, although changes in FA may be caused by many factors.

Three intuitive measures are C_L, C_P, and C_S, which are the linear, planar, and spherical shape measures.[37,44] They describe whether the shape of diffusion is similar to a cigar (linear), pancake (planar), or sphere (spherical).

$$C_L = \frac{\lambda_1 - \lambda_2}{\lambda_1} \quad (3)$$

$$C_P = \frac{\lambda_2 - \lambda_3}{\lambda_1} \quad (4)$$

$$C_S = \frac{\lambda_3}{\lambda_1} \quad (5)$$

In voxels with high planar or spherical measure, the principal eigenvector will not always match an underlying fiber tract direction (where tracts cross the eigenvector may point to neither one). However, if the largest eigenvalue is much larger than the other two eigenvalues, the linear measure will be large, indicating the presence of a single fiber tract. These measures can be normalized by λ_1, by the trace, or by $\sqrt{\lambda_1^2 + \lambda_2^2 + \lambda_3^2}$.

Although FA measures how far the tensor is from a sphere, another complementary measure discriminates between linear and planar anisotropy. This information is given by the mode, a quantity that is mathematically orthogonal to the FA measure and relates to the skewness of the eigenvalues.[45]

mode

$$= \frac{(-\lambda_1 - \lambda_2 + 2\lambda_3)(2\lambda_1 - \lambda_2 - \lambda_3)(-\lambda_1 + 2\lambda_2 - \lambda_3)}{2(\lambda_1^2 + \lambda_2^2 + \lambda_3^2 - \lambda_1\lambda_2 - \lambda_1\lambda_3 - \lambda_2\lambda_3)^{3/2}} \quad (6)$$

The parallel diffusivity measure, also called the *axial diffusivity*, is equal to the largest eigenvalue. The perpendicular diffusivity measure, also called the *radial diffusivity*, is equal to the average of the two smaller eigenvalues. These measures are interpreted as diffusivity parallel and perpendicular to a white matter fiber tract, and therefore make the most sense in regions of coherently oriented axons with no fiber crossings.

Often in scientific studies, the reported measures from the diffusion tensor are not independent. However, complete sets of orthogonal (mathematically independent) scalars have been defined.[45,46]

Colors Derived from DTI

Another type of image can represent the major eigenvector field using a mapping to colors (**Fig. 5**). The color scheme most commonly used to represent the orientation of the major eigenvector works as follows: blue is superior–inferior, red is left–right, and green is anterior–posterior.[47] To enhance visualization of the white matter and suppress information outside of it, the brightness of the color is usually controlled by tensor anisotropy (FA).

Glyphs Derived from DTI

Small three-dimensional objects called *glyphs* can be used to display information from each tensor eigensystem. Example glyphs include "sticks" representing the orientation of the major eigenvector, ellipsoids related to the diffusion isoprobability surfaces,[6] and superquadric tensor glyphs.[48]

Tractography

The word *tractography* refers to any method for estimating the trajectories of the fiber tracts in the white matter. Ciccarelli and colleagues[15] provide a clinical and technical overview of tractography in neurologic disorders. Tractography techniques, including explanations of common tractography artifacts and a comparison of methods, are reviewed elsewhere.[49,50] Many methods have been proposed for tractography, and the results will vary enormously depending on the chosen method.

The most common approach is streamline tractography (**Fig. 6**),[51–54] which is closely related to an earlier method for visualization of tensor fields, known as *hyperstreamlines*.[55] This method produces as output discrete curves or trajectories that are also referred to by terms such as *tracts*, *fibers*, and *traces*. The streamline tract-tracing approach works by successively stepping in the direction of the principal eigenvector (the direction of fastest diffusion). The eigenvectors are thus tangent to the trajectory that is produced. A fixed step size of 1 mm or less (smaller than a voxel) is generally used for DTI data.

Several computational methods can be used to perform basic streamline tractography, including Euler's method (following the eigenvector or tangent for a fixed step size), second-order Runge-Kutta (also known as the *midpoint method*, in which the tangent is followed for half a step, then a new tangent is calculated at the midpoint of the interval and used to take the full step), and

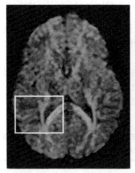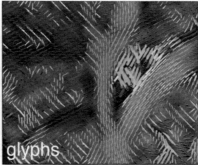

Fig. 5. An example using glyphs and colors for diffusion tensor magnetic resonance imaging visualization. On the left an axial image plane, showing the average diffusion-weighted image with semitransparent color overlay indicating the major eigenvector orientation, and a white square indicating the zoomed-in area (*right image*). In both images, the color red indicates right–left orientation, blue is superior–inferior, and green is anterior–posterior. The right image contains glyphs representing major eigenvector orientations (and scaled by the largest eigenvalue) in the region of the corpus callosum (*yellow* and *red*) and right lateral ventricle. The cingulum can be seen in blue, and the posterior limb of the internal capsule in green.

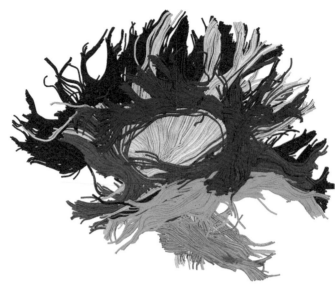

Fig. 6. Whole-brain streamline DTI tractography. Colors were assigned automatically according to an atlas-based tractography segmentation method. (*Data from* O'Donnell LJ, Westin CF. Automatic tractography segmentation using a high-dimensional white matter atlas. IEEE Trans Med Imaging 2007;26:1562–75.)

fourth-order Runge-Kutta (in which the weighted average of four estimated tangents to the curve is used when taking each step).[56] Basser and colleagues[51] and Conturo and colleagues[52] explored application of the Euler and Runge-Kutta methods to white matter tractography. Another popular method is called fiber assessment by continuous tracking.[53] Some related methods attempt to introduce inertia when tracking through regions of planar anisotropy (likely fiber crossings). These methods modulate the incoming tangent direction by the tensor instead of directly using the major eigenvector of the tensor.[37,54,57,58]

Processing DTI data to display fiber tracts of interest requires expert knowledge or an automatic algorithm. After performing streamline tractography, the fiber trajectories of interest can be interactively selected through virtual dissection, in which inclusion/exclusion regions are defined and used to select trajectories.[3,59,60] Automated methods for atlas-based tractography segmentation, which use prior knowledge to select trajectories, have also been developed.[61–67]

In addition to streamline tractography, many other methods are available,[49,50] including probabilistic tractography that outputs connection strengths or probabilities,[68,69] optimization methods that use graph theory or physical models,[70,71] region-growing and wavefront evolution methods,[72] tractography using advanced models for fiber crossings,[73–76] and tractography meta-analysis methods that perform clustering or fit more sophisticated tract models.[61,77–79]

Tractography methods can produce false-positive and -negative results (discussed in next section); however, clinical validations of streamline tractography have shown accurate reconstructions (true-positive results). Tract end points, especially of the corticospinal or motor tract, have been compared with electrocortical stimulation during neurosurgery[80,81] with good correspondence. In a study of 238 neurosurgical patients with gliomas involving the motor tract who were randomized to study or control groups, DTI was shown to increase survival and reduce postoperative motor deficits.[33]

ISSUES IN INTERPRETING DTI DATA

This section presents two issues that are relevant to the clinical interpretation or meaning of the DTI data. Jones and Cercignani[4] have provided a more thorough discussion, including additional information about scanning and processing pitfalls.

Scale of Diffusion Measurements Versus Axons

The measured diffusion effects are averaged over a voxel (three-dimensional pixel), complicating the biophysical interpretation of the diffusion tensor.[40,82] For example, in scientific studies FA is often interpreted as "white matter integrity"; however, many factors (eg, cell death, change in myelination, increase in extracellular or

Table 1
The scale of diffusion tensor magnetic resonance imaging and the brain: neuron sizes and quantities, and water diffusion times and distances

Quantity	Measurement	References
Axon packing density (pyramidal tract)	60,000–70,000/mm^2	11
Axon packing density (corpus callosum)	338,000/mm^2	11
Axon diameter (pyramidal tract)	26 μm	11
Axon diameters in central nervous system	0.2–20 μm	83
Neuron cell body diameter	≥50 μm	83
Typical voxel size in diffusion MRI	2.5 × 2.5 × 2.5 mm	
Typical diffusion time in diffusion tensor magnetic resonance imaging	30–100 ms	34,42
Mean water diffusion distance	1–15 μm (in 50–100 ms)	42
Number of neurons in human brain	100 billion (10^{11})	83
Synaptic connections per axon	Up to 1,000	83

intracellular water) may cause changes in FA. Overall, this difficulty in interpreting DTI is because the scale at which diffusion is measured with DTI is very different from the size scale of individual axons. To illustrate the complexity of the human brain and the size/time scales of the diffusion imaging experiment, **Table 1** lists relevant quantities, such as the number of neurons in the brain (10^{11}) and the distance over which water diffuses during an imaging experiment (1–15 μm, a distance similar to the diameter of an axon).

False-Positive or -Negative Tractography

Because the tensor model is only able to represent one major fiber direction in a voxel, DTI tractography can be confounded by regions of crossing fibers, as shown schematically in **Fig. 7**. A significant fraction of white matter voxels in the brain contain multiple fiber bundles oriented in different directions, where the diffusion tensor model is not reliable.[73] Other factors can confound tractography. Partial volume effects, in which two types of

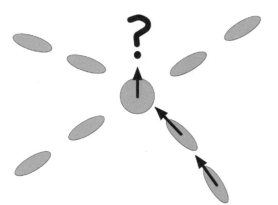

Fig. 7. The major eigenvector may not be aligned with a fiber tract in the case of crossing fibers.

tissue are present in a voxel, can produce a tensor that represents neither tissue well.[82] Also, crossing, "kissing," and "fanning" fiber tracts[12] are not represented well at the voxel level by the diffusion tensor. Finally, in standard streamline tractography, all decisions are made locally, and therefore errors can accumulate.

These issues may cause false-positive and -negative connections (**Figs. 8** and **9**). Common false-positive connections include trajectories from the corona radiata that cross the corpus callosum, and trajectories from the corona radiata that cross at the pons and ascend in the corona radiata of the other hemisphere. Common false-negatives with DTI tractography are the lateral lip/hand connections of the corticospinal tract[49,73] and lateral connections of the corpus callosum.[74]

The particular errors depend strongly on the tractography algorithm used, and on the type of diffusion data used (DTI vs higher-order models). However, no perfect method exists, and perfect tractography is unlikely to be possible because even perfect diffusion MRI data would not solve the peak selection problem. At each step, a direction must be chosen to follow for the next step, and with a more detailed model than the tensor, this requires some logical heuristic, such as choosing the closest direction to the current direction.

ADVANCES BEYOND THE DIFFUSION TENSOR

New diffusion models, scanning paradigms, and analysis methods are continually being developed for diffusion MRI.

High angular resolution diffusion imaging (HARDI) includes methods that acquire diffusion data using many more than 6 diffusion directions (eg, ≥ 32).[84] These methods generally use a higher

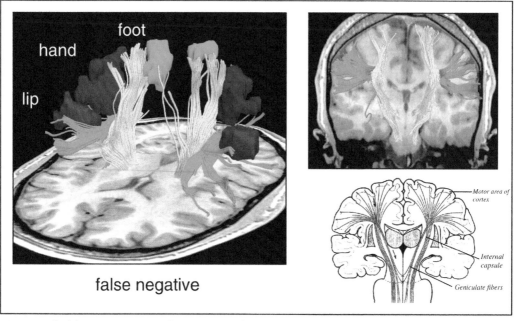

Fig. 8. Example false-negative streamline tractography error. The motor fibers (*yellow*) do not reach all functional magnetic resonance (fMRI) motor activations (*aqua*, *blue*, and *pink*) due to the presence of the superior longitudinal fasciculus (*green*) that runs perpendicular to the motor tract. In the right column are coronal views of the typical streamline tractography result (*top*) and expected anatomy (*bottom*).

b-value than the standard 1000 for DTI, or multiple b-values (multiple "shells" of data). Multi-shell acquisitions enable description of the full diffusion function using measures such as displacement, zero-probability, and kurtosis that are highly sensitive to myelin.[85,86] Another type of multiple b-value acquisition is diffusion spectrum imaging (DSI).[87] Diffusion models that go beyond DTI have been proposed to extract important biomarkers, such as compartmentalization[13,82,88,89] and axon diameter.[90] Higher-rank tensor models have been proposed to extend DTI.[91] Use of multiple pairs of diffusion gradients (double pulsed field gradient diffusion MRI) has been shown to increase sensitivity to small size scales.[92,93] Diffusion MRI data analysis has benefited from the introduction of novel tractography methods, many types of white matter atlas,[61–67] advanced tract-based quantification methods,[77–79,94] new visualization methods,[95] and new scalar measures.[45,96]

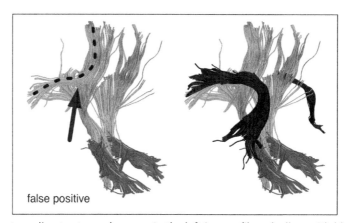

Fig. 9. False-positive streamline tractography error. In the left image, fibers (*yellow with black dotted line*) have traced parts of two anatomic structures by incorrectly crossing from one to the other (*at arrow*). In the right image, both structures (arcuate fasciculus in *magenta* and corona radiata in *yellow*) can be seen.

SUMMARY

DTI is an increasingly prevalent and popular imaging modality that has been applied to numerous scientific studies and clinical problems since its invention a little more than 15 years ago. The field is expected to benefit from many future advances in diffusion imaging and analysis.

REFERENCES

1. Johansen-Berg H, Behrens Timothy EJ, editors. Diffusion MRI: from quantitative measurement to in-vivo neuroanatomy. 1st edition. Elsevier Academic Press; May 4, 2009.
2. Jellison BJ, Field AS, Medow J, et al. Diffusion tensor imaging of cerebral white matter: a pictorial review of physics, fiber tract anatomy, and tumor imaging patterns. AJNR Am J Neuroradiol 2004;25:356–69.
3. Oishi K, Faria AV, Zijl Peter CM, et al. MRI atlas of human white matter. Elsevier Academic Press; 2010.
4. Jones DK, Cercignani M. Twenty-five pitfalls in the analysis of diffusion MRI data. NMR Biomed 2010; 23:803–20.
5. Basser PJ, Mattiello J, LeBihan D. Estimation of the effective self-diffusion tensor from the NMR spin echo. J Magn Reson B 1994;103:247–54.
6. Basser PJ, Mattiello J, LeBihan D. MR diffusion tensor spectroscopy and imaging. Biophys J 1994;66:259–67.
7. Le Bihan D, Breton E, Lallemand D, et al. MR imaging of intravoxel incoherent motions: application to diffusion and perfusion in neurologic disorders. Radiology 1986;161:401–7.
8. Le Bihan D, Basser PJ. Diffusion and perfusion magnetic resonance imaging: applications to functional MRI chapter. Molecular diffusion and nuclear magnetic resonance. Raven Press; 1995. p. 5–17.
9. LeBihan D. Molecular diffusion nuclear magnetic resonance imaging. Magn Reson Q 1991;7:1–30.
10. Beaulieu C, Allen PS. Water diffusion in the giant axon of the squid: implications for diffusion-weighted MRI of the nervous system. Magn Reson Med 1994;32: 579–83.
11. Pierpaoli C, Jezzard P, Basser PJ, et al. Diffusion tensor MR imaging of the human brain. Radiology 1996;201:637.
12. Wiegell MR, Larsson HB, Wedeen VJ. Fiber crossing in human brain depicted with diffusion tensor MR imaging1. Radiology 2000;217:897–903.
13. Tuch DS. High angular resolution diffusion imaging reveals intravoxel white matter fiber heterogeneity. Magn Reson Med 2002;48:577–82.
14. Horsfield MA, Jones DK. Applications of diffusion-weighted and diffusion tensor MRI to white matter diseases—a review. NMR Biomed 2002;15:570–7.
15. Ciccarelli O, Catani M, Johansen-Berg H, et al. Diffusion-based tractography in neurological disorders:

concepts, applications, and future developments. Lancet Neurol 2008;7:715–27.
16. Assaf Y, Pasternak O. Diffusion tensor imaging (DTI)-based white matter mapping in brain research: a review. J Mol Neurosci 2008;34:51–61.
17. Kubicki M, McCarley R, Westin CF, et al. A review of diffusion tensor imaging studies in schizophrenia. J Psychiatr Res 2007;41:15–30.
18. Maller JJ, Thomson RH, Lewis PM, et al. Traumatic brain injury, major depression, and diffusion tensor imaging: making connections. Brain Res Rev 2010; 64:213–40.
19. Inglese M, Bester M. Diffusion imaging in multiple sclerosis: research and clinical implications. NMR Biomed 2010;23:865–72.
20. Filippi M, Agosta F. Imaging biomarkers in multiple sclerosis. J Magn Reson Imaging 2010;31:770–88.
21. Lange N, DuBray MB, Lee JE, et al. Atypical diffusion tensor hemispheric asymmetry in autism. Autism Res 2010;3(6):350–8.
22. Westlye LT, Walhovd KB, Dale AM, et al. Life-span changes of the human brain white matter: diffusion tensor imaging (DTI) and volumetry. Cereb Cortex 2010;20:2055–68.
23. Catani M, Jones DK, ffytche DH. Perisylvian language networks of the human brain. Ann Neurol 2005;57:8–16.
24. Glasser MF, Rilling JK. DTI tractography of the human brain's language pathways. Cereb Cortex 2008;18:2471–82.
25. Jahanshad N, Lee AD, Barysheva M, et al. Genetic influences on brain asymmetry: a DTI study of 374 twins and siblings. Neuroimage 2010;52:455–69.
26. Schotten Thiebaut M, Ffytche DH, Bizzi A, et al. Atlasing location, asymmetry and inter-subject variability of white matter tracts in the human brain with MR diffusion tractography. Neuroimage 2011; 54:49–59.
27. Sporns O, Tononi G, Kotter R. The human connectome: a structural description of the human brain. PLoS Comput Biol 2005;1:e42.
28. Honey CJ, Sporns O, Cammoun L, et al. Predicting human resting-state functional connectivity from structural connectivity. Proc Natl Acad Sci U S A 2009;106(6):2035–40.
29. Talos IF, O'Donnell L, Westin CF, et al. Diffusion tensor and functional MRI fusion with anatomical MRI for image-guided neurosurgery. Presented at: Sixth International Conference on Medical Image Computing and Computer-Assisted Intervention-MICCAI; November 15–18, 2003; Montreal, Canada; 407–15.
30. Nimsky C, Ganslandt O, Fahlbusch R. Implementation of fiber tract navigation. Neurosurgery 2006; 58:ONS-292–303.
31. Bello L, Gambini A, Castellano A, et al. Motor and language DTI fiber tracking combined with

intraoperative subcortical mapping for surgical removal of gliomas. Neuroimage 2008;39:369–82.

32. Golby AJ, Kindlmann G, Norton I, et al. Interactive diffusion tensor tractography visualization for neurosurgical planning. Neurosurgery 2011;68(2):496–505.

33. Wu JS, Zhou LF, Tang WJ, et al. Clinical evaluation and follow-up outcome of diffusion tensor imaging-based functional neuronavigation: a prospective, controlled study in patients with gliomas involving pyramidal tracts. Neurosurgery 2007;61:935.

34. Beaulieu C. The basis of anisotropic water diffusion in the nervous system—a technical review. NMR Biomed 2001;15:435–55.

35. Sen PN, Basser PJ. A model for diffusion in white matter in the brain. Biophys J 2005;89:2927–38.

36. Basser PJ. Inferring microstructural features and the physiological state of tissues from diffusion-weighted images. NMR Biomed 1995;8:333–44.

37. Westin CF, Maier SE, Mamata H, et al. Processing and visualization of diffusion tensor MRI. Med Image Anal 2002;6:93–108.

38. Goodlett C, Fletcher PT, Lin W, et al. Quantification of measurement error in DTI: theoretical predictions and validation. In: Proceedings of the 10th International Conference on Medical image Computing and Computer-Assisted Intervention—Volume Part I. Springer-Verlag; 2007:10–7.

39. Le Bihan D, Mangin JF, Poupon C, et al. Diffusion tensor imaging: concepts and applications. J Magn Reson Imaging 2001;13:534–46.

40. Basser PJ, Jones DK. Diffusion-tensor MRI: theory, experimental design and data analysis—a technical review. NMR Biomed 2002;15:456–67.

41. Schlaug G, Siewert B, Benfield A, et al. Time course of the apparent diffusion coefficient (ADC) abnormality in human stroke. Neurology 1997;49:113–9.

42. Le Bihan D. Looking into the functional architecture of the brain with diffusion MRI. Nat Rev Neurosci 2003;4:469–80.

43. Basser PJ, Pierpaoli C. Microstructural and physiological features of tissues elucidated by quantitative-diffusion-tensor MRI. J Magn Reson B 1996;111:209–19.

44. Westin CF, Peled S, Gudbjartsson H, et al. Geometrical diffusion measures for MRI from tensor basis analysis. In: ISMRM 97 Vancouver, Canada; 1997: p. 1742.

45. Ennis DB, Kindlmann G. Orthogonal tensor invariants and the analysis of diffusion tensor magnetic resonance images. Magn Reson Med 2006;55:136–46.

46. Kindlmann G, Ennis DB, Whitaker RT, et al. Diffusion tensor analysis with invariant gradients and rotation tangents. IEEE Trans Med Imaging 2007;26:1483–99.

47. Pajevic S, Pierpaoli C. Color schemes to represent the orientation of anisotropic tissues from diffusion tensor data: application to white matter fiber tract

mapping in the human brain. Magn Reson Med 1999;42(3):526–40. [Erratum in: Magn Reson Med 2000;43(6):921].

48. Kindlmann G. Superquadric tensor glyphs. In: IEEE Transactions on Visualization and Computer Graphics/EG Symposium on Visualization; 2004. p. 147–54.

49. Jones DK. Studying connections in the living human brain with diffusion MRI. Cortex 2008;44:936–52.

50. Lazar M. Mapping brain anatomical connectivity using white matter tractography. NMR Biomed 2010;23:821–35.

51. Basser PJ, Pajevic S, Pierpaoli C, et al. In vivo fiber tractography using DT–MRI data. Magn Reson Med 2000;44:625–32.

52. Conturo TE, Lori NF, Cull TS, et al. Tracking neuronal fiber pathways in the living human brain. Neurobiology 1999;96:10422–7.

53. Mori S, Crain BJ, Chacko VP, et al. Three dimensional tracking of axonal projections in the brain by magnetic resonance imaging. Ann Neurol 1999;45:265–9.

54. Westin CF, Maier SE, Khidhir B, et al. Image processing for diffusion tensor magnetic resonance imaging. In: Medical Image Computing and Computer-Assisted Intervention, Lecture Notes in Computer Science; 1999. p. 441–52.

55. Delmarcelle T, Hesselink L. Visualization of second order tensor fields and matrix data. In: Proceedings of IEEE Visualization '92; 1992. p. 316–23.

56. Press WH, Teukolsky SA, Vetterling WT, et al. Numerical recipes in C: the art of scientific computing. Cambridge University Press; 1992.

57. Weinstein D, Kindlmann G, Lundberg E. Tensorlines: advection-diffusion based propagation through diffusion tensor fields. In: Proceedings of IEEE Visualization '99; 1999. p. 249–53.

58. Lazar M, Weinstein DM, Tsuruda JS, et al. White matter tractography using diffusion tensor deflection. Hum Brain Mapp 2003;18:306–21.

59. Conturo TE, Lori NF, Cull TS, et al. Tracking neuronal fiber pathways in the living human brain. Proc Natl Acad Sci U S A 1999;96:10422.

60. Catani M, Howard RJ, Pajevic S, et al. Virtual in vivo interactive dissection of white matter fasciculi in the human brain. Neuroimage 2002;17:77–94.

61. O'Donnell LJ, Westin CF. Automatic tractography segmentation using a high-dimensional white matter atlas. IEEE Trans Med Imaging 2007;26:1562–75.

62. Goodlett C, Davis B, Jean R, et al. Improved correspondence for DTI population studies via unbiased atlas building. Proceedings of Med Image Comput Comput Assist Interv 2006;9(Pt 2):260–67.

63. Yushkevich PA, Zhang H, Simon T, et al. Gee structure-specific statistical mapping of white matter tracts. Neuroimage 2008;41(2):448–61.

64. Mori S, Oishi K, Jiang H, et al. Stereotaxic white matter atlas based on diffusion tensor imaging in an ICBM template. Neuroimage 2008;40:570–82.

65. Maddah M, Grimson WE, Warfield SK, et al. A unified framework for clustering and quantitative analysis of white matter fiber tracts. Med Image Anal 2008;12:191–202.

66. Catani M, Schotten T. A diffusion tensor imaging tractography atlas for virtual in vivo dissections. Cortex 2008;44:1105–32.

67. Hagler DJ Jr, Ahmadi ME, Kuperman J, et al. Automated white-matter tractography using a probabilistic diffusion tensor atlas: application to temporal lobe epilepsy. Hum Brain Mapp 2009;30:1535.

68. Behrens TE, Woolrich MW, Jenkinson M, et al. Characterisation and propagation of uncertainty in diffusion weighted MR imaging. Magn Reson Med 2003;50:1077–88.

69. Behrens TE, Johansen-Berg H, Woolrich MW, et al. Non-invasive mapping of connections between human thalamus and cortex using diffusion imaging. Nat Neurosci 2003;6:750–7.

70. O'Donnell L, Haker S, Westin CF. New approaches to estimation of white matter connectivity in diffusion tensor MRI: elliptic PDEs and Geodesics in a tensor-warped space. In: Dohi T, Kikinis R, editors. Medical Image Computing and Computer-Assisted Intervention (MICCAI). Tokyo (Japan): 2002. p. 459–66.

71. Kreher BW, Mader I, Kiselev VG. Gibbs tracking: a novel approach for the reconstruction of neuronal pathways. Magn Reson Med 2008;60:953–63.

72. Melonakos J, Mohan V, Niethammer M, et al. Finsler tractography for white matter connectivity analysis of the cingulum bundle. In: Proceedings of the 10th International Conference on Medical Image Computing and Computer-Assisted Intervention—Volume Part IMICCAI'07. Berlin, Heidelberg: Springer-Verlag; 2007:36–43.

73. Behrens TE, Berg HJ, Jbabdi S, et al. Probabilistic diffusion tractography with multiple fibre orientations: what can we gain? Neuroimage 2007;34: 144–55.

74. Wedeen VJ, Wang RP, Schmahmann JD, et al. Diffusion spectrum magnetic resonance imaging (DSI) tractography of crossing fibers. Neuroimage 2008; 41:1267–77.

75. Qazi AA, Radmanesh A, O'Donnell L, et al. Resolving crossings in the corticospinal tract by two-tensor streamline tractography: method and clinical assessment using fMRI. Neuroimage 2008;47(Suppl 2): T98–106.

76. Malcolm JG, Shenton ME, Rathi Y. Filtered multi-tensor tractography. IEEE Trans Med Imaging 2010;29:1664–75.

77. Yushkevich PA, Zhang H, Simon TJ, et al. Structure-specific statistical mapping of white matter tracts. Neuroimage 2008;41:448–61.

78. O'Donnell L, Golby AJ, Westin CF. Tract-based morphometry for white matter group analysis. Neuroimage 2009;45:832–44.

79. Sherbondy A, Rowe M, Alexander D. MicroTrack: an algorithm for concurrent projectome and microstructure estimation. In: Jiang T, Navab N, Pluim J, et al, editors. Medical image computing and computer-assisted intervention: MICCAI 2010. Springer; 2010. p. 183–90.

80. Kamada K, Todo T, Ota T, et al. The motor-evoked potential threshold evaluated by tractography and electrical stimulation. J Neurosurg 2009;111:785–95.

81. Bello L, Castellano A, Fava E, et al. Intraoperative use of diffusion tensor imaging fiber tractography and subcortical mapping for resection of gliomas: technical considerations. Neurosurg Focus 2010;28:E6.

82. Alexander AL, Hasan KM, Lazar M, et al. Analysis of partial volume effects in diffusion-tensor MRI. Magn Reson Med 2001;45:770–80.

83. Kandel Eric R, Schwartz James H, Jessel Thomas M. Principles of neural science. McGraw-Hill; 2000.

84. Tuch DS. Q-ball imaging. Magn Reson Med 2004; 52:1358–72.

85. Bar-Shir A, Duncan ID, Cohen Y. QSI and DTI of excised brains of the myelin-deficient rat. Neuroimage 2009;48:109–16.

86. Wu EX, Cheung MM. MR diffusion kurtosis imaging for neural tissue characterization. NMR Biomed 2010;23:836–48.

87. Wedeen VJ, Hagmann P, Tseng WI, et al. Mapping complex tissue architecture with diffusion spectrum magnetic resonance imaging. Magn Reson Med 2005;54:1377–86.

88. Assaf Y, Basser PJ. Composite hindered and restricted model of diffusion (CHARMED) MR imaging of the human brain. Neuroimage 2005;27: 48–58.

89. Peled S, Friman O, Jolesz F, et al. Geometrically constrained two-tensor model for crossing tracts in DWI. Magn Reson Imaging 2006;24:1263–70.

90. Assaf Y, Blumenfeld-katzir T, Yovel Y, et al. AxCaliber: a method for measuring axon diameter distribution from diffusion MRI. Magn Reson Med 2008;59: 1347–54.

91. Ozarslan E, Vemuri Baba C, Mareci Thomas H. Higher rank tensors in diffusion MRI. In: Weickert J, Hagen H, editors. Visualization and processing of tensor fields. Mathematics and visualization. Berlin: Springer; 2006. p. 177–87.

92. Ozarslan E, Basser PJ. Microscopic anisotropy revealed by NMR double pulsed field gradient experiments with arbitrary timing parameters. J Chem Phys 2008;128:154511.

93. Shemesh N, Ozarslan E, Komlosh ME, et al. From single-pulsed field gradient to double-pulsed field

gradient MR: gleaning new microstructural information and developing new forms of contrast in MRI. NMR Biomed 2010;23:757–80.

94. Smith SM, Jenkinson M, Johansen-Berg H, et al. Tract-based spatial statistics: voxelwise analysis of multi-subject diffusion data. Neuroimage 2006;31: 1487–505.

95. Kindlmann G, Westin CF. Diffusion tensor visualization with glyph packing. In: Proceedings Visualization/Information Visualization. IEEE Transactions on Visualization and Computer Graphics 2006;12:1329–35.

96. Savadjiev P, Kindlmann G, Bouix S, et al. Local white matter geometry from diffusion tensor gradients. Neuroimage 2010;49:3175–86.

Multimodal Image Registration for Preoperative Planning and Image-Guided Neurosurgical Procedures

Petter Risholm, MSc[a,*], Alexandra J. Golby, MD[a,b],
William Wells III, PhD[a]

KEYWORDS

• Brain • Registration • Functional information • Tumor

Image registration is the process of transforming images acquired at different time points, or with different imaging modalities, into the same coordinate system. It is an essential part of any neurosurgical planning and navigation system because it facilitates combining images with important complementary, structural, and functional information to improve the information based on which a surgeon makes critical decisions.

Magnetic resonance imaging (MRI) can be used to generate both structural and functional neurologic images and thus plays an important role in planning neurosurgical procedures. High-resolution anatomic magnetic resonance (MR) images can be used to discriminate between healthy and pathologic tissue, functional MRI (fMRI) can be used to identify the location, and extent, of important cognitive areas of the brain, whereas diffusion tensor imaging (DTI) can be used to identify the white matter connectivity of the brain (**Fig. 1**). If important cognitive areas are injured or removed during surgery, it can have an adverse effect on the patient's quality of life after surgery.

It is especially important to put these complementary images into the same coordinate system when functional areas are located adjacent to a tumor. A map of important anatomic structures and surrounding functional areas can then be built and used by the surgeon to plan the surgical procedure.[1] Because the brain is enclosed by the skull, a rigid transformation that consists of a translation and rotation is adequate to align these images. The importance of fMRI in planning tumor resections is underlined by the findings of Petrella and colleagues[2] who studied the effect of therapeutic decision making in patients with brain tumors. Treatment plans before and after fMRI differed in 19 of 49 patients, with a more aggressive approach recommended after imaging in 18 patients. The availability of fMRI resulted in reduced surgical time in 22 patients who underwent surgery, a more aggressive resection in 6 patients, and a smaller resection in 2 patients.

Other modalities have been and are also currently being used in neurosurgical navigation systems. Positron emission tomography (PET) allows the function and metabolism of the brain to

This work was supported by the grants R01CA138419, P41RR13218, P41RR19703 from National Institutes of Health.

The authors have nothing to disclose.

[a] Department of Radiology, Brigham and Women's Hospital and Harvard Medical School, 75 Francis Street, Boston, MA 02115, USA

[b] Department of Neurosurgery, Brigham and Women's Hospital, Harvard Medical School, Boston, MA, USA

* Corresponding author.

E-mail address: pettri@bwh.harvard.edu

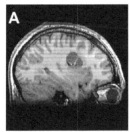
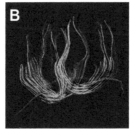
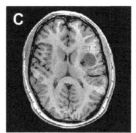
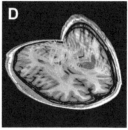

Fig. 1. Anatomic and functional MRI information acquired preoperatively.[48] (*A*) An anatomic T1 scan of a patient with a lesion in the left frontal region. (*B*) Extracted white matter tracts using tractography from diffusion tensor imaging (DTI). (*C*) Speech areas found with functional MRI (fMRI) overlaid on an axial anatomic slice. Note that one of the speech centers is adjacent to the tumor and should be conserved during surgery. (*D*) Composite view of the anatomic magnetic resonance image and functional DTI and fMRI.

be analyzed. It is mainly used to localize the most malignant parts of brain tumors but has also been used to locate eloquent areas of the cortex. However, it does not provide useful structural information and is therefore combined with high-resolution structural imaging, such as MRI and computed tomography (CT), to accurately locate the functional areas in relation to anatomic structures.[3] For planning of neurosurgical procedures, PET images are usually combined with those of MRI because they provide the best tissue contrast. fMRI has now superseded PET as a functional imaging modality for locating eloquent cortex because it eliminates any radiation exposure.

Registration also plays an important role in other neurosurgical guidance applications besides tumor removal, for instance, in resection of suspected epileptogenic centers. The epileptogenic centers are located using information from subdural electrodes, and the location of these electrodes is extracted from CT. By registering CT with structural MRI, the centers can be precisely located within the brain anatomy and used to plan the resection.[4]

Because of brain shift, tissue resection, and retraction, the preoperative image information does not necessarily reflect the intraoperative anatomy the surgeon sees during surgery, even after rigid registration. Brain shift, a deformation of the brain tissue that occurs after the craniotomy and opening of the dura mater, is caused by various combined factors: cerebrospinal fluid (CSF) leakage, gravity, edema, tumor mass effect, and administration of osmotic diuretics.[5,6] A clinical example of brain shift is shown in **Fig. 2**. Reported deformations of the brain tissue caused by brain shift measure up to 24 mm,[7–9] and further deformations may be induced because of tissue manipulation during the resection.[5,10]

For acquiring up-to-date anatomic information during surgery, intraoperative MRI has been introduced into the surgical workflow.[11,12] Intraoperative imaging during neurosurgical procedures helps identify any residual tumor tissue and leads

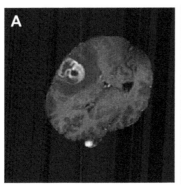
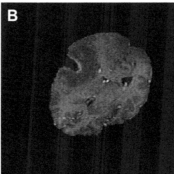
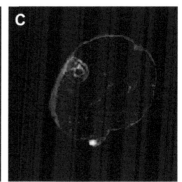

Fig. 2. Preoperative and intraoperative magnetic resonance images showing brain shift and resection. (*A*) Preoperative image. (*B*) Intraoperative image showing the cavity that is a result of the tumor resection. (*C*) Absolute difference image of the images in (*A*) and (*B*). Note the large intensity differences around the tumor site. Large image gradients and image intensity differences are often the driving force in image registration methods. However, in the case of resections, these image forces should be contained to prevent them from driving the registration into false minima.

to a significant increase in the extent of tumor removal and survival times.[13] However, intraoperative images are often of a degraded quality compared with the preoperative images. Many factors lead to the reduced quality of intraoperative MR images: fast acquisition protocols, which are used to reduce the surgical time, intraoperative MRI scanners that often operate on lower magnetic field strengths than diagnostic MRI scanners, use of surface coils instead of head coils, and disturbances to the main magnetic field caused by the surgery.

Ultrasonography (US) is another imaging modality used to acquire up-to-date images during neurosurgery.[14] Compared with MRI, acquisition is faster with US and does not require the patient to move, but image quality and soft tissue discrimination is reduced. US can identify functional information such as blood flow but not areas of cognitive functions, such as motor, visual, and language cortices. Reliable and accurate acquisition of intraoperative fMR images is, in general, not feasible because of factors such as time constraint, the requirement that the patient be conscious during acquisition of fMR image, and disturbances of the magnetic field from the surgical procedure.[1]

How then can we accurately and robustly provide the surgeon with the location of these important eloquent areas in relation to the intraoperative anatomy? Nonrigid transformations have a high degree of freedom and are capable of accommodating the local brain deformations that occur during surgery. Nonrigid intraoperative registration has therefore been introduced as a way of mapping the preoperative functional information into the intraoperative space. In practice, a transformation cascade is constructed to facilitate intraoperative navigation of the preoperative image data (Fig. 3). First, the functional images, typically those of fMRI and DTI, are rigidly registered to a high-resolution preoperative anatomic image. Next, the preoperative anatomic image is nonrigidly registered with the intraoperative image. Finally, to facilitate navigation of these images, the intraoperative image is registered with the physical patient space by estimating a rigid transformation from corresponding (fiducial) landmarks identified in the image and on the patient. Most commercial neurosurgical navigation systems register the preoperative images to the intraoperative space using fiducial markers and rigid registration and do not take into account the nonrigid deformations caused by brain shift.[15]

Brigham and Women's Hospital (BWH), an affiliate of Harvard Medical School, has been one of the pioneers in developing intraoperative registration methods for aligning preoperative and intraoperative images of the brain.[12] This article presents an overview of intraoperative registration and highlights some of the recent developments at BWH. The rest of the article is organized as follows. First, patient-to-image registration is introduced followed by a discussion of the error

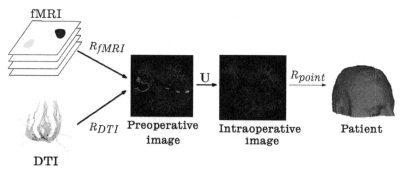

Fig. 3. Transformation cascade. Three steps are needed to map the functional images of fMRI and DTI into the intraoperative physical space. First, the rigid, or affine, transforms R_{fMRI} and R_{DTI} are estimated to align the functional images with the preoperative anatomic image. A rigid transform is generally adequate because the brain is still enclosed in the skull and assumed to move rigidly up until the start of the surgery. Second, a nonrigid transform U is estimated to align the anatomic preoperative image with the anatomic intraoperative image. A nonrigid transform is required to capture the nonlinear movements caused by, for instance, brain shift. A rigid transform R_{point} is estimated from homologous points extracted from the patient space and the intraoperative image. In some intraoperative MRI scanners, for instance, the GE Signa SP 0.5T (GE Healthcare, Milwaukee, WI, USA) that was in use at Brigham and Women's Hospital until 2007, the physical tracking space and the image space were aligned, and the estimation of R_{point} was unnecessary. Consequently, points X in the preoperative functional space can be mapped to the patient (physical) space with the following transformation cascade: $R_{point}(U[R_{fMRI}(X)])$. This step enables navigation of the functional images in a neurosurgical navigation system.

involved in such estimations. Next, an introduction of image-to-image registration and the specific challenges of intraoperative registration are provided. Finally, an overview of the research that has been performed to handle these challenges is presented.

PATIENT-TO-IMAGE REGISTRATION

The primary requirement of a neurosurgical navigation system is to relate both preoperative and intraoperative images to the physical patient space, that is, to ensure that when the surgeon points a tracked device to an easily identifiable structure on the patient, the navigation system shows the pointer at the correct location in the images. The common approach is to identify a set of homologous points in the 2 spaces the image space and the physical patient space. One example is to record the positions, $f = \{f_1, ...,f_n\}$, of a set of n fiducial markers attached to the skull as located using a tracking device and the corresponding set of points, $m = \{m_1, ...,m_n\}$, in the image. The transformation is established by finding a rigid body transformation R_{point}, which minimizes the root-mean-square (RMS) distances between the homologous points.

$$\arg \min_{R_{point}} \sqrt{\frac{\sum_{i=1}^{n} \left(f_i - R_{point}(m_i) \right)^2}{n}}$$

Because the skull is a rigid object, this transformation is generally considered to be rigid consisting of a translation and rotation.

It is important to understand that errors and uncertainties are involved in such calculations. For point-based registration, the error is usually separated into 3 parts[16]:

1. Fiducial localization error (FLE) is the error in localizing the fiducials in both physical and image space.
2. Fiducial registration error (FRE) is the RMS error between corresponding points after registration.
3. Target registration error (TRE) is the distance between homologous points, other than the fiducials used to compute FRE, after registration.

FRE is the only error that is easily computed because it is the minimum of the cost function that is minimized. The expected value of FRE depends on the number of fiducials and the squared value of FLE but is independent of the fiducial configuration. A more critical measure, the TRE, can provide some information on the error around the site that will be operated on. However, in contrast to FRE, the expected value of TRE does in some way depend on the fiducial configuration. Recent results by Shamir and Joskowicz[17] showed that for realistic configurations of the FLE, the TRE and FRE are uncorrelated, regardless of the target location and the number and configuration of fiducials. Although it could be assumed that the FRE is less than its expected value, according to Fitzpatrick,[18] it is not possible to assume that the TRE will also be less than its expected value. Thus, Fitzpatrick argues, the FRE for a given patient does not provide useful information about the true registration accuracy (TRE) and should be warily used as a measure for registration accuracy.

INTRAOPERATIVE IMAGE-TO-IMAGE REGISTRATION

Although current commercial image-guided navigation systems use rigid registration to establish the mapping between the preoperative and intraoperative spaces, there is a shift toward nonrigid registration, which is necessary to accommodate the nonrigid movement of brain tissue, for example, that is caused by brain shift.[19] Reasons for the late adoption of nonrigid registration in image-guided neurosurgical systems are the strict constraints and tough challenges that intraoperative registration faces:

1. Brain shift: the craniotomy and opening of the dura mater may induce a considerable high-dimensional warp of the brain tissue.
2. Time constraints: a registration algorithm should not, in general, affect the surgical workflow or extend the total surgical time. Hence, only a limited period is available to register the preoperative into the intraoperative images. It should, in general, not exceed the time taken to get the patient ready for surgery after acquiring the intraoperative images, which is approximately 5 to 10 minutes.
3. Resection and retraction: manipulation of the brain tissue by the surgeon leads to discontinuities in the movement of tissue because of retraction of tissue and to a nonbijective mapping because of missing tissue due to resection.
4. Uncertainty: registration uncertainty is a nearly neglected topic in the nonrigid registration community. The surgeon is provided with registered images but never with an estimate of how much the registered image data can be trusted, that is, the uncertainty of the estimated transformation. The authors believe that it will be mandatory for intraoperative registration methods to report the registration uncertainty alongside the

registered data because critical surgical decisions are taken based on the registered data.

In the following sections, image registration is defined and the different components that make up a registration method are introduced with a focus on brain shift. Next, there is a discussion on methods for accommodating resection and retraction followed by methods for quantifying the registration uncertainty.

BASIC IMAGE-TO-IMAGE REGISTRATION

Given 2 images f and m, the goal of a registration algorithm is to find a transformation u that spatially aligns homologous structures in the 2 images. A distance (similarity) function D is used to estimate how well points in the images overlap given a transformation, whereas a regularization function R generally reduces the space of permissible transformations to physically realistic ones. Basically, the transformation u that minimizes $D[f, u(m)] + \alpha R(u)$ is expected. The constant α controls the relative importance of the regularization term versus the distance function. A high-level diagram of a general registration algorithm is shown in **Fig. 4**, and general image registration surveys can be found in Maintz and Viergever[20] and Zitova and Flusser.[21]

DISTANCE MEASURES IN IMAGE REGISTRATION

Much of the early work in image-to-image registration was in registering brain images of the same patient (intrasubject) acquired with different imaging modalities (intramodality). Researchers were especially focused on finding robust distance (similarity) measures for aligning images acquired from different modalities in which there is not necessarily a simple relationship between intensities in the images. Woods and colleagues[22] presented some early work registering PET-MRI by minimizing the standard deviation of the PET pixel values that correspond to each MRI pixel value. Today, however, most intermodality registration is based on different variants of mutual information,[23] which was introduced in 1996. Mutual information is a generally applicable similarity measure because it only assumes a probabilistic relationship between intensities and has been used for registering a variety of different modalities.[24] Sometimes, the intensity differences are not of a global character, which is often seen in intraoperative MR images because of disturbances in the magnetic field. Clatz and colleagues[25] introduced a block-matching algorithm that was robust to local intensity changes by estimating local displacements and from them estimating a global transformation in which local displacements that diverged from permissible global transformations were discarded. Some investigators have totally circumvented the direct use of intensities by registering sparsely measured displacements instead (eg, cortex and ventricle surfaces extracted from images).[26]

TRANSFORMATION

Depending on the situation, the transformation can range from a simple rigid transformation (translation and rotation) to a nonrigid transformation. Before the introduction of intraoperative imaging, a rigid body approximation was adequate to estimate the movement of the brain in intrasubject registration because there is minimal change to the brain shape and position within the skull between scans.[22] However, registering preoperative with intraoperative images requires high-dimensional transformation models that allow local movements of the brain. Popular high-dimensional transformation models used in registration of the brain include splines,[27] finite element models (FEMs),[25] and optical flow–based methods.[28] Spline-based models determine a globally smooth deformation field by interpolating displacements defined at control points in the image (eg, corresponding landmarks). The main disadvantage of spline methods is that special measures are sometimes required to prevent folding of the deformation field. FEMs divide the image into cells and provide a high degree of freedom in defining the granularity of the deformation. In areas where highly local

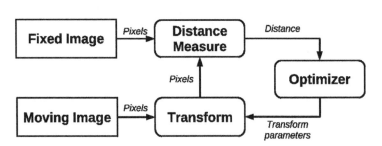

Fig. 4. General flow of a registration algorithm. It is generally an iterative process in which the transformation parameters are estimated to minimize the distance between 2 images. The distance measure can measure anything from image intensities to the distance between homologous points in the 2 images.

deformations are expected, many degrees of freedom can be used, whereas areas that are assumed to move rigidly (eg, bones) can be modeled with few degrees of freedom. Optical flow methods are usually used when speed is important and can provide highly localized deformations but their main disadvantage is that they are not robust with regard to intensity differences.

REGULARIZATION

Images only partially constrain the transformation. For transformations with many degrees of freedom, regularization is used to constrain the transformation to mimic underlying physical properties of the tissue being registered. Depending on the tissue, such properties can include smoothness, volume preservation, or elasticity. State-of-the-art nonrigid registration methods for registering brain images use physically based regularization. These methods use biomechanical models for including patient-specific modeling (eg, mechanical properties of different biologic tissues). In the context of intraoperative registration, deformation of brain tissue is often well approximated with linear elastic models.[25,29] Elastic models allow the use of different material properties, such as stiffness and compressibility, for the different tissue type models. Methods that use the linear elastic model can be divided into 2 groups, those that exclusively use image information as the driving force in the registration[25,26] and those that use externally measured displacements, for instance, laser scanners,[30] stereovision,[31] or some combination of intensities and landmarks.[32] More sophisticated physical models such as hyperelastic models, hyperviscoelastic[33] models, or coupling of fluid and elastic[34] models have also been investigated. However, Wittek and colleagues[35] have shown that using more advanced models rather than linear elastic models may not affect the estimated results significantly enough to justify the added complexity and computational time.

A substantial uncertainty is involved in determining exact values for the material properties of brain tissue, and consequently, the reported estimates of material parameters are divergent.[36] In addition, medication, radiation, and other factors related to the surgical procedure may significantly change the material parameters. Because the literature reports divergent values for the material parameters, most investigators make more or less qualified guesses as for the values of these parameters. The authors have recently introduced a probabilistic registration framework.[37] Instead of using point estimates for the material parameters, this framework is modeled with broad prior distributions

and the posterior distribution over deformations and the material parameters are jointly estimated. The authors showed that the deformation could be accurately recovered and also that the plausible material parameters for CSF and gray and white matter could be recovered.

MODELING RESECTION AND RETRACTION

When a tumor is located deep in the brain, it is necessary to retract brain tissue to create an access channel to the tumor. This process is commonly performed by making an incision in the brain tissue down to the tumor, inserting a device called a retractor, and pulling the brain tissue apart to leave an open space through which the surgeon can resect the tumor. Most intraoperative images are acquired some time after the start of the resection, either to check that all tumor tissue has been resected or to confirm that important functional or structural areas are not compromised. Because of the resected, or missing, tissue, there is no longer a one-to-one (bijective) correspondence between the preoperative and intraoperative anatomy. Consequently, a discontinuous and nonbijective deformation model is required to capture the motion of the brain tissue.[10]

One result of the resection, especially in intensity-based registration approaches, is that unwanted image forces are likely to occur in the nonbijective areas because of large image gradients and image intensity differences. Most nonrigid registration methods assume a bijective deformation field and regularize the deformation field accordingly. With a few notable exceptions, researchers have usually not included models for accommodating the nonbijectivity that is caused by retraction and resection. Periaswamy and Farid[38] proposed a registration framework that handles missing data by applying the expectation maximization method to alternately estimate the missing data and the registration parameters. Miga and colleagues[39] introduced a biomechanical FEM that explicitly handles resection and retraction. The FEM mesh was split along the retraction, while nodes in the area of resection were decoupled from the FEM computations. No automatic means of determining the resected and retracted areas were included because they needed to be manually delineated. The main drawback of using a conventional FEM for modeling retraction and resection is that it requires remeshing, which is a complex and time-consuming process.

Nonphysically based registration methods are computationally efficient and robust, provide straightforward implementations, and require minimal manual interaction. However, the main drawback with nonphysically based methods is that they do not include any domain-specific modeling to encourage realistic deformations of biologic tissues. The Demons method is a widely used nonphysically based nonrigid registration method based on optical flow.[28] It is an iterative method in which each iteration consists of a 2-step procedure. First, an unconstrained update to the transformation is estimated to improve the distance measure. Second, the updated transformation is regularized by applying a gaussian smoothing filter. The Demons method has proved to be fast enough for intraoperative use but is, in general, constrained to intramodal registration. A version of the method that could handle affine intensity correspondences was introduced by Guimond and colleagues[40] but at the cost of a considerable increase in computation time. In their recent work,[41,42] the authors have extended the Demons method to handle both retraction and resection by adapting the regularization step of the method to accommodate discontinuities and missing data. They reached speeds adequate for intraoperative registration and achieved increased registration accuracy near the resection compared with traditional Demons based methods.

Another approach by Toews and Wells[43] focused on automatically identifying and registering informative local image features between preoperative MR and intraoperative US images. The goal is to robustly determine a sparse set of image-to-image correspondences if underlying tissues may not be present or visible in both the images to be registered due to either resection or modality-specific characteristics. The correspondences identified can potentially be useful in constraining further registration or analysis of more difficult, less informative image regions.

REGISTRATION UNCERTAINTY

Registration uncertainty is another important, but mostly neglected, topic in nonrigid image registration. Most investigators focus on finding the most likely estimate of their registration problem and disregard any treatment of uncertainty in their estimate. In the case of intraoperative registration, it is likely that the registration uncertainty increases around the tumor because of intensity differences caused by contrast enhancement, degraded image quality, and missing data due to resection. Registration uncertainty is closely tied to surgical risk. Registration uncertainty means the lack of complete certainty, that is, the existence of more than 1

possible transformation that will align 2 images. A surgical risk exists whenever a set of possible transformations that might lead to an undesirable outcome. In the case of intraoperative registration, one of the possible transformations might lead the surgeon to think that resecting a certain part of the brain will not affect any cognitive areas, whereas another possible outcome might indicate the opposite. Hence, it is critical that intraoperative registration reports the registration uncertainty to increase the surgeon's confidence level and ability to make better intraoperative decisions that are less risky.

In point-based rigid body registration, registration uncertainty has been studied extensively to quantify the distribution of the TRE,[44] which can be important information to the surgeon, for example, during image-guided biopsies.

However, few investigators have reported methods for quantifying nonrigid registration uncertainty. Hub and colleagues[45] developed a heuristic method for quantifying uncertainty in B-spline image registration by perturbing the B-spline control points and analyzing the effect on the similarity criterion. Kybic[46] considers images to be random processes and proposed a general bootstrapping method to compute statistics on registration parameters. This is a computationally intensive approach but is applicable to a large set of minimization-based registration algorithms.

Another approach by the authors introduced a bayesian registration framework to characterize the posterior distribution over deformation parameters instead of estimating the conventional point estimates.[47] The posterior distribution contains information about the modes, and the corresponding uncertainty, of the transformation parameters. The authors introduced methods for summarizing the marginal posterior distributions on deformation parameters and showed how these summaries can be visualized in a clinical and meaningful way. An example is included in **Fig. 5**.

DISCUSSION

Neurosurgical navigation systems depend on image registration methods to relate images acquired from different sources or time points. Most registration methods that are available in commercial systems are point based and constrained to rigid transformations. It is important to understand the limitations of these methods and the error associated with the registration. The point-based methods commonly report the FRE, which is the distance between the fiducials after registration. This article points out that the FRE is not necessarily a good estimate of the

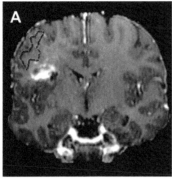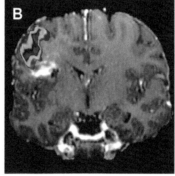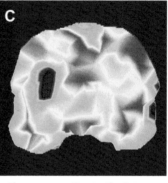

Fig. 5. Effect of registration uncertainty on mapping of functional areas from the preoperative to the intraoperative space. The anatomic image is a postoperative image, acting as a proxy for an intraoperative image, acquired from the same patient as the preoperative images in **Fig. 1**. (*A*) A coronal MRI slice with the estimated boundary of a speech-activated functional area after registration. (*B*) This method takes into account the registration uncertainty, and rather than visualizing the point estimate as in (*A*), it visualizes the marginal probability that a certain voxel is inside the functional area (*purple* denotes a probability of 1 that decreases normal to the isocontours down to red, which is close to a zero probability). If it is assumed that the hyperintense area is the site of the resection, then it can be concluded with a small probability that the functional area was touched during surgery because the outer rim of the color map touches the resected area. (*C*) An uncertainty map. The uncertainty is measured as the dispersion of the marginal posterior distribution over deformation parameters. High uncertainty is colored purple; low uncertainty, red. It can be seen that the registration uncertainty is higher closer to the resection than away from it. However, a high uncertainty in the registration does not necessarily mean that the registration is inaccurate, but the chance that it is less accurate is higher.

TRE and should be used warily as a measure of registration error.

Rigid registration methods cannot account for the highly nonrigid warps caused by, for example, brain shift. Nonrigid registration methods have not reached a level of maturity, especially with regard to handling the tough challenges of intraoperative registration, to be routinely used in commercial registration systems. Some of the remaining challenges are to handle discontinuities and missing data in the registration algorithms caused by, for example, retraction and resection and to meet the time requirements of intraoperative registration. However, it is most important to develop methods that not only provide registration results but also report the uncertainty associated with registration results because such methods increase the surgeon's confidence level in the registered image data and help reduce the risk involved in making important clinical decisions.

REFERENCES

1. Tharin S, Golby A. Functional brain mapping and its applications to neurosurgery. Neurosurgery 2007;4: 185–201.

2. Petrella JR, Shah LM, Harris KM, et al. Preoperative functional MR imaging localization of language and motor areas: effect on therapeutic decision making in patients with potentially resectable brain tumors. Radiology 2006;240(3):793–802.

3. Nabavi A, Kacher DF, Gering DT, et al. Neurosurgical procedures in a 0.5 tesla, open-configuration intraoperative MRI: planning, visualization and navigation. Automedica 2001;00:1–35.

4. Ken S, Di Gennaro G, Giulietti G. Quantitative evaluation for brain CT/MRI coregistration based on maximization of mutual information in patients with focal epilepsy investigated with subdural electrodes. Magn Reson Imaging 2007;25(6):883–8.

5. Hartkens T, Hill DL, Catellano-Smith AD, et al. Measurement and analysis of brain deformation during neurosurgery. IEEE Trans Med Imaging 2003;22(1):82–92.

6. Nimsky C, Ganslandt O, Cerny S, et al. Quantification of, visualization of, and compensation for brain shift using intraoperative magnetic resonance imaging. Neurosurgery 2000;47(5):1070–9.

7. Hastreiter P, Rezk-Salama C, Soza G, et al. Strategies for brain shift evaluation. Med Image Anal 2004;8(4):447–64.

8. Nabavi A, Black PM, Gering DT, et al. Serial intraoperative MR imaging of brain shift. Neurosurgery 2001;48(4):787–98.

9. Roberts DW, Hartov A, Kennedy FE, et al. Intraoperative brain shift and deformation: a quantitative analysis of cortical displacement in 28 cases. Neurosurgery 1998;43(4):749–58.

10. Platenik L, Miga M, Roberts D, et al. In vivo quantification of retraction deformation modeling for updated image-guidance during neurosurgery. IEEE Trans Biomed Eng 2002;49(8):823–35.

11. Claus E, Horlacher A, Hsu L, et al. Survival rates in patients with low-grade glioma after intra-operative magnetic resonance image guidance. Cancer 2005;103(6):1227–33.

12. Warfield S, Haker S, Talos I, et al. Capturing intraoperative deformations: research experience at Brigham and Women's Hospital. Med Image Anal 2005; 9(2):145–62.

13. Wirtz CR, Knauth MA, Subert MM, et al. Clinical evaluation and follow-up results for intraoperative magnetic resonance imaging in neurosurgery. Neurosurgery 2000;46(5):1112–20.

14. Rasmussen IA, Lindseth F, Rygh OM, et al. Functional neuronavigation combined with intraoperative 3D ultrasound: initial experiences during surgical resections close to eloquent brain areas and future directions in automatic brain shift compensation of preoperative data. Acta neurochir (Wien) 2006;149(4):365–78.

15. Shamir RR, Joskowicz L, Spektor S, et al. Localization and registration accuracy in image guided neurosurgery: a clinical study. Int J Comput Assist Radiol Surg 2009;4(1):45–52.

16. Fitzpatrick JM, West JB. The distribution of target registration error in rigid body point-based registration. IEEE Trans Med Imaging 2001;20(9): 917–27.

17. Shamir RR, Joskowicz L. Geometrical analysis of registration errors in point-based rigid-body registration using invariants. Med Image Anal 2011; 15(1):85–95.

18. Fitzpatric JM. Fiducial registration error and target registration error are uncorrelated. SPIE Medical Imaging 2009;7261:726102.

19. Archip N, Clatz O, Whalen S, et al. Non-rigid alignment of pre-operative MRI, fMRI and DT-MRI with intra-operative MRI for enhanced visualization and navigation in image-guided neurosurgery. Neuroimage 2007;35(2):609–24.

20. Maintz J, Viergever M. A survey of medical image registration. Med Image Anal 1998;2(1):1–36.

21. Zitova B, Flusser J. Image registration methods: a survey. Image Vis Comput 2003;21(11):977–1000.

22. Woods RP, Mazziotta JC, Cherry SR. MRI-PET registration with automated algorithm. J Comput Assist Tomogr 1993;17:536–46.

23. Wells WM, Viola P, Atsumi H, et al. Multi-modal volume registration by maximization of mutual information. Med Image Anal 1996;1(1):35–51.

24. Pluim JP, Maintz JB, Viergever MA. Mutual information based registration of medical images: a survey. IEEE Trans Med Imaging 2003;22(8): 986–1004.

25. Clatz O, Delingette H, Talos IF, et al. Robust nonrigid registration to capture brain shift from intraoperative MRI. IEEE Trans Med Imaging 2005; 24(11):1417–27.

26. Vigneron LM, Boman RC, Ponthot JP, et al. Enhanced FEM-based modeling of brain shift deformation in image guided neurosurgery. J Comput Appl Math 2010;234(7):2046–53.

27. Holden M, Schnabel JA, Hill DL. Quantification of small cerebral ventricular volume changes in treated growth hormone patients using non-rigid registration. IEEE Trans Med Imaging 2002;21:1292–301.

28. Thirion JP. Image matching as a diffusion process: an analogy with Maxwell's demons. Med Image Anal 1998;2(3):243–60.

29. Ferrant M, Nabavi A, Macq B, et al. Serial registration of intraoperative MR images of the brain. Med Image Anal 2002;6(4):337–59.

30. Miga MI, Sinha TK, Cash DM, et al. Cortical surface registration for image-guided neurosurgery using laser-range scanning. IEEE Trans Med Imaging 2003;22(8):973–85.

31. Skrinjar O, Nabavi A, Duncan J. Model-driven brain shift compensation. Med Image Anal 2002;6(4): 361–73.

32. Paul P, Morandi X, Jannin P. A surface registration method for quantification of intra-operative brain deformations in image-guided neurosurgery. IEEE Trans Inf Technol Biomed 2009;13(6):976–83.

33. Wittek A, Miller K, Kikinis R, et al. Patient-specific model of brain deformation: application to medical image registration. J Biomech 2007;40(4):919–29.

34. Hagemann A, Rohr K, Stiehl HS. Coupling of fluid and elastic models for biomechanical simulations of brain deformations using FEM. Med Image Anal 2002;6(4):375–88.

35. Wittek A, Hawkins T, Miller K. On the unimportance of constitutive models in computing brain deformation for image guided surgery. Biomech Model Mechanobiol 2009;8(1):77–84.

36. Hagemann A, Rohr K, Stiehl H, et al. Biomechanical modeling of the human head for physically based nonrigid image registration. IEEE Trans Image Process 1999;18(10):875–84.

37. Risholm P, Samset E, Wells WM. Bayesian estimation of deformation and elastic parameters in non-rigid registration. LNCS, Springer Berlin/Heidelberg. Biomedical Image Registration 2010;6204:104–15.

38. Periaswamy S, Farid H. Medical image registration with partial data. Med Image Anal 2006;10(3):452–64.

39. Miga M, Roberts DW, Kennedy FE, et al. Modeling of retraction and resection for intraoperative updating of images. Neurosurgery 2001;49(1):75–85.

40. Guimond A, Roche A, Ayache N, et al. Three-dimensional brain warping using the Demons algorithm and adaptive intensity corrections. IEEE Trans Med Imaging 2001;20(1):58–69.

41. Risholm P, Samset E, Talos I, et al. A non-rigid registration framework that accommodates resection and retraction. LNCS, Springer Berlin/Heidelberg vol. 5636. Inf Process Med Imaging 2009;21:447–58.

42. Risholm P, Samset E, Wells WM. Validation of a non-rigid registration framework that accommodates tissue resection. SPIE Medical Imaging 2010;7623: 762319.

43. Toews M, Wells WM. Bayesian registration via local image regions: information, selection and marginalization. LNCS, Springer Berlin/Heidelberg vol. 5636. Inf Process Med Imaging 2009;21:435–46.

44. Moghari M, Abolmaesumi P. Distribution of target registration error for anisotropic and inhomogeneous fiducial localization error. IEEE Trans Med Imaging 2009;28(6):799–813.

45. Hub M, Kessler M, Karger C. A stochastic approach to estimate the uncertainty involved in B-spline image registration. IEEE Trans Med Imaging 2009; 28(11):1708–16.

46. Kybic J. Bootstrap resampling for image registration uncertainty estimation without ground truth. IEEE Trans Image Process 2010;19(1):64–73.

47. Risholm P, Pieper S, Samset E, et al. Summarizing and visualizing uncertainty in non-rigid registration. LNCS, Springer Berlin/Heidelberg vol. 6362. Med Image Comput Comput Assist Interv 2010;13:554–61.

48. Pace D, Hata N. Image guided therapy in slicer3: planning for image guided neurosurgery. 2008. Surgical planning laboratory, Brigham and Women's Hospital. Available at: http://www.spl.harvard.edu/publications/item/view/1608. Accessed December 3, 2010.

Motor and Sensory Mapping

Andrei I. Holodny, MD[a,b,]*, Nina Shevzov-Zebrun[a],
Nicole Brennan, BA[a], Kyung K. Peck, PhD[a]

KEYWORDS

- Brain tumors • Functional MRI • Motor and sensory
- Paradigm

Functional magnetic resonance imaging (fMRI) has been used to enhance the understanding of neuroanatomy and functions of the brain and is becoming an accepted brain-mapping tool for clinicians, researchers, and basic scientists alike. A noninvasive procedure with no known risks, fMRI has an ever-growing list of clinical applications, including presurgical mapping of motor, language, and memory functions.[1] By superimposing fMRI data onto high-resolution anatomic magnetic resonance images, the location of eloquent cortices relative to a lesion can be determined.[2] This information gives the neurosurgeon the opportunity to make more informed decisions regarding the approach to the tumor and the necessity for invasive mapping procedures. fMRI data can also guide intraoperative mapping techniques, such as direct cortical stimulation and somatosensory evoked potentials. This article reviews the applicability of fMRI to clinical neurosurgical practice, describes the optimization of paradigm design and delivery, and illustrates artifacts and other clinically relevant pitfalls of fMRI.

CLINICAL IMPORTANCE

The use of fMRI in the clinical setting benefits patients insomuch as it allows neurosurgeons to be aware of and to navigate the precise location of patient-specific eloquent cortices and any structural anomalies that may have developed from a tumor.[2] This anatomic/functional preview facilitates the creation of more effective patient-specific treatment plans. Before the use of fMRI, the preoperative location of eloquent cortices and their relationship to the lesion was determined based on the historical localization of function and performing intraoperative mapping using direct cortical stimulation. However, direct cortical stimulation has several drawbacks. First, this procedure requires a craniotomy. Hence, an adjustment of the operative plan and possible expected complications may ensue, should intraoperative mapping reveal a relationship of the eloquent cortex to the lesion than is different from what was assumed using historical data. Further, in the authors' experience, patients occasionally have difficulty cooperating with task performance during cortical stimulation, especially when attempting to map higher function, such as language. As a result, operations can be terminated early because of inadequate intraoperative mapping results that might have been foreseen and avoided with a reliable preoperative mapping technique such as fMRI. A lack of preoperative functional information may also cause a lesion to be unnecessarily deemed inoperable.[2] In addition, mapping is restricted to the exposed surface of the brain and as a result, the cortex in the deep sulci cannot be mapped. Lastly, invasive mapping procedures, such as cortical stimulation, do not aid the neurosurgeon in presurgical risk assessment and patient counseling.

The authors have nothing to disclose.

[a] Functional MRI Laboratory, Department of Radiology, Memorial Sloan-Kettering Cancer Center, 1275 York Avenue, New York, NY 10065, USA

[b] Department of Radiology, Weill Medical College of Cornell University, 1300 York Avenue, New York, NY 10065, USA

* Corresponding author. Functional MRI Laboratory, Department of Radiology, Memorial Sloan-Kettering Cancer Center, 1275 York Avenue, New York, NY 10065.

E-mail address: holodnya@mskcc.org

Preoperative fMRI, however, by defining eloquent motor, language, and/or memory areas, allows a surgeon optimize perioperative planning to maximize tumor resection[2–5] while minimizing damage to surrounding areas (**Fig. 1**). Planning a surgical resection relies heavily on the anatomic location of a tumor relative to the eloquent cortices. However, the locations of the functional cortices vary with individuals and may be affected by the lesion itself and/or associated cortical reorganization and thus may not match the predicted anatomic locations.[2,5–9] fMRI allows for the clarification of anatomy in specific patients and detection of any irregularities. These details may become even more important when the eloquent cortices are infiltrated by a tumor.[10]

In addition, fMRI data can help a surgeon decide either for or against resection by providing information about tumors in high-risk locations (involving Broca's area, Wernicke's area, and so on) without invasive mapping (in some cases), sparing the patient awake anesthesia and associated potential complications. If a surgeon decides to perform surgery, fMRI helps the surgeon to choose the best trajectory for resection (eg, taking a more posterior approach to bypass an important functional area).[2] Other benefits of using fMRI before surgery include gathering data to guide intraoperative direct cortical stimulation (or other mapping procedures) and decreasing the operation time.[2] In patients for whom invasive mapping is not an option, fMRI provides a safe alternative,

affording an opportunity for better comparable care.[11]

fMRI can also mitigate the consequences of failed intraoperative cortical stimulation. Such failures may result from the limited time available for various testing paradigms or the inability of the patient to cooperate with the paradigms while conscious and undergoing cortical stimulation with an exposed cariotomy.[2] Optimum sedation for an open craniotomy may prove difficult to achieve, and patients may not be able to follow instructions. If awake mapping fails, previously acquired fMRI data can offer information to the surgeon.[2]

Coregistration to Neuronavigational Systems

The application of fMRI to guide neurosurgical procedures has been greatly facilitated by the ability to register fMRI with high-resolution MRI data and to display this coregistered information in the operating room in real time. Coregistration of fMRI onto high-resolution anatomic images[2,12] allows for better visualization of lesions when compared with the quality of images from low-resolution fMRI (T2*-weighted images). Typical in-plane resolution for functional images is lower than that of routine magnetic resonance images (for example, 64 × 64 matrix vs 256 × 256 matrix). After analyzing the fMRI data and determining active voxels in an fMR image, these low-resolution data are coregistered onto high-resolution images to

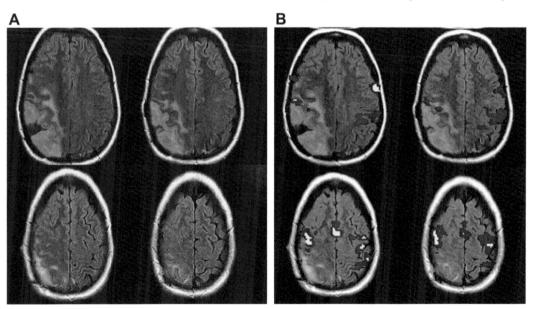

Fig. 1. fMRI motor map of a 38-year-old woman with a low-grade glioma in which motor fMRI was essential in the identification of the motor gyrus. (*A*) FLAIR image showing mass effect and ambiguous precentral gyrus location. (*B*) Motor gyrus is localized using a bilateral finger-tapping protocol and coregistered with relevant FLAIR anatomic image. FLAIR, fluid-attenuated inversion recovery.

reveal the precise location in the brain in which these signal changes occurred. The coregistered images are then downloaded to the neurosurgical navigational system in the operating room, which allows the neurosurgeon to view the relationship of the lesion to the adjacent eloquent cortex in real time intraoperatively. This whole process can be accomplished using commercially available software packages.[12] Using the coregistered data, the neurosurgeon can also envision the 3-dimensional relationship between the lesion and adjacent eloquent cortices during the resection itself, allowing for more precise patient-specific functional localization.

Verification of fMRI Results

The accuracy of fMRI results, in general, has been validated by a variety of techniques. For instance, magnetoencephalography (MEG), which is based on electric activity, has shown excellent concordance.[12,13] When compared with results of the sodium amobarbital procedure (also known as the Wada test), fMRI has shown good concordance with determinations of hemispheric dominance.[14] Studies have also shown that data collected by both intraoperative electrocorticography and direct cortical stimulation are comparable to those collected by fMRI for motor mapping.[12,15–17] In a study by Jack and colleagues,[15] 100% of subjects had concordant fMRI and direct cortical stimulation results regarding sensory/motor areas.

Integration with Other Techniques

fMRI used in conjunction with electroencephalography (EEG) or magnetoencephalography (MEG) may allow for the tracking of neural networks[18] and a better understanding of the relationships, or connections, between brain areas used to perform a task.[19] Whereas both EEG and MEG are best in the temporal domain (timing resolution <1 millisecond),[20] fMRI has superior spatial resolution (as small as 1.5 mm). In this way, the techniques can be complimentary. Also, it is significant that fMRI and EEG can be performed simultaneously, allowing for more extensive data acquisition related to one-time events, such as seizures.[18] The combination of methods, therefore, lends complimentary information that allows for a more complete and clinically useful picture of brain function.

PARADIGM SELECTION AND PATIENT PREPARATION
Neuroanatomic Review

A brief review of basic anatomy of the motor and sensory system facilitates the discussion of paradigm selection. The motor and sensory systems both have a topographic organization; in other words, motor and sensory functions are mapped to specific locations on the cortex.[1] The foot and leg are represented along the interhemispheric fissure, the hand lateral to that of the foot and leg, and the tongue and face lateral to that of the hand (**Fig. 2**).

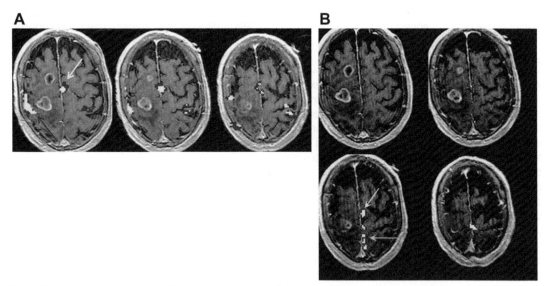

Fig. 2. fMRI motor maps showing basic neuroanatomy of the sensory and motor system. (*A*) Position of the hand motor area (bilateral activation, *red arrow*) and SMA (superior frontal gyrus, *yellow arrow*). (*B*) Location of the foot motor area (*orange arrow*). Note: foot motor area (*orange arrow*) is posterior to the more anterior supplementary motor area (*yellow arrow*). SMA, supplementary motor area.

Voluntary movement is performed through a network of different motor areas: the primary motor cortex (M1), the supplementary motor area (SMA), the lateral premotor cortex, and the superior parietal lobules.[21] M1 is involved in actually performing movement, whereas the SMA is involved in motor planning and organization.[21,22] SMA, located in the superior frontal gyrus, consists of 2 parts: the rostral pre-SMA and the caudal SMA proper. The pre-SMA functions in cognitive tasks and language, whereas the SMA proper, which is anatomically closer to primary motor and sensory areas, is involved in sensory and motor planning and word articulation.[21–26]

The role of the motor strip in language processes, although not completely understood,[27–30] should be acknowledged in preoperative fMRI/planning because it has been shown that silent speech paradigms, most commonly used for language mapping, may reveal only negligible inferior motor area activity, primarily showing only activation of the dominant inferior frontal gyrus (frontal speech areas).[27] Vocalized speech fMRI paradigms may help better estimate the network responsible for speech production (both silent and vocalized speech production), allowing patients to retain normal speech capacity after surgery.[27] This result is particularly true given that the surgeon measures speech localization in terms of speech disruption of vocalized speech rather than speech production. This finding again reinforces the complementarity of fMRI and direct cortical stimulation. fMRI identifies speech production, whereas direct cortical stimulation delineates speech arrest, which are clearly related but not equivalent.[27]

Paradigm Design

With the most commonly requested fMRI examinations being language and sensory/motor related,[1] it is important to consider the aforementioned neuroanatomy (specifically the anatomy of the motor homunculus) in light of the lesion's location in selecting paradigms. Paradigms should be designed according to certain guidelines. First, paradigms should help neurosurgeons and neurologists offer the best care to patients by providing physicians with critical information that they can use to consider the benefits and risks of neurosurgery and other treatments. Second, paradigms should be selected based on the position of the tumor[2] and the surrounding functional areas (eg, language, motor and sensory, memory). Lastly, paradigms should be chosen such that the task can be performed by the patient adequately while in the MRI scanner, taking into account the

patient's age, neurologic deficits, and general medical history.[1,2,31,32]

Common paradigm designs include block and event-related paradigms. To acquire meaningful results, a patient typically performs the fMRI task (the "ON" state) 3 to 10 times, with breaks, or "OFF" states, between each ON state.[2] When performing a block paradigm, patients alternate between ON and OFF periods of equal or unequal duration (nonperiodic task delivery). To identify the hand motor area, for instance, a block paradigm might consist of alternating finger-tapping and resting periods, each lasting 20 seconds.[2,12] Nonperiodic task delivery often proves effective in decreasing noise from the scanner, heartbeat, and breathing.[2,33]

In an event-related paradigm, a patient performs a single event (such as swallowing or clenching a fist), which lasts much shorter than the ON period in the block design. The OFF period lasts the same duration as in the block paradigm. This type of paradigm is used to investigate the neuronal or hemodynamic response to a specific single event.[1,12] In event-related paradigms, statistical power for the events being measured is compromised; hence, these designs typically require more images to regain the statistical power obtained with a block paradigm.[1,34] However, the advantage of event-related paradigms is that the hemodynamic parameters such as the time to peak, full width half maximum, and return to baseline can be estimated in a way that is not possible with block designs.[34] These more advanced parameters allow one to study complicated neurologic phenomena, such as cortical reorganization.

Regardless of the paradigm used, it is important that it be designed to minimize any type of unwanted head or body motion to achieve ideal results. A toe paradigm, for example, should be performed with no ankle motion, and tongue paradigms should be performed with a closed mouth.[12,35,36] Another method of limiting motion is using pillows under the knees or behind the neck.[2]

Sensory and Motor Mapping

Sensory and motor mapping often entails simple paradigms that use the previously described ON/OFF method.[2,31] Mapping of the motor cortex involves finger, toe, and/or tongue movement paradigms that help identify the relative locations of the lesion and regions of the motor homunculus[12]; paradigms chosen should determine the position of the lesion with regard to the different areas of the motor strip. For lesions close to the midline, leg or foot paradigms are used[2] (because the foot and leg motor areas are represented along the interhemispheric fissure).

Sensory paradigms can identify the sensory cortex or can be used to determine the location of the motor cortex in paretic patients. A sensory paradigm may include brushing, squeezing, or touching the patient's foot or hand.[31] Because there is significant reciprocity between the motor and sensory gyri, such a sensory paradigm often elicits M1 activation as well (**Fig. 3**). Even without motor homunculus fMRI activation during a sensory paradigm, the location of the motor gyrus can often be deduced from the sensory information. This can serve as a useful trick in a neurologically compromised patient.

Patient Preparation and Scanning Optimization

Another crucial step in obtaining optimal results is patient preparation to ensure proper paradigm delivery and patient compliance. Many difficulties that may occur during an fMRI scan can be avoided through a thorough preprocedure screening and paradigm explanation. This procedure is especially true for more complex paradigms and in neurologically compromised patients.[1,2,31] Patients should arrive early to receive an explanation of the fMRI procedure and the timing of the paradigms. They should then practice paradigms that they will be asked to perform because this will help to foresee possible complications. Paradigms may also be modified to better suit the patient's neurologic limitations.[1,2,31] It is difficult for some neurologically impaired patients to follow instructions and actually perform the paradigms; hence, patient progress and performance should be continuously monitored to achieve meaningful and helpful results.[1,2]

It is important to properly position the patient in the scanner and to properly select the scanning plane. For motor paradigms, the scanning plane is usually parallel to the axial plane, intersecting the anterior and posterior commissures (AC-PC line). If the scanning plane is not properly oblique to the AC-PC line, the motor gyrus will be artifactually pushed back on the image, making anatomic judgments (even with functional information) difficult.

CORTICAL PLASTICITY/REORGANIZATION

fMRI can provide an insight into cortical plasticity/reorganization, a phenomenon that can add new layers of complexity to the analysis of fMRI data and to the planning and resection of brain lesions. Cortical reorganization is thought to occur when an area of the brain is no longer able to complete its function, which causes another area of the brain to attempt to compensate in an effort to maintain function.[11,31] Cortical reorganization is an area of intense investigation both in the basic science and clinical arenas and there is much debate about the mechanism. It is likely that the details of the injury, the type of injury (eg, tumor vs stroke), the extent of brain damage, and the function affected greatly affect the resultant pattern of interhemispheric or intrahemispheric compensation.[2] Plasticity is important to consider in light of presurgical fMRI as there is evidence suggesting that

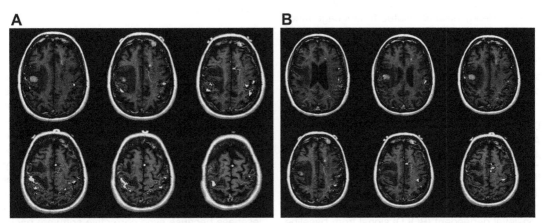

Fig. 3. A 77-year-old woman with metastatic adenocarcinoma. Both hand motor and passive hand sensory paradigms were performed. The passive hand sensory task result (*A*) is more specific, clearly showing both motor and sensory gyri, whereas the hand motor task response (*B*) is somewhat less robust in the patient. The hand motor task fMRI is also distorted by head motion caused by the patient's hemiparesis. Note the significant motor gyrus activation in the passive sensory task, making it a reasonable choice to localize the motor gyrus in compromised patients.

tumor growth may elicit reorganization.[31] Of course, any atypical functional organization would be surgically relevant. However, the extent to which this changing fMRI map represents translocation of function or just struggling cortical adaptation that is not clinically relevant is unknown and a topic of current research.[37]

When a primary motor area is damaged, for example, other areas (such as the SMA) may start to play a larger role in normal motor function and movement execution.[21] Studies have shown that in normal humans, the SMA does in fact activate (temporally) before M1.[21,38–41] Interestingly, the SMA was shown to assume a larger role in motor planning and movement execution, classically thought of as an M1 function, in patients with tumor for whom high-grade tumors were affecting normal M1 function. A shift in SMA's hemodynamic response "time to peak" toward that of the affected M1 suggests cortical reorganization, with the SMA's response looking temporally more like that of the expected M1 hemodynamics.[21] The mechanism by which such reorganization occurs in the motor strip is being investigated but may involve a decrease in the ipsilateral functional activity and an increased activity in the contralateral hemisphere.[2,31]

In addition to tumor-induced motor compensation involving the SMA, dynamic reorganization can also result from strokes. fMRI aids in the understanding of poststroke cortical reorganization, an important factor to consider in stroke recovery therapy.[31] fMRI studies have shown that damage to M1 can induce cortical plasticity.[42,43] Indeed, a main aspect of this natural recovery may include enhanced motor network activity (which can include a larger role for the SMA).[21] Reorganization related to language function has also been documented. In one case,[44] a tumor infiltrating Broca's area resulted in the translocation of Broca's area to the right hemispheric homolog. Such translocation has also been documented as a result of a stroke.[2,45,46]

DATA ANALYSIS, CORRECTION, AND INTERPRETATION
Analysis Overview

fMRI data analysis seeks to determine active areas through identification of voxels in the brain with statistically significant changes in blood oxygenation–level dependent (BOLD) signal from baseline to activation.[11] The goal is to pinpoint voxels that show changes in signal related to the paradigm performed (the timing of the ON/OFF periods).[11,12] Surgeons can then consider the locations of such active areas when planning surgery. Signal

changes, however, are very small, between 0.5% and 5.0%.[12] With such a small margin for error, false-positive and false-negative results can easily mar results, making data analysis more difficult. Analysis software packages (either provided by vendors or available on the Internet) can improve data usefulness by correcting for artifacts (eg, extraneous motion, artifacts from prior surgery), making more accurate results available promptly. However, when interpreting fMRI data or planning an operation based on such data, it is essential to understand that such artifacts exist and can occasionally lead to spurious results.

fMRI: BOLD Effect

fMRI creates functional maps derived from changes in cerebral blood flow (CBF), cerebral blood volume, and cerebral metabolic rate of oxygen, which occur secondary to an increase in neuronal activity. Changes in these vascular parameters together yield the BOLD effect.[47] An increase in neuronal activity (due to the performance of a specific task or paradigm) is accompanied by relative increases in both oxygen consumption and CBF. The BOLD effect is a phenomenon resulting from an overshoot in the amount of diamagnetic oxyhemoglobin (from the increase in CBF in response to task-related demand) relative to paramagnetic deoxyhemoglobin (from the increase in oxygen consumption). Alone, the paramagnetic deoxyhemoglobin produced due to oxygen use would cause a drop in fMRI signal strength. However, as the deoxyhemoglobin is diluted by the overshoot in diamagnetic oxyhemoglobin, fMRI signal actually increases in the active area. fMRI signal, therefore, is derived from the relative differences in the magnetic susceptibility of these 2 states of hemoglobin.

ARTIFACTS AND OTHER PITFALLS IN CLINICAL fMRI

Artifacts from various sources can affect the results of fMRI data. Unwanted movement can produce motion artifacts; such motion can include larger head or body movement or simple periodic fluctuations in heart rate and respiration (pulsatile artifact).[12,31] Often leading to false-negative/false-positive results, head motion can inadvertently move voxels of a high signal intensity to locations of low signal intensity.[31] Patient comfort must also be ensured to minimize extra motion and restlessness because even corrective software packages cannot eliminate all effects of motion. In fact, whereas types of motion can be compensated for by software, stimulus-correlated motion (eg, when the patient bobs his/her head in time with a finger-tapping paradigm) often cannot be compensated for because the artifactual signal looks deceptively similar to real fMRI signal. Therefore, any measure that minimizes head motion during the fMRI examination is valuable.

The magnetic resonance sequences used to acquire fMRI data (usually, the echoplanar imaging sequence) are used to maximize the subtle difference in susceptibility between oxyhemoglobin and deoxyhemoglobin. An unfortunate consequence is that these sequences also maximize susceptibility artifacts, which can cause signal dropout or distortions due to field inhomogeneities, masking the BOLD signal from the active site.[2] Such false-negative results can lead to inaccuracies and need to be acknowledged for the purpose of neurosurgical planning.

In patients without prior surgery, susceptibility artifacts are usually located at air-tissue interfaces, near cavities, or near moving tissues (**Fig. 4**).[19] Susceptibility artifacts pose an even larger issue for patients who have previously had neurosurgery; staples, titanium plates, and residue from skull drills increase the risk of susceptibility artifact and may affect the accuracy of the fMRI data.[2,47] A recent study considered how susceptibility artifacts from prior surgery affect the accuracy of BOLD signal in fMRI results.[48] The study

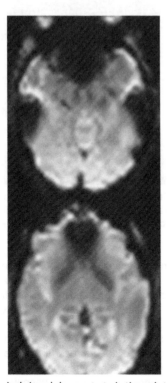

Fig. 4. Typical signal dropout at air-tissue interfaces at the base of the frontal and temporal lobes. Images are T2* weighted and are taken at 128 × 128 on a 3T magnet.

compared the M1 activation volumes (using a finger-tapping paradigm) in 43 patients with tumor, 13 of whom had undergone previous surgery and 30 of whom had not. In patients who underwent previous surgery, there was a decrease in the volume of activation in the ipsilateral M1. Inspection of the T2*-weighted images (the raw data, which is analyzed to produce the fMR images) suggested that this decrease was likely caused by susceptibility artifacts from previous surgery—the artifacts caused signal dropout (incurring false-negative results). This study also suggested that compared with tumor neovasculature, artifacts from previous surgery may have a greater effect on fMRI results than (**Fig. 5**).[48]

fMRI has limitations that at times can make it difficult to acquire consistent, accurate, and meaningful data. It is more difficult, for instance, to obtain reliable data from certain parts of the brain: a well-known area of susceptibility artifact is near the areas of bone-air interface. Notorious areas for artifactual signal dropout are the temporal lobes, which are adjacent to the air and bone of the petrous apices. Such a signal dropout limits accurate evaluation of the hippocampi and fMRI tests for memory. The high frontoparietal convexities, on the other hand, are generally devoid of such limiting artifacts and are optimal for evaluation by fMRI.

Further, signal variance is greater in areas around moving tissues (such as the eyes).[19] In addition, such use of the BOLD effect does not guarantee equal consideration of all the areas involved in the performance of the paradigm because some areas are more reliably measured than others.[11]

Another issue encountered in analyzing fMRI data is the distinction between the signal from large draining veins and the microvasculature near the active area.[2,31,49] The problem in this case is that the BOLD signal in fMRI registers both the changes in oxyhemoglobin/deoxyhemoglobin as activation. The BOLD activation of the microvasculature accurately depicts the site of neuronal firing, whereas the BOLD activation in the draining veins is at some (rather small) distance from the actual neuronal firing. It is thought that these 2 activations can be distinguished by the differences in time between their relative signal increases. The increase in signal (corresponding to activation) from the draining veins is delayed relative to that of the venules around the activated site.[31] However, in practice for neurosurgical planning, in which the mandate is biased toward a less statistically restricted and more conservative map of function (ie, larger more inclusive activations), contributions from draining veins are usually not a factor.

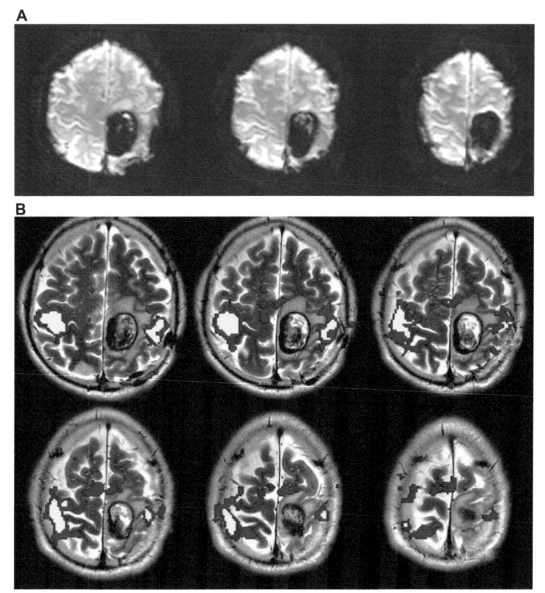

Fig. 5. A 37-year-old man with a frontoparietal glioblastoma multiforme. (*A*) T2* dropout caused by artifacts from paramagnetic blood products and previous surgery (*black areas*). Functional localization in this case was limited to hand motor regions. (*B*) T2*-weighted image resulting from a bilateral finger-tapping paradigm.

Neurovascular Decoupling

Studies have also shown that tumor neovasculature itself leads to a decrease in fMRI activation volume (specifically in areas next to high-grade lesions, such as glioblastoma multiforme). BOLD fMRI is based on the principle of neurovascular coupling—an increase in neuronal activation leads to changes in blood flow, which lead to the BOLD effect. In malignant brain tumors, the tumor neovasculature loses the ability to autoregulate. Hence, an increase in neuronal activity does not lead to an increase in blood flow, which eliminates the basis for the BOLD effect. The tumor neovasculature may cause decoupling, or delinking, of neuronal activity and the subsequent CBF response related specifically to that activity.[50] Increased CBF to an area causes an increase in signal because of the increase in oxyhemoglobin (and decrease in deoxyhemoglobin) concentration, and hence, a tumor neovasculature does not behave like a healthy neovasculature and may alter the reliability of the BOLD response. In addition, especially in areas of hypoxia in malignant brain tumors, the vasculature may already be maximally dilated and therefore would not be able to further increase the CBF in response to an increase in neuronal activity.

Applications in Treatment and Therapy

It has been suggested that neuroimaging may be used to lead to new methods of therapy and pain management and to better understand existing methods.[13,51] Maks and colleagues[52] showed that neuroimaging located the areas in which deep brain stimulation (DBS) delivered the most effective therapy for patients with Parkinson disease. Although each patient must be considered individually before DBS therapy, overall stimulation of the tissue that is dorsal, lateral, and posterior to the centroid of the subthalamic nucleus[52] is thought to have best therapeutic results. fMRI can be used to examine areas active in response to pain and pain relief from therapy.[13] There is evidence of specific cortical activity related to pain and relief by a peripheral nerve block, demonstrating a possible use for fMRI to study the brain's response to various methods of pain management and to explore new treatments and therapies.[13]

fMRI can aid in the investigation of the physiologic basis for neurologic disorders such as cerebellar dysfunction, neglect syndrome,[13] and epilepsy. fMRI data allow for the tracking of neural networks and mechanisms associated with such disorders[11,13,53,54] and suggest possible clinical uses of fMRI pertaining to them as well. In fact, fMRI has proved to be helpful in localizing seizures and mapping the involved brain regions[13] as well as in investigating seizure progression and progression of neurologic diseases in general.[11] Also, regarding epilepsy treatment and planning, fMRI may ultimately be able to replace the invasive Wada test for language/memory dominance.[31]

In addition to assisting in more precise delineation of the areas of the brain concerned with complex tasks, such as language formation and higher cognition,[13] fMRI may also be helpful in areas of rehabilitation, diagnosis, and clinical decision making. First, fMRI may ultimately facilitate the prediction of both positive and negative effects of treatment of certain neurologic diseases;[11,55] it can also provide more precise direct measurements of treatment response, as previously discussed regarding DBS. Second, fMRI may be used in tests to validate the diagnoses of various functional disorders (eg, conversion syndrome),[11,56] encouraging safer prompter treatment and may even provide insights into the development of new drugs. In addition, fMRI can be used to identify targets for functional neurosurgery, in which direct stimulation of certain areas is used to allay symptoms; this is an often-difficult task because the location of targets varies with individuals and are often deeply seated in the brain.[11]

The ability of fMRI to provide individualized care[57] for patients is an exciting prospect and is currently being investigated. Such tailoring of treatment and the fMRI procedure itself (eg, modify paradigms) would not only supply neurosurgeons with information about patient-specific atypical functional organization but also allow patients to make important lifestyle decisions regarding brain functions that they would or would not be willing to sacrifice in resection.

APPLICATIONS FOR MOTOR AND SENSORY MAPPING: CURRENT AND FUTURE RESEARCH
Current Research for Future Applications

Current research with fMRI is revealing exciting future applications for enhanced use in presurgical planning and areas of treatment/rehabilitation. With increased use and understanding of the technique, fMRI-guided presurgical planning concerning atypical anatomy[13] (eg, disruptions caused by tumors and tumor neovasculature) will improve and become more reliable. In patients with gliosis, for example, in whom functional areas surrounding the lesion may be distorted due to mass effect,[12] presurgical planning guided by fMRI data permits for a map of shifted eloquent anatomy. Additionally, fMRI is also proving to be an important tool in studies of cortical plasticity, especially important in the clinical setting, providing neurosurgeons with valuable information that may influence their decision on whether or not to perform surgery.[2,31]

Research has addressed the possible role of fMRI in the treatment of epileptic patients as well as patients with tumor. A study[58] on nearly 50 patients sought to determine how fMRI is used in various stages of treatment, namely, presurgical planning, decisions regarding resection, and assessment of the necessity for invasive mapping. In 32 of 46 patients with tumor or epileptic patients, fMRI was able to locate the functional central sulcus on the same side as the lesion. Such fMRI results were used in the treatment of 91% of the epileptic patients and 89% of the patients with tumor, leading to the conclusion that fMRI is helpful not only in resection planning and decision making but also in epilepsy surgery.

Another area of active fMRI research relevant to neurosurgical planning is the body specificity of fMRI data, that is, how an individual's movement habits, motor experiences, and medical history affect the results of motor imagery fMRI.[59] This 2009 study concluded that because the imagination of movement is most likely to be envisioned based on the way one would normally perform a motion, motor imagery fMRI results reflect one's lifestyle (including handedness, movement habits, and patterns).[59] Such knowledge can help in the designing of more appropriate patient-specific paradigms, allowing for the creation of motor maps that successfully identify eloquent cortices.

SUMMARY

fMR is important to the understanding of brain function, structure, and mechanism as well as to the localization of critical motor, speech, and cognitive function. It has many advantages when compared with other methods of neuroimaging and functional mapping: it is noninvasive, it does not entail the use of radioactive isotopes, it is easily repeatable, and it has no known risks.[2] Its use in presurgical mapping, such as locating motor, sensory, language, and/or memory functional areas in relation to a lesion, is becoming increasingly widespread and accepted,[27] and current research is investigating other exciting uses of the technique, such as more patient-specific functional mapping.

REFERENCES

1. Brennan NP. Preparing the patient for the fMRI Study and optimization of paradigm selection and delivery. In: Holodny AI, editor. Functional neuroimaging: a clinical approach. New York: Informa Healthcare USA, Inc; 2008. p. 13–21.
2. Bogomolny DL, Petrovich NM, Hou BL, et al. Functional MRI in the brain tumor patient. Top Magn Reson Imaging 2004;15(5):325–35.
3. Maldjian JA, Schulder M, Liu WC, et al. Intraoperative functional MRI using a real-time neurosurgical navigation system. J Comput Assist Tomogr 1997; 21(6):910–2.
4. Schulder M, Maldjian JA, Liu WC, et al. Functional image-guided surgery of intracranial tumors located in or near the sensorimotor cortex. J Neurosurg 1998;89(3):412–8.
5. Rezai AR, Hund M, Kronberg E, et al. The interactive use of magnetoencephalography in stereotactic image-guided neurosurgery. Neurosurgery 1996; 39(1):92–102.
6. Orrison WW Jr, Rose DF, Hart BL, et al. Noninvasive preoperative cortical localization by magnetic source imaging. AJNR Am J Neuroradiol 1992;13(4):1124–8.
7. Bucholz RD. The central sulcus and surgical planning. AJNR Am J Neuroradiol 1993;14(4):926–7.
8. Sobel DF, Gallen CC, Schwartz BJ, et al. Locating the central sulcus: comparison of MR anatomic and magnetoencephalographic functional methods. AJNR Am J Neuroradiol 1993;14(4):915–25.
9. Seitz RJ, Huang Y, Knorr U, et al. Large-scale plasticity of the human motor cortex. Neuroreport 1995; 6(5):742–4.
10. Wilkinson ID, Romanowski CA, Jellinek DA, et al. Motor functional MRI for pre-operative and intraoperative neurosurgical guidance. Br J Radiol 2003; 76(902):98–103.
11. Matthews PM, Honey GD, Bullmore ET. Applications of fMRI in translational medicine and clinical practice. Nat Rev Neurosci 2006;7(9):732–44.
12. Kesavadas C, Thomas B. Clinical applications of functional MRI in epilepsy. Indian J Radiol Imaging 2008;18(3):210–7.
13. (PICS) CUMCPflaCS. About functional MRI (general). Available at: http://www.fmri.org/fmri.htm. Accessed June 25, 2010.
14. Kesavadas C, Thomas B, Sujesh S, et al. Real-time functional MR imaging (fMRI) for presurgical evaluation of paediatric epilepsy. Pediatr Radiol 2007; 37(10):964–74.
15. Jack CR Jr, Thompson RM, Butts RK, et al. Sensory motor cortex: correlation of presurgical mapping with functional MR imaging and invasive cortical mapping. Radiology 1994;190(1):85–92.
16. Lehericy S, Duffau H, Cornu P, et al. Correspondence between functional magnetic resonance imaging somatotopy and individual brain anatomy of the central region: comparison with intraoperative stimulation in patients with brain tumors. J Neurosurg 2000;92(4):589–98.
17. Puce A, Constable RT, Luby ML, et al. Functional magnetic resonance imaging of sensory and motor cortex: comparison with electrophysiological localization. J Neurosurg 1995;83(2):262–70.
18. Liu Z, Ding L, He B. Integration of EEG/MEG with MRI and fMRI in functional neuroimaging. IEEE Eng Med Biol Mag 2006;25(4):46–53.
19. Ramsey NF. Direct comparison of functional MRI and PET. In: Moonen CT, Bandettini PA, editors. Functional MRI. Berlin: Springer-Verlag; 2000. p. 421–31.
20. Barkley GL, Baumgartner C. MEG and EEG in epilepsy. J Clin Neurophysiol 2003;20(3):163–78.
21. Peck KK, Bradbury MS, Hou BL, et al. The role of the supplementary motor area (SMA) in the execution of primary motor activities in brain tumor patients: functional MRI detection of time-resolved differences in the hemodynamic response. Med Sci Monit 2009; 15(4):MT55–62.
22. Peck KK, Bradbury M, Psaty EL, et al. Joint activation of the supplementary motor area and presupplementary motor area during simultaneous motor

and language functional MRI. Neuroreport 2009;
20(5):487–91.

23. Picard N, Strick PL. Motor areas of the medial wall: a review of their location and functional activation. Cereb Cortex 1996;6(3):342–53.

24. Roland PE, Zilles K. Functions and structures of the motor cortices in humans. Curr Opin Neurobiol 1996;6(6):773–81.

25. Vorobiev V, Govoni P, Rizzolatti G, et al. Parcellation of human mesial area 6: cytoarchitectonic evidence for three separate areas. Eur J Neurosci 1998;10(6): 2199–203.

26. Alario FX, Chainay H, Lehericy S, et al. The role of the supplementary motor area (SMA) in word production. Brain Res 2006;1076(1):129–43.

27. Petrovich N, Holodny AI, Tabar V, et al. Discordance between functional magnetic resonance imaging during silent speech tasks and intraoperative speech arrest. J Neurosurg 2005;103(2): 267–74.

28. Larner AJ, Robinson G, Kartsounis LD, et al. Clinical-anatomical correlation in a selective phonemic speech production impairment. J Neurol Sci 2004; 219(1–2):23–9.

29. Quinones-Hinojosa A, Ojemann SG, Sanai N, et al. Preoperative correlation of intraoperative cortical mapping with magnetic resonance imaging landmarks to predict localization of the Broca area. J Neurosurg 2003;99(2):311–8.

30. Riecker A, Ackermann H, Wildgruber D, et al. Articulatory/phonetic sequencing at the level of the anterior perisylvian cortex: a functional magnetic resonance imaging (fMRI) study. Brain Lang 2000; 75(2):259–76.

31. Peck KK, Holodny AI. fMRI clinical applications. In: Reiser MF, Semmler W, Hricak H, editors. Magnetic resonance tomography. Berlin: Springer Verlag; 2007. p. 1308–31.

32. Bartsch AJ, Homola G, Biller A, et al. Diagnostic functional MRI: illustrated clinical applications and decision-making. J Magn Reson Imaging 2006; 23(6):921–32.

33. Veltman DJ, Mechelli A, Friston KJ, et al. The importance of distributed sampling in blocked functional magnetic resonance imaging designs. Neuroimage 2002;17(3):1203–6.

34. Birn RM, Cox RW, Bandettini PA. Detection versus estimation in event-related fMRI: choosing the optimal stimulus timing. Neuroimage 2002;15(1): 252–64.

35. Hoeller M, Krings T, Reinges MH, et al. Movement artefacts and MR BOLD signal increase during different paradigms for mapping the sensorimotor cortex. Acta Neurochir (Wien) 2002;144(3):279–84 [discussion: 284].

36. Krings T, Reinges MH, Erberich S, et al. Functional MRI for presurgical planning: problems, artefacts,

37. Holodny AI. Cortical plasticity. In: Holodny AI, editor. Functional neuroimaging: a clinical approach. New York: Informa Healthcare, Inc; 2008.

38. Peck KK, Sunderland A, Peters AM, et al. Cerebral activation during a simple force production task: changes in the time course of the haemodynamic response. Neuroreport 2001;12(13):2813–6.

39. Weilke F, Spiegel S, Boecker H, et al. Time-resolved fMRI of activation patterns in M1 and SMA during complex voluntary movement. J Neurophysiol 2001;85(5):1858–63.

40. Wildgruber D, Erb M, Klose U, et al. Sequential activation of supplementary motor area and primary motor cortex during self-paced finger movement in human evaluated by functional MRI. Neurosci Lett 1997;227(3):161–4.

41. Richter W, Andersen PM, Georgopoulos AP, et al. Sequential activity in human motor areas during a delayed cued finger movement task studied by time-resolved fMRI. Neuroreport 1997;8(5): 1257–61.

42. Wang L, Yu C, Chen H, et al. Dynamic functional reorganization of the motor execution network after stroke. Brain 2010;133(Pt 4):1224–38.

43. Nudo RJ. Functional and structural plasticity in motor cortex: implications for stroke recovery. Phys Med Rehabil Clin N Am 2003;14(Suppl 1):S57–76.

44. Holodny AI, Schulder M, Ybasco A, et al. Translocation of Broca's area to the contralateral hemisphere as the result of the growth of a left inferior frontal glioma. J Comput Assist Tomogr 2002;26(6):941–3.

45. Thulborn KR, Carpenter PA, Just MA. Plasticity of language-related brain function during recovery from stroke. Stroke 1999;30(4):749–54.

46. Weiller C, Isensee C, Rijntjes M, et al. Recovery from Wernicke's aphasia: a positron emission tomographic study. Ann Neurol 1995;37(6):723–32.

47. Ogawa S, Lee TM, Kay AR, et al. Brain magnetic resonance imaging with contrast dependent on blood oxygenation. Proc Natl Acad Sci U S A 1990;87(24):9868–72.

48. Kim MJ, Holodny AI, Hou BL, et al. The effect of prior surgery on blood oxygen level-dependent functional MR imaging in the preoperative assessment of brain tumors. AJNR Am J Neuroradiol 2005;26(8):1980–5.

49. Kaufman JF, Maldjian JA. Fact or artifact? In: Holodny AI, editor. Functional neuroimaging: a clinical approach. New York: Informa Healthcare USA, Inc; 2008. p. 37–49.

50. Hou BL, Bradbury M, Peck KK, et al. Effect of brain tumor neovasculature defined by rCBV on BOLD fMRI activation volume in the primary motor cortex. Neuroimage 2006;32(2):489–97.

51. Jech R. Functional imaging of deep brain stimulation: fMRI, SPECT, and PET. In: Tarsy D, Vitek JL, Starr PA, editors. Deep brain stimulation in neurological and psychiatric disorders. Totowa (NJ): Humana Press; 2008. p. 179–201.

52. Maks CB, Butson CR, Walter BL, et al. Deep brain stimulation activation volumes and their association with neurophysiological mapping and therapeutic outcomes. J Neurol Neurosurg Psychiatry 2009; 80(6):659–66.

53. Tracey I. Nociceptive processing in the human brain. Curr Opin Neurobiol 2005;15(4):478–87.

54. Borsook D, Ploghaus A, Becerra L. Utilizing brain imaging for analgesic drug development. Curr Opin Investig Drugs 2002;3(9):1342–7.

55. Paulus MP, Tapert SF, Schuckit MA. Neural activation patterns of methamphetamine-dependent subjects during decision making predict relapse. Arch Gen Psychiatry 2005;62(7):761–8.

56. Werring DJ, Weston L, Bullmore ET, et al. Functional magnetic resonance imaging of the cerebral response to visual stimulation in medically unexplained visual loss. Psychol Med 2004;34(4):583–9.

57. Bernad DM, Doyon J. The role of noninvasive techniques in stroke therapy. Int J Biomed Imaging 2008;2008:672582.

58. Lee CC, Ward HA, Sharbrough FW, et al. Assessment of functional MR imaging in neurosurgical planning. AJNR Am J Neuroradiol 1999;20(8): 1511–9.

59. Willems RM, Toni I, Hagoort P, et al. Body-specific motor imagery of hand actions: neural evidence from right- and left-handers. Front Hum Neurosci 2009;3:39.

Preoperative Prediction of Verbal Episodic Memory Outcome Using fMRI

Jeffrey R. Binder, MD

KEYWORDS
- fMRI • Memory • Epilepsy • Temporal lobectomy

Interest in functional imaging of memory systems stems from 2 clinical problems. The first of these is localization of seizure foci in temporal lobe epilepsy (TLE). TLE often arises from the medial temporal lobe (MTL),[1–3] and structural and functional abnormalities in the MTL can provide important evidence regarding seizure localization. Asymmetric sclerosis and volume loss in TLE can be detected with good sensitivity and specificity using structural MRI.[4–7] Positron emission tomography (PET) may reveal interictal MTL hypometabolism and associated hypoperfusion in patients with TLE.[8–10] The memory portion of the Wada test, which assesses episodic encoding during unilateral cerebral anesthesia, can detect asymmetric dysfunction of the MTL, which can be used to infer the laterality of a seizure focus.[11–15] One potential application of fMRI, therefore, is to provide evidence about seizure focus laterality by measuring asymmetry of activation in the MTL. In addition to assisting in seizure focus identification, asymmetry of activation might be useful for predicting seizure outcome after anterior temporal lobe (ATL) surgery. When functional asymmetry consistent with the side of seizure focus is demonstrated on PET or on the Wada memory test, for example, seizure control is better than when no asymmetry or reversed asymmetry is observed.[8,10,15–18] Although several fMRI studies suggest that MTL activation asymmetry may be correlated with side of seizure focus and seizure outcome in TLE,[19–22] sample sizes in these studies have been small, and no studies have yet examined whether fMRI contributes additional predictive value beyond ictal EEG, ictal semiology, and structural MRI.

The present article focuses on an equally important neurosurgical problem for which functional imaging may have a role. Temporal lobe epilepsy surgery typically involves removal of much of the anterior MTL, including portions of the hippocampus and parahippocampus, which are known to be critical for encoding and retrieval of long-term episodic memories.[23] Verbal episodic memory decline after left ATL resection is a consistent finding in group studies and is observed in 30% to 60% of such patients.[24–39] In contrast, nonverbal memory decline after right ATL resection is less consistently observed in both groups and individuals.[25,34,35,39] One main focus of the preoperative evaluation in ATL surgery candidates is, therefore, to estimate risk of verbal memory decline, particularly in patients undergoing left ATL resection.

The Wada memory test was originally developed for the purpose of predicting global amnesia after ATL resection,[40] although its reliability for this purpose has often been questioned.[41–47] Studies of its ability to predict relative verbal memory decline have been inconsistent, with several suggesting good predictive value[29,33,36,38,48] and others showing little or none, particularly when used in combination with noninvasive tests.[25,35,39,49–51] Other presurgical tests of MTL functional or anatomic asymmetry are modestly predictive of memory outcome, including

Department of Neurology, Medical College of Wisconsin, 9200 West Wisconsin Avenue, Milwaukee, WI 53226, USA
E-mail address: jbinder@mcw.edu

Neurosurg Clin N Am 22 (2011) 219–232
doi:10.1016/j.nec.2010.12.002
1042-3680/11/$ – see front matter © 2011 Elsevier Inc. All rights reserved.

structural MRI of the hippocampus[35,39,52–54] and interictal PET.[55] Preoperative neuropsychological testing also has predictive value, in that patients with good memory abilities before surgery are more likely to decline than patients with poor preoperative memory.[24,25,27,30–32,35,39,56–58] Given the availability of these other known predictors, the value of fMRI depends not only on its ability to predict memory outcome in isolation, but also on its ability to contribute additional predictive value beyond other noninvasive measures.

A key point often neglected in discussion of these topics is that the goals of seizure focus lateralization and memory outcome prediction call for fundamentally different methodological considerations. In the case of seizure focus lateralization, the ideal fMRI procedure is probably one that activates the MTL symmetrically in healthy people, thus allowing optimal detection of deviation from normal symmetry in either direction. In contrast, prediction of verbal memory outcome requires an fMRI procedure that specifically identifies verbal memory processes. Because many stimuli are encoded into memory in both verbal and nonverbal forms, MTL activation resulting from such stimuli cannot be assumed to represent verbal memory processes. Stimuli that are dually encoded, such as pictures, might be ideal for producing bilateral MTL activation and thus for detecting seizure focus lateralization, whereas these same activation patterns, because they represent a mix of verbal and nonverbal processes, may predict little or nothing about verbal memory outcome.

VARIETIES OF MEMORY

Memory refers to the ability to store and retrieve information. The human brain performs 4 essentially different kinds of memory processes, distinguished by the type of information stored and the length of time over which storage persists. At one end of the spectrum is *procedural memory*, which refers to knowing how to do motor and sensory tasks. Common examples include walking, eating, throwing a ball, tying a tie, and riding a bike. The information stored involves complex sensory-motor sequences that are largely outside conscious awareness and cannot be described in detail. Another notable example of procedural memory is talking, which involves very complex sequences of tongue, lip, vocal cord, and diaphragm movements of which perfectly fluent speakers are largely unaware. *Semantic memory* refers to knowing facts about the world, such as the color of a banana, the capital of France, or the meaning of a word. Semantic memory allows us to recognize and name objects, produce and comprehend sentences, form opinions, and plan the future. Like procedural memory, information in semantic memory typically persists over an entire lifetime, although loss of semantic memory is a characteristic feature of some forms of dementia. At the other end of the spectrum, *short-term memory* refers to the ability to hold information in consciousness for seconds or a few minutes, usually by active mental recitation. Short-term memory allows us to hold in mind otherwise meaningless sequences like telephone numbers long enough to complete a task for which they are needed. The transient nature of short-term memory is illustrated by the fact that distraction of attention typically causes the information to rapidly fade, and by the common use of semantic memory in the form of "mnemonic devices" to allow longer maintenance of otherwise meaningless sequences.

The focus of the present review is *episodic memory*, which refers to the ability to update and maintain a conscious record of personal experiences. Episodic memory can include both verbal and nonverbal information, such as the content of recent conversations, names of new friends, personally experienced events and their order of occurrence, or the location of one's car in a parking lot. Information in episodic memory can persist for hours, days, or years depending on factors such as the meaningfulness or emotional significance of the event and the frequency with which the event is recalled. Episodic memory was first linked conclusively with the MTL after cases of severe episodic memory loss, labeled amnesia, were reported from temporal lobe damage involving the MTL bilaterally.[59,60] Such patients are unable to form new memories of events or learn new verbal information (anterograde amnesia), and may also lose partial memory of events experienced before the MTL damage (retrograde amnesia). In contrast, knowledge about objects and previously learned facts about the world are spared, as are motor skills and the ability to hold information through active recitation, indicating relative preservation of semantic, procedural, and short-term memory.

A LITTLE BIT OF THEORY

Episodic memory plays a vital role in everyday life. The purpose of having an ongoing, constantly updated record of personal events is so that we can accomplish the basic tasks of survival. Without such a record, we would be unable to keep track of our current needs, the steps already taken to meet these needs, or the plans for meeting them.

We could not keep track of imminent threats or new information about potential threats. We could not maintain a record of common experience that forms the basis for human discourse.

Given these vital functions of episodic memory, it should not be surprising that the episodic memory system has evolved a method for preferentially storing events that are meaningful and of personal significance. A typical meaningful event (say, a conversation about an upcoming trip) includes processing of sensory information (eg, speech sounds), retrieval of semantic information (eg, word meanings, factual knowledge), cognitive responses (eg, conversational exchanges), and emotional responses (eg, excitement, pleasure). Thus, a meaningful event typically elicits a complex, sequential cascade of neural activations throughout the cortex that are specific to the event. Research suggests that the essential role of the hippocampus is to bind these sensory, semantic, executive, and affective responses into unique, indexable event configurations.[61–63] Recall of the event is accompanied by a partial recreation of the spatial-temporal sequence of neural activity that occurred during the original event. Events that are more meaningful to the individual (emotionally or intellectually) elicit more widespread semantic, executive, and affective processing, and are thus more easily recalled.[64] This simple principle accounts for a wide range of phenomena observed in experimental studies of verbal episodic memory, such as the greater ease of learning lists of words compared with nonsense words, familiar relative to unfamiliar words, semantically encoded compared with phonologically encoded words, concrete compared with abstract words, semantically related compared with unrelated words, and stories compared with sequences of unrelated sentences.[64–72]

Two interesting and important aspects of episodic memory are often overlooked despite their particular relevance to imaging studies. The first is the ongoing, continuous nature of this process. We remember events without specifically trying to, and without instruction beforehand to do so. Except for periods during sleep, we do not have long gaps in our recent memory record. If the evolutionary purpose of episodic memory is to maintain a record of events, it makes sense that the "recorder keeps running" whenever we are awake. A complementary point is that events recorded in episodic memory need not be physical events occurring in the external world. Mental events, too, can induce extensive semantic processing, executive responses, and emotional responses. Lying in an MRI scanner during periods

of "rest" in an fMRI study, it is not hard to imagine a patient thinking about the experience and how it feels, or composing a list of things to do when the study is over. After the study, it would be surprising indeed if the patient could not recall how the experience felt or the to-do list he or she composed. The ability to do so indicates that these mental events are every bit as "encoded" into episodic memory as are external physical events.

fMRI OF THE MEDIAL TEMPORAL LOBE

MTL activation during memory encoding and retrieval tasks has been a subject of intense research with fMRI (for reviews, see[73–79]). Hippocampal activation has been demonstrated using a variety of task paradigms (eg,[80–100]), although fMRI of this region is not without technical challenges. The hippocampal formation is small relative to typical voxel sizes used in fMRI. Within-voxel averaging of signals from active and inactive structures may thus impair detection of hippocampal activity. Loss of MRI signal in the medial ATL because of macroscopic field inhomogeneity can affect the amygdala and occasionally the anterior hippocampus.[82,101,102] Finally, the baseline condition used in subtraction analyses is of critical importance. Hippocampal encoding processes continue beyond the duration of external stimuli,[103] and human imaging evidence suggests that the hippocampus is relatively activated in the "resting" state.[91,97,104,105] Stark and Squire,[97] for example, showed that the hippocampus and parahippocampus both show higher BOLD signals during "rest" than during active perceptual discrimination tasks. Activation of these MTL regions during encoding of pictures was detected using the perceptual discrimination tasks as a baseline, but not when "rest" was used as a baseline.

MTL fMRI paradigms generally use 1 of 3 approaches. The first of these involves a contrast between encoding novel and repeated stimuli, based on earlier electrophysiological studies showing that the hippocampus responds more strongly to novel than to repeated stimuli.[106–109] The encoding task might involve explicit memorization for later retrieval testing or a decision task designed to produce implicit encoding. Such novelty contrasts mainly activate the posterior parahippocampus and adjacent fusiform gyrus, with involvement of the posterior hippocampus in some but not all studies.[80,101,110–114] The second approach involves manipulating the degree of associative/semantic processing that occurs during encoding. As noted previously, hippocampal encoding is thought to involve the creation of configural representations that tie together sensory, semantic, affective, and other codes activated by an event.[61-63] External events that are meaningful and activate semantic and emotional associations engage the hippocampus more robustly and are thus more effectively recorded.[64] Thus, many fMRI studies have demonstrated hippocampal activation using contrasts between a stimulus or task that engages associative/semantic processing (eg, a word or picture) and a stimulus or task that engages only sensory processing (eg, a nonword or unrecognizable visual form).[80,81,83,88-92,95,96,100,115-117] Finally, a third approach uses subsequent recognition performance as a direct index of MTL activity during encoding. Items encoded during the fMRI scan are sorted according to whether they were later remembered, and a contrast is made between successfully and unsuccessfully encoded items. These studies consistently show greater MTL activation during subsequently remembered compared with subsequently forgotten stimuli, although the precise MTL regions showing this effect have varied considerably.[82,83,85,92,94,99,112,117-121]

Finally, the lateralization of MTL activation detected by fMRI depends on the type of stimulus material encoded. MTL activation is left-lateralized for word stimuli, symmetric for scene stimuli, and generally right-lateralized for face stimuli.[26,80,81,91,92,122-126]

MEDIAL TEMPORAL LOBE fMRI AS A PREDICTOR OF VERBAL MEMORY OUTCOME

The relationship between preoperative MTL activation and memory outcome after ATL surgery has been explored in a number of studies (**Table 1**). Rabin and colleagues[22] examined 23 patients undergoing ATL resection (10 left, 13 right) using a scene-encoding task that activates the posterior MTL bilaterally.[122] Patients were tested for delayed recognition of the same pictures immediately after scanning. Delayed picture recognition was then tested again after surgery, and the change on this recognition task was used as the primary memory outcome variable. About half of the patients in both surgery groups declined on this measure. Preoperative fMRI activation lateralization toward the side of surgery was correlated with decline, as was the extent of activation on the side of surgery. These results were the first to demonstrate a relationship between preoperative fMRI activation asymmetry and outcome, yet they are of limited relevance to the problem of predicting verbal memory outcome. In the left ATL

patients studied by Rabin and colleagues,[22] neither Wada memory nor fMRI activation asymmetry predicted verbal memory decline as measured by standard verbal memory tests.

Powell, and colleagues[127] and Richardson and colleagues[128,129] studied correlations between hippocampal activation and verbal memory outcome in three small studies. Patients performed a semantic decision task with words during the fMRI scan and then took a recognition test after scanning. Words that were subsequently recognized were contrasted with words that were judged to be familiar but not recognized. The aim of these studies was to ascertain whether activation or activation asymmetry in any region of the MTL was related to outcome, rather than to predict outcome per se. Rather than defining an a priori region of interest (ROI), the investigators searched the MTL image space for any voxels where activation, or activation asymmetry, was correlated with memory change scores. The results, although somewhat inconsistent across the studies, suggested that preoperative fMRI activation maps contain information related to memory outcome. It is important to note, however, that the ROIs in these studies were defined post hoc using a group analysis and have varied in location across studies. It is not clear how this method of extracting activation values could be applied to a newly encountered patient.

Frings and colleagues[130] studied the relationship between preoperative hippocampal activation asymmetry and verbal memory outcome in a small sample of patients undergoing left or right ATL resection. The fMRI protocol used a task in which patients viewed a virtual-reality environment containing colored geometric shapes and either memorized the location of these objects or performed a recognition decision following memorization. These "memory tasks" were contrasted with a control task in which patients saw 2 versions of a geometric object and indicated which one was larger. This fMRI contrast had been shown previously to activate posterior MTL regions (mainly posterior parahippocampus) bilaterally. A lateralization index was computed using the entire hippocampus as the ROI. Verbal memory change was marginally correlated (1-tailed $P = .077$) with preoperative laterality index (LI) in the left ATL surgery group, but not in the right surgery group. A significant correlation (1-tailed $P<.05$) was obtained when the groups were combined, indicating greater verbal memory decline with increasing lateralization of activation toward the side of surgery.

Köylü and colleagues[131] examined correlations between preoperative MTL activation and verbal

Table 1
fMRI studies of verbal memory outcome prediction in ATL surgery

Author	Year	N	fMRI Contrast	Memory Measure	Summary
Rabin et al[22]	2004	10 L 13 R	Indoor/outdoor decision on visual scenes vs Passive viewing of scrambled scenes	Recognition of scenes encoded during fMRI; standardized verbal memory tests	MTL laterality index (LI) predicts change in scene memory in both surgery groups, but not change in verbal memory
Richardson et al[129]	2004	10 L	Subsequently Recognized vs Familiar but not recognized words encoded during a semantic decision task	Word list learning and story recall (Adult Memory and Information Processing Battery)	Activation asymmetry in part of the hippocampus is correlated with memory outcome
Richardson et al[128]	2006	12 L	Same as Richardson et al (2004)[129]	Same as Richardson et al (2004)[129]	Unilateral activation in both left and right hippocampus is correlated with memory outcome
Binder et al[25]	2008	60 L	Semantic decision on auditory words vs Sensory decision on tones	Word list learning and delayed recall (Selective Reminding Test)	Language LI predicts verbal memory outcome, adds value beyond other predictors
Frings et al[130]	2008	9 L 10 R	Memorizing and recognizing object locations vs Comparing size of two objects	Word list learning (Verbaler Lern- & Merkfaehigkeitstest)	Hippocampal LI predicts verbal memory outcome, mainly in left group
Köylü et al[131]	2008	14 L 12 R	Semantic decision on auditory words vs Sensory decision on tones	Word list learning and delayed recall (Münchner Gedächtnistest)	MTL activation correlates with pre- and postoperative memory
Powell et al[127]	2008	7 L 8 R	Subsequently Recognized vs Forgotten words and faces encoded during a semantic decision task	Word list learning and visual design learning	Unilateral activation in dominant-side hippocampus is correlated with memory outcome in dominant resection
Binder et al[132]	2010	30 L 37 R	Indoor/outdoor decision on visual scenes vs Perceptual matching of scrambled scenes	Word list learning and delayed recall (Selective Reminding Test)	Hippocampal LI for scenes does not predict verbal memory outcome
Bonelli et al[26]	2010	29 L 25 R	Same paradigm as in Powell et al (2008)[127] for MTL activation Verbal fluency task for frontal lobe language LI	Same as Powell et al (2008)[127]	Anterior and posterior MTL LIs from the word encoding condition predict verbal memory outcome Language LI predicts verbal memory outcome, but less strongly than MTL LIs

memory performance before and after ATL surgery. Average fMRI activation produced by a semantic decision–tone decision contrast was measured in left and right MTL ROIs including the hippocampus and parahippocampus. The investigators observed correlations between MTL activation and both preoperative and postoperative verbal memory. In the left ATL surgery group, postoperative memory was positively correlated with preoperative activation in the right MTL. Unfortunately, the analyses examined only pre- and postoperative scores in isolation and not pre- to postoperative change, which is the primary issue of clinical interest.

Binder and colleagues[132] measured hippocampal activation asymmetry in 30 left and 37 right ATL surgery patients using a scene encoding task. An anterior hippocampal ROI was defined using a probabilistic atlas in standard stereotaxic space. When contrasted with a perceptual matching task, this paradigm activates the anterior hippocampus bilaterally.[80] Activation asymmetry was correlated with side of seizure focus ($P = .004$) and with Wada memory testing performed in the same patients ($P = .009$). This activation asymmetry, however, did not predict verbal memory outcome.

In the most significant study on this topic to date, Bonelli and colleagues[26] examined verbal and nonverbal memory outcome in 29 patients undergoing left ATL surgery. The fMRI paradigm used the subsequent recognition contrast with words and faces developed by Powell and colleagues.[125,127] The investigators operationally defined ROIs in each individual as the location where activation asymmetry was highest. An "asymmetry image" was created in each individual by contrasting activation levels in mirror-symmetric voxels in the left and right temporal lobe. A small sphere around the voxel with the highest asymmetry value was used as the ROI. Two such ROIs were created in each patient, one in the anterior MTL and one in the posterior MTL. The main finding was a strong correlation ($R^2 = 0.23$, $P = .008$) between anterior MTL ROI asymmetry during word encoding and verbal memory change scores, such that the greater the asymmetry toward the left, the greater the decline in verbal memory. Interestingly, there was a significant correlation ($R^2 = 0.14$, $P = .04$) in the opposite direction for the posterior MTL ROI, such that greater asymmetry toward the left was associated with *less* verbal memory decline. Given that the posterior hippocampus is typically spared in ATL resections, the investigators interpret the latter finding as evidence that intrahemispheric recruitment of the posterior left hippocampus in left TLE is important for preservation of verbal memory processes.

These studies are informative in several ways. Three studies[22,130,132] used scene encoding tasks that activate the MTL bilaterally on fMRI, a pattern that suggests activation of both verbal and nonverbal memory encoding systems. Prediction of verbal memory outcome using these paradigms appears to be weak at best. In contrast, the verbal memory fMRI paradigms used by Richardson and colleagues,[128,129] Powell and colleagues,[127] and Bonelli and colleagues[26] provide better predictive information regarding verbal memory outcome. These results provide further support for the long-standing concept of material-specific encoding in the episodic memory system. The results of Bonelli and colleagues,[26] although based on a relatively small sample, are particularly promising and should be confirmed prospectively in a larger group of patients.

LANGUAGE LATERALIZATION AS A PREDICTOR OF VERBAL MEMORY OUTCOME

Binder and colleagues[25] studied the relationship between preoperative language lateralization and verbal memory outcome. The premise underlying this approach is that the verbal episodic memory encoding system is likely to be co-lateralized with language. More generally, the investigators proposed that the type of material encoded by the left or right MTL depends on the type of information it receives from the ipsilateral neocortex. According to this model, language lateralization should be a reliable indicator of verbal memory lateralization and thus should predict verbal memory outcome.

The study included 60 patients who underwent left ATL resection and a control group of 63 right ATL resection patients. The fMRI paradigm used a contrast between an auditory semantic decision task and a nonlinguistic tone decision task. Verbal memory was measured preoperatively and 6 months after surgery using the Selective Reminding Test, a word-list learning and delayed recall test.[133] Testing also included several measures of nonverbal learning and memory. Language LIs were computed from the fMRI data using a large region of interest covering the lateral two-thirds of each hemisphere.[134] All patients also underwent preoperative Wada language and memory testing.

The left ATL surgery group showed substantial changes in verbal memory, with an average raw score decline of 43% on word list learning and 45% on delayed recall of the word list. Of the individual patients, 33% declined significantly on the learning measure and 55% on the delayed recall measure. In contrast, the right ATL surgery group improved slightly on both measures. Neither group showed significant changes on any nonverbal memory tests. The strongest predictor of verbal memory change in the left surgery group was the preoperative score (r = 0.662 for list learning, r = 0.654 for delayed recall). The next strongest predictor was fMRI language LI (r = 0.432 for list learning, r = 0.316 for delayed recall). Wada memory asymmetry was only marginally predictive (r = 0.331 for list learning, r = 0.135 for delayed recall).

In applying these results to real clinical situations, the main questions to resolve are: which tests make a significant independent contribution to predicting outcome, and how should results from these tests be optimally combined? Binder and colleagues[25] addressed these questions in a series of stepwise multiple regression analyses. The first variables entered in all analyses were preoperative test performance and age at onset of epilepsy, as these variables can be obtained at relatively little cost and at no risk to the patient. Next, the fMRI language LI was added, followed by simultaneous addition of both the Wada memory and Wada language asymmetry scores. The rationale for adding fMRI in the second step is that fMRI is noninvasive and carries less risk than the Wada test. The 2 Wada scores were added together in the final step because these measures are typically obtained together.

Preoperative score and age at onset of epilepsy together accounted for 49% of the variance in list learning outcome and 54% of the variance in delayed recall outcome. The fMRI LI explained an additional 10% of the variance in list learning outcome (P = .001) and 7% of the variance in delayed recall outcome (P = .003). Addition of the Wada language and memory data did not improve the predictive power in either case. Used together in a multivariate regression formula, the preoperative score, age at onset, and fMRI LI showed 90% sensitivity and 80% specificity for predicting significant decline on list learning, and 81% sensitivity and 100% specificity for predicting decline on delayed recall.

These results are interesting for several reasons. Most intriguing is the finding that *language* lateralization, whether measured by fMRI or the Wada test, is a better predictor of verbal *memory* outcome than Wada memory testing. The explanation for this apparent paradox rests on 2 hypotheses. One, mentioned previously, is that verbal memory encoding processes tend to co-lateralize with language processes. The second hypothesis is that many tests of memory lateralization do not specifically assess verbal memory

encoding. Visual stimuli, such as objects and pictures, can be dually encoded as both names and visual objects. Wada memory procedures that use such stimuli (including the Wada test used by Binder and colleagues[25]) therefore do not provide a measure of verbal memory lateralization, but rather a measure of overall memory lateralization that includes both verbal and nonverbal encoding processes. Thus, verbal memory lateralization is more tightly linked with language lateralization than with Wada memory asymmetry. Of greatest concern are patients who show marked declines in verbal memory postoperatively despite preoperative Wada testing showing lateralization of memory to the right side. The explanation for these cases is simple: overall memory as measured by the Wada was lateralized to the right, but *verbal* memory remained on the left, a fact that cannot be determined by object memory testing.

Further confirmation of a link between language lateralization and verbal memory outcome comes from the recent study by Bonelli and colleagues,[26] who reported a correlation of r = 0.331 between fMRI language LI and verbal memory change in 29 left ATL surgery patients. Language LI was measured in a frontal ROI using a word generation task contrasted with rest. As noted previously, the investigators also examined activation asymmetry in the MTL during word encoding, which produced a stronger correlation with verbal memory outcome (r = 0.480) than the frontal language LI. Preoperative scores, duration of epilepsy, and left hippocampal volume were all uncorrelated with outcome. In a multivariate regression analysis, MTL activation asymmetry was the only significant predictor, with all other variables, including language LI, failing to contribute additional predictive power. In a final analysis, however, the investigators report that the specificity of an outcome prediction "algorithm" improved from 41% to 86%, and the positive predictive value increased from 35% to 70%, by adding language lateralization and preoperative memory data, suggesting substantial additional predictive value from these variables.

SUMMARY

Two recent studies provide the first strong evidence that preoperative fMRI is clinically useful for predicting verbal memory outcome in left ATL surgery. The larger study used preoperative language dominance to predict verbal memory outcome,[25] whereas the second study used MTL activation asymmetry during word encoding.[26] Both methods predicted about 20% of the variance in outcome when used alone, and both added independent predictive power when combined with other noninvasive measures. The language LI approach of Binder and colleagues[25] is based on activation over a very large ROI, thus the LI might be more stable and reproducible than an LI based on a small MTL ROI, and less susceptible to signal dropout that can affect the MTL. From an economical standpoint, the language LI can also be used to predict naming outcome in left ATL surgery,[135] thus this approach addresses two clinical questions with a single protocol. The advantage of the MTL approach is that it could in theory have higher predictive value, because it lateralizes verbal encoding processes directly rather than indirectly. Results of the MTL approach are still based on a relatively small sample of patients and need to be confirmed in future studies. Future studies should also compare the MTL and language LI approaches in larger samples.

The goal of the studies reviewed here has been to develop methods for quantitative prediction of cognitive risk from ATL surgery. The quantitative nature of these predictions represents something of a paradigm shift, in that traditional predictive models using the Wada test tended to be implemented as a dichotomous "pass or fail" judgment. In addition to examining the role of fMRI, recent studies have increasingly used multivariate models to optimize predictions and to compute predicted change scores (**Fig. 1**). These quantitative predictions provide a much more realistic picture of the actual outcomes, which are not

dichotomous, but vary smoothly along a continuum. Ultimately, of course, the decision whether to undergo surgery is a categorical one, but the categorical nature of the decision does not obviate the need for precision regarding the factors that enter into the decision. A patient disabled by frequent seizures may be willing to tolerate a substantial memory decline for seizure control, whereas a patient who depends on such cognitive abilities for his or her livelihood may be willing to risk a small decline but not a large one.

The availability of fMRI for predicting memory outcome raises further questions about the role of Wada testing in the presurgical epilepsy evaluation.[136,137] fMRI is a safe, noninvasive test that improves prediction accuracy relative to other noninvasive measures. In the study by Binder and colleagues, Wada memory asymmetry was a relatively weak predictor of memory outcome and did not improve prediction accuracy relative to available noninvasive tests, confirming several previous studies that also examined multivariate prediction models.[35,39,49–51] These results call into question the routine use of the Wada test for predicting material-specific verbal memory outcome, particularly if a validated fMRI test is available. Some practitioners use the Wada test to assess risk for global amnesia, which may occur after bilateral MTL damage.[40,60,138,139] According to this theory, anesthetization of the to-be-resected MTL is necessary to discover whether the contralateral hemisphere is healthy enough to support memory on its own. Empirical

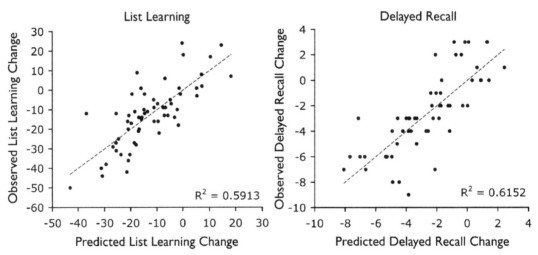

Fig. 1. Predicted versus observed individual memory change scores in 60 left ATL surgery patients on tests of word list learning and delayed recall. Predicted list learning change scores were computed from the formula: 17.67 − 0.704(Preoperative Score) − 0.280(Age at Onset) − 12.19(fMRI LI). Predicted delayed recall change scores were computed from the formula: 3.76 − 0.688(Preoperative Score) − 0.093(Age at Onset) − 2.14(fMRI LI). (*Adapted from* Binder JR, Sabsevitz DS, Swanson SJ, et al. Use of preoperative functional MRI to predict verbal memory decline after temporal lobe epilepsy surgery. Epilepsia 2008;49:1377–94; with permission.)

observations, however, provide little support for such an approach. Cases of global amnesia following unilateral temporal lobe resection, especially modern, well-documented cases, appear to be rare in the extreme.[41,44,46,47,140,141] Furthermore, there is ample evidence that contralateral hemisphere "memory failure" on the Wada test suffers from poor test-retest reliability and does not reliably predict amnesia.[41–47,142,143] Given the availability of fMRI for predicting material-specific verbal memory outcome, perhaps use of the Wada test should be reserved only for those patients at greatest risk for global amnesia, ie, patients undergoing unilateral ATL resection who have structural or functional evidence of damage to the contralateral MTL. Because it is noninvasive and requires fewer personnel, fMRI is also likely to be substantially less costly than the Wada test.[144]

An important caveat to keep in mind is that fMRI is a complex test of higher brain function, which will produce high-quality results only if high-quality methods are used. Unlike a structural imaging study, the patient is required to perform a specific mental task or tasks during fMRI, must understand fully what to do, and must be monitored for compliance during the study. The task conditions must be designed to reliably and specifically identify the mental processes of interest, based on modern scientific evidence about these processes rather than on folk psychology or 19th century neurology. These challenges can best be met through close involvement of cognitive scientists in the design of task protocols and by direct involvement of clinicians with expertise in cognitive testing to provide patient instruction and performance assessment during scanning (see **Fig. 1**).

ACKNOWLEDGMENTS

Thanks to Linda Allen, Thomas Hammeke, Wade Mueller, Conrad Nievera, Ed Possing, Manoj Raghavan, David Sabsevitz, Sara Swanson, and other personnel at the Froedtert-MCW Comprehensive Epilepsy Center for assistance with this research, which was also supported by National Institute of Neurologic Diseases and Stroke grant R01 NS35929, National Institutes of Health General Clinical Research Center grant M01 RR00058, and the Charles A. Dana Foundation.

REFERENCES

1. Babb TL, Lieb JP, Brown WJ, et al. Distribution of pyramidal cell density and hyperexcitability in the epileptic human hippocampal formation. Epilepsia 1984;25:721–8.

2. Cook MJ, Fish DR, Shorvon SD, et al. Hippocampal volumetric and morphometric studies in frontal and temporal lobe epilepsy. Brain 1992;115:1001–5.

3. Van Paesschen W, Connelly A, King MD, et al. The spectrum of hippocampal sclerosis: a quantitative magnetic resonance imaging study. Ann Neurol 1997;41:41–51.

4. Bronen RA, Fulbright RK, King D, et al. Qualitative MRI imaging of refractory temporal lobe epilepsy requiring surgery: correlation with pathology and seizure outcome after surgery. AJR Am J Roentgenol 1997;169:875–82.

5. Cascino GD, Trenerry MR, So EL, et al. Routine EEG and temporal lobe epilepsy: relation to long-term EEG monitoring, quantitative MRI, and operative outcome. Epilepsia 1996;37:651–6.

6. Jack CR, Sharbrough FW, Twomey CK, et al. Temporal lobe seizures: lateralization with MR volume measurements of the hippocampal formation. Radiology 1990;175:423–9.

7. Van Paesschen W, Sisodiya S, Connelly A, et al. Quantitative hippocampal MRI and intractable temporal lobe epilepsy. Neurology 1995;45:2233–40.

8. Manno EM, Sperling MR, Ding X, et al. Predictors of outcome after anterior temporal lobectomy: positron emission tomography. Neurology 1994;44:2331–6.

9. Spencer S. The relative contributions of MRI, SPECT, and PET imaging in epilepsy. Epilepsia 1994;35(Suppl 6):S72–89.

10. Weinand ME, Carter LP. Surface cortical cerebral blood flow monitoring and single photon emission computed tomography: prognostic factors for selecting temporal lobectomy candidates. Seizure 1994;3:55–9.

11. Alpherts WC, Vermeulen J, van Veelen CW. The Wada test: prediction of focus lateralization by asymmetric and symmetric recall. Epilepsy Res 2000;39:239–49.

12. Kanemoto K, Kawasaki J, Takenouchi K, et al. Lateralized memory deficits on the Wada test correlate with the side of lobectomy only for patients with unilateral medial temporal lobe epilepsy. Seizure 1999;8:471–5.

13. Loring DW, Lee GP, Bowden SC, et al. Diagnostic utility of Wada memory asymmetries: sensitivity, specificity, and likelihood ratio characterization. Neuropsychology 2009;23:687–93.

14. Loring DW, Murro AM, Meador KJ, et al. Wada memory testing and hippocampal volume measurements in the evaluation for temporal lobectomy. Neurology 1993;43:1789–93.

15. Perrine K, Westerveld M, Sass KJ, et al. Wada memory disparities predict seizure laterality and postoperative seizure control. Epilepsia 1995;36:851–6.

16. Lancman ME, Banbadis S, Geller E, et al. Sensitivity and specificity of asymmetric recall on Wada

test to predict outcome after temporal lobectomy. Neurology 1998;50:455–9.

17. Loring DW, Meador KJ, Lee GP, et al. Wada memory performance predicts seizure outcome following anterior temporal lobectomy. Neurology 1994;44:2322–4.

18. Sperling MR, Saykin AJ, Glosser G, et al. Predictors of outcome after anterior temporal lobectomy: the intracarotid amobarbital test. Neurology 1994; 44:2325–30.

19. Golby AJ, Poldrack RA, Illes J, et al. Memory lateralization in medial temporal lobe epilepsy assessed by functional MRI. Epilepsia 2002;43: 855–63.

20. Jokeit H, Okujava M, Woermann FG. Memory fMRI lateralizes temporal lobe epilepsy. Neurology 2001; 57:1786–93.

21. Killgore WDS, Glosser G, Casasanto D, et al. Functional MRI and the Wada test provide complementary information for predicting post-operative seizure control. Seizure 2000;8:450–5.

22. Rabin ML, Narayan VM, Kimberg DY, et al. Functional MRI predicts post-surgical memory following temporal lobectomy. Brain 2004;127:2286–98.

23. Squire LR. Memory and the hippocampus: a synthesis from findings with rats, monkeys, and humans. Psychol Rev 1992;99:195–231.

24. Baxendale S, Thompson P, Harkness W, et al. Predicting memory decline following epilepsy surgery: a multivariate approach. Epilepsia 2006; 47:1887–94.

25. Binder JR, Sabsevitz DS, Swanson SJ, et al. Use of preoperative functional MRI to predict verbal memory decline after temporal lobe epilepsy surgery. Epilepsia 2008;49:1377–94.

26. Bonelli SB, Powell RHW, Yogarajah M, et al. Imaging memory in temporal lobe epilepsy: predicting the effects of temporal lobe resection. Brain 2010;133:1186–99.

27. Chelune GJ, Naugle RI, Lüders H, et al. Prediction of cognitive change as a function of preoperative ability level among temporal lobectomy patients at six months follow-up. Neurology 1991;41:399–404.

28. Chelune GJ, Naugle RI, Lüders H, et al. Individual change after epilepsy surgery: practice effects and base-rate information. Neuropsychology 1993;7: 41–52.

29. Chiaravalloti ND, Glosser G. Material-specific memory changes after anterior temporal lobectomy as predicted by the intracarotid amobarbital test. Epilepsia 2001;42:902–11.

30. Gleissner U, Helmstaedter C, Schramm J, et al. Memory outcome after selective amygdalohippocampectomy in patients with temporal lobe epilepsy: one-year follow-up. Epilepsia 2004;45: 960–2.

31. Helmstaedter C, Elger CE. Cognitive consequences of two-thirds anterior temporal lobectomy on verbal memory in 144 patients: a three-month follow-up study. Epilepsia 1996;37:171–80.

32. Hermann BP, Seidenberg M, Haltiner A, et al. Relationship of age at onset, chronologic age, and adequacy of preoperative performance to verbal memory change after anterior temporal lobectomy. Epilepsia 1995;36:137–45.

33. Kneebone AC, Chelune GJ, Dinner DS, et al. Intracarotid amobarbital procedure as a predictor of material-specific memory change after anterior temporal lobectomy. Epilepsia 1995;36:857–65.

34. Lee TMC, Yip JTH, Jones-Gotman M. Memory deficits after resection of left or right anterior temporal lobe in humans: a meta-analytic review. Epilepsia 2002;43:283–91.

35. Lineweaver TT, Morris HH, Naugle RI, et al. Evaluating the contributions of state-of-the-art assessment techniques to predicting memory outcome after unilateral anterior temporal lobectomy. Epilepsia 2006;47:1895–903.

36. Loring DW, Meador KJ, Lee GP, et al. Wada memory asymmetries predict verbal memory decline after anterior temporal lobectomy. Neurology 1995;45:1329–33.

37. Martin RC, Sawrie SM, Roth DL, et al. Individual memory change after anterior temporal lobectomy: a base rate analysis using regression-based outcome methodology. Epilepsia 1998;39: 1075–82.

38. Sabsevitz DS, Swanson SJ, Morris GL, et al. Memory outcome after left anterior temporal lobectomy in patients with expected and reversed Wada memory asymmetry scores. Epilepsia 2001;42: 1408–15.

39. Stroup E, Langfitt JT, Berg M, et al. Predicting verbal memory decline following anterior temporal lobectomy (ATL). Neurology 2003;60:1266–73.

40. Milner B, Branch C, Rasmussen T. Study of short-term memory after intracarotid injection of sodium amytal. Trans Am Neurol Assoc 1962;87:224–6.

41. Kubu CS, Girvin JP, McLachlan RS, et al. Does the intracarotid amobarbital procedure predict global amnesia after temporal lobectomy? Epilepsia 2000;41:1321–9.

42. Lee GP, Loring DW, Smith JR, et al. Intraoperative hippocampal cooling and Wada memory testing in the evaluation of amnesia risk following anterior temporal lobectomy. Arch Neurol 1995;52:857–61.

43. Loddenkemper T, Morris HH, Lineweaver TT, et al. Repeated intracarotid amobarbital tests. Epilepsia 2007;48:553–8.

44. Loring DW, Lee GP, Meador KJ, et al. The intracarotid amobarbital procedure as a predictor of memory failure following unilateral temporal lobectomy. Neurology 1990;40:605–10.

45. Martin RC, Grote CL. Does the Wada test predict memory decline following epilepsy surgery. Epilepsy Behav 2002;3:4–15.

46. Novelly RA, Williamson PD. Incidence of false-positive memory impairment in the intracarotid amytal procedure. Epilepsia 1989;30:711.

47. Simkins-Bullock J. Beyond speech lateralization: a review of the variability, reliability, and validity of the intracarotid amobarbital procedure and its nonlanguage uses in epilepsy surgery candidates. Neuropsychol Rev 2000;10:41–74.

48. Bell BD, Davies KG, Haltiner AM, et al. Intracarotid amobarbital procedure and prediction of postoperative memory in patients with left temporal lobe epilepsy and hippocampal sclerosis. Epilepsia 2000;41:992–7.

49. Chelune GJ, Najm IM. Risk factors associated with postsurgical decrements in memory. In: Luders HO, Comair Y, editors. Epilepsy surgery. 2nd edition. Philadelphia: Lippincott; 2000. p. 497–504.

50. Kirsch HE, Walker JA, Winstanley FS, et al. Limitations of Wada memory asymmetry as a predictor of outcomes after temporal lobectomy. Neurology 2005;65:676–80.

51. Lacruz ME, Alarcon G, Akanuma N, et al. Neuropsychological effects associated with temporal lobectomy and amygdalohippocampectomy depending on Wada test failure. J Neurol Neurosurg Psychiatry 2004;75:600–7.

52. Cohen-Gadol AA, Westerveld M, Alvarez-Carilles J, et al. Intracarotid amytal memory test and hippocampal magnetic resonance imaging volumetry: validity of the Wada test as an indicator of hippocampal integrity among candidates for epilepsy surgery. J Neurosurg 2004;101:926–31.

53. Trenerry MR, Jack CRJ, Ivnik RJ, et al. MRI hippocampal volumes and memory function before and after temporal lobectomy. Neurology 1993;43:1800–5.

54. Wendel JD, Trenerry MR, Xu YC, et al. The relationship between quantitative T2 relaxometry and memory in nonlesional temporal lobe epilepsy. Epilepsia 2001;42:863–9.

55. Griffith HR, Perlman SB, Woodard AR, et al. Preoperative FDG-PET temporal lobe hypometabolism and verbal memory after temporal lobectomy. Neurology 2000;54:1161–5.

56. Baxendale S, Thompson P, Harkness W, et al. The role of the intracarotid amobarbital procedure in predicting verbal memory decline after temporal lobe resection. Epilepsia 2007;48:546–52.

57. Davies KG, Bell BD, Bush AJ, et al. Prediction of verbal memory loss in individuals after anterior temporal lobectomy. Epilepsia 1998;39:820–8.

58. Jokeit H, Ebner A, Holthausen H, et al. Individual prediction of change in delayed recall of prose passages after left-sided anterior temporal lobectomy. Neurology 1997;49:481–7.

59. Milner B. Amnesia following operations on the temporal lobes. In: Whitty CMW, Zangwill OL, editors. Amnesia. London: Butterworth; 1966. p. 109.

60. Scoville WB, Milner B. Loss of recent memory after bilateral hippocampal lesions. J Neurol Neurosurg Psychiatry 1957;20:11–21.

61. Cohen NJ, Eichenbaum H. Memory, amnesia, and the hippocampal system. Cambridge (MA): MIT Press; 1993.

62. McClelland JL, McNaughton BL, O'Reilly RC. Why are there complementary learning systems in the hippocampus and neocortex: insights from the success and failures of connectionist models of learning and memory. Psychol Rev 1995;102:409–57.

63. O'Reilly RC, Rudy JW. Conjunctive representations in learning and memory: principles of cortical and hippocampal function. Psychol Rev 2001;108:311–45.

64. Craik FIM, Lockhart RS. Levels of processing: a framework for memory research. Journal of Verbal Learning and Verbal Behavior 1972;11:671–84.

65. Einstein GO, McDaniel MA, Bowers CA, et al. Memory for prose: the influence of relational and proposition-specific processing. J Exp Psychol Learn Mem Cogn 1984;10:133–43.

66. Kintsch W, Kozminsky E, Streby WJ, et al. Comprehension and recall of text as a function of content variables. Journal of Verbal Learning and Verbal Behavior 1975;14:196–214.

67. Paivio A. Abstractness, imagery, and meaningfulness in paired-associate learning. Journal of Verbal Learning and Verbal Behavior 1965;4:32–8.

68. Paivio A. A factor-analytic study of word attributes and verbal learning. Journal of Verbal Learning and Verbal Behavior 1968;7:41–9.

69. Postman L. Effects of word frequency on acquisition and retention under conditions of free-recall learning. Q J Exp Psychol 1970;22:185–95.

70. Smith MC, Theodor L, Franklin PE. The relationship between contextual facilitation and depth of processing. J Exp Psychol Learn Mem Cogn 1983;9:697–712.

71. Smith SW, Rebok GW, Smith WR, et al. Adult age differences in the use of story structure in delayed free recall. Exp Aging Res 1983;9:191–5.

72. Winnick WA, Kressel K. Tachistoscopic recognition thresholds, paired-associate learning, and immediate recall as a function of abstractness-concreteness and word frequency. J Exp Psychol 1965;70:163–8.

73. Gabrieli JDE. Functional imaging of episodic memory. In: Cabeza R, Kingstone A, editors. Handbook of functional neuroimaging of cognition. Cambridge (MA): MIT Press; 2001. p. 253–91.

74. Hwang DY, Golby AJ. The brain basis for episodic memory: insights from functional MRI, intracranial EEG, and patients with epilepsy. Epilepsy Behav 2006;8:115–26.

75. Paller KA, Wagner AD. Observing the transformation of experience into memory. Trends Cogn Sci 2002;6:93–102.

76. Rugg MD, Otten LJ, Henson RNA. The neural basis of episodic memory: evidence from functional neuroimaging. Philos Trans R Soc Lond B Biol Sci 2002;357:1097–110.

77. Schacter DL, Addis DR. The cognitive neuroscience of constructive memory: remembering the past and imagining the future. Philos Trans R Soc Lond B Biol Sci 2007;362:773–86.

78. Schacter DL, Wagner AD. Medial temporal lobe activations in fMRI and PET studies of episodic encoding and retrieval. Hippocampus 1999;9:7–24.

79. Vilberg KL, Rugg MD. Memory retrieval and the parietal cortex: a review of evidence from a dual-process perspective. Neuropsychologia 2008;46:1787–99.

80. Binder JR, Bellgowan PSF, Hammeke TA, et al. A comparison of two fMRI protocols for eliciting hippocampal activation. Epilepsia 2005;46:1061–70.

81. Binder JR, Frost JA, Hammeke TA, et al. Human brain language areas identified by functional MRI. J Neurosci 1997;17:353–62.

82. Constable RT, Carpentier A, Pugh K, et al. Investigation of the hippocampal formation using a randomized event-related paradigm and z-shimmed functional MRI. Neuroimage 2000;12:55–62.

83. Davachi L, Wagner AD. Hippocampal contributions to episodic memory: insights from relational and item-based learning. J Neurophysiol 2002;88:982–90.

84. Eldridge LL, Knowlton BJ, Furmanski CS, et al. Remembering episodes: a selective role for the hippocampus during retrieval. Nat Neurosci 2000;3:1149–52.

85. Fernandez G, Weyerts H, Schrader-Bölsche M, et al. Successful verbal encoding into episodic memory engages the posterior hippocampus: a parametrically analyzed functional magnetic resonance imaging study. J Neurosci 1998;18:1841–7.

86. Greene AJ, Gross WL, Elsinger CL, et al. An fMRI analysis of the human hippocampus: inference, context, and task awareness. J Cogn Neurosci 2006;18:1156–73.

87. Hassabis D, Kumaran D, Maguire EA. Using imagination to understand the neural basis of episodic memory. J Neurosci 2007;27:14365–74.

88. Henke K, Buck A, Weber B, et al. Human hippocampus establishes associations in memory. Hippocampus 1997;7:249–56.

89. Kensinger EA, Clarke RJ, Corkin S. What neural correlates underlie successful encoding and retrieval? A functional magnetic resonance imaging study using a divided attention paradigm. J Neurosci 2003;23:2407–15.

90. Killgore WD, Casasanto DJ, Yurgelun-Todd DA, et al. Functional activation of the left amygdala and hippocampus during associative encoding. Neuroreport 2002;11:2259–63.

91. Martin A. Automatic activation of the medial temporal lobe during encoding: lateralized influences of meaning and novelty. Hippocampus 1999;9:62–70.

92. Otten LJ, Henson RNA, Rugg MD. Depth of processing effects on neural correlates of memory encoding. Relationship between findings from across- and within-task comparisons. Brain 2001;124:399–412.

93. Parsons MW, Haut MW, Lemieux SK, et al. Anterior medial temporal lobe activation during encoding of words: fMRI methods to optimize sensitivity. Brain Cogn 2006;60:253–61.

94. Prince SE, Tsukiura T, Cabeza R. Distinguishing the neural correlates of episodic memory encoding and semantic memory retrieval. Psychol Sci 2007;18:144–51.

95. Small SA, Nava AS, Perera GM, et al. Circuit mechanisms underlying memory encoding and retrieval in the long axis of the hippocampal formation. Nat Neurosci 2001;4:442–9.

96. Sperling RA, Bates JF, Cocchiarella AJ, et al. Encoding novel face-name associations: a functional MRI study. Hum Brain Mapp 2001;14:129–39.

97. Stark CE, Squire LR. When zero is not zero: the problem of ambiguous baseline conditions in fMRI. Proc Natl Acad Sci U S A 2001;98:12760–6.

98. Vincent JL, Snyder AZ, Fox MD, et al. Coherent spontaneous activity identifies a hippocampal-parietal memory network. J Neurophysiol 2006;96:3517–31.

99. Weis S, Klaver P, Reul J, et al. Temporal and cerebellar brain regions that support both declarative memory formation and retrieval. Cereb Cortex 2004;14:256–67.

100. Zeinah MM, Engel SA, Thompson PM, et al. Dynamics of the hippocampus during encoding and retrieval of face-name pairs. Science 2003;299:577–80.

101. Fransson P, Merboldt KD, Ingvar M, et al. Functional MRI with reduced susceptibility artifact: high-resolution mapping of episodic memory encoding. Neuroreport 2001;12:1415–20.

102. Morawetz C, Holz P, Lange C, et al. Improved functional mapping of the human amygdala using a standard functional magnetic resonance imaging sequence with simple modifications. Magn Reson Imaging 2008;26:45–53.

103. Alvarez P, Squire LR. Memory consolidation and the medial temporal lobe: a simple network model. Proc Natl Acad Sci U S A 1994;91:7041–5.

104. Andreasen NC, O'Leary DS, Cizadlo T, et al. Remembering the past: two facets of episodic memory explored with positron emission tomography. Am J Psychiatry 1995;152:1576–85.

105. Binder JR, Frost JA, Hammeke TA, et al. Conceptual processing during the conscious resting state: a functional MRI study. J Cogn Neurosci 1999;11: 80–93.

106. Grunwald T, Lehnertz K, Heinze HJ, et al. Verbal novelty detection within the human hippocampus proper. Proc Natl Acad Sci U S A 1998;95:3193–7.

107. Knight RT. Contribution of the human hippocampal region to novelty detection. Nature 1996;383:256–9.

108. Li L, Miller EK, Desimone R. The representation of stimulus familiarity in anterior inferior temporal cortex. J Neurophysiol 1993;69:1918–29.

109. Riches IP, Wilson FAW, Brown MW. The effects of visual stimulation and memory on neurones of the hippocampal formation and neighboring parahippocampal gyrus and inferior temporal cortex of the primate. J Neurosci 1991;11:1763–79.

110. Gabrieli JDE, Brewer JB, Desmond JE, et al. Separate neural bases of two fundamental memory processes in human medial temporal lobe. Science 1997;276:264–6.

111. Hunkin NM, Mayes AR, Gregory LJ, et al. Novelty-related activation within the medial temporal lobes. Neuropsychologia 2002;40:1456–64.

112. Kirchhoff BA, Wagner AD, Maril A, et al. Prefrontal-temporal circuitry for episodic encoding and subsequent memory. J Neurosci 2000;20:6173–80.

113. Stern CE, Corkin S, González RG, et al. The hippocampal formation participates in novel picture encoding: evidence from functional magnetic resonance imaging. Proc Natl Acad Sci U S A 1996;93:8660–5.

114. Tulving E, Markowitsch HJ, Crail FIM, et al. Novelty and familiarity activations in PET studies of memory encoding and retrieval. Cereb Cortex 1996;6:71–9.

115. Bartha L, Brenneis C, Schocke M, et al. Medial temporal lobe activation during semantic language processing: fMRI findings in healthy left- and right-handers. Brain Res Cogn Brain Res 2003;17:339–46.

116. Henke K, Weber B, Kneifel S, et al. Human hippocampus associates information in memory. Proc Natl Acad Sci U S A 1999;96:5884–9.

117. Wagner AD, Schacter DL, Rotte M, et al. Building memories: remembering and forgetting of verbal experiences as predicted by brain activity. Science 1998;281:1188–91.

118. Brewer JB, Zhao Z, Desmond JE, et al. Making memories: brain activity that predicts how well visual experience will be remembered. Science 1998;281:1185–8.

119. Buckner RL, Wheeler ME, Sheridan MA. Encoding processes during retrieval tasks. J Cogn Neurosci 2001;13:406–15.

120. Prince SE, Daselaar SM, Cabeza R. Neural correlates of relational memory: successful encoding and retrieval of semantic and perceptual associations. J Neurosci 2005;25:1203–10.

121. Uncapher MR, Rugg MD. Encoding and durability of episodic memory: a functional magnetic resonance imaging study. J Neurosci 2005;25: 7260–7.

122. Detre JA, Maccotta L, King D, et al. Functional MRI lateralization of memory in temporal lobe epilepsy. Neurology 1998;50:926–32.

123. Golby AJ, Poldrack RA, Brewer JB, et al. Material-specific lateralization in the medial temporal lobe and prefrontal cortex during memory encoding. Brain 2001;124:1841–54.

124. Kelley WM, Miezin FM, McDermott KB, et al. Hemispheric specialization in human dorsal frontal cortex and medial temporal lobe for verbal and nonverbal memory encoding. Neuron 1998;20: 927–36.

125. Powell HW, Koepp MJ, Symms MR, et al. Material-specific lateralization of memory encoding in the medial temporal lobe: blocked versus event-related design. Neuroimage 2005;48:1512–25.

126. Reber PJ, Wong EC, Buxton RB. Encoding activity in the medial temporal lobe examined with anatomically constrained fMRI analysis. Hippocampus 2002;12:363–76.

127. Powell HWR, Richardson MP, Symms MR, et al. Preoperative fMRI predicts memory decline following anterior temporal lobe resection. J Neurol Neurosurg Psychiatry 2008;79:686–93.

128. Richardson MP, Strange BA, Duncan JS, et al. Memory fMRI in left hippocampal sclerosis. Optimizing the approach to predicting postsurgical memory. Neurology 2006;66:699–705.

129. Richardson MP, Strange BA, Thompson PJ, et al. Pre-operative verbal memory fMRI predicts postoperative memory decline after left anterior temporal lobe resection. Brain 2004;127:2419–26.

130. Frings L, Wagner K, Halsband U, et al. Lateralization of hippocampal activation differs between left and right temporal lobe epilepsy patients and correlates with postsurgical verbal learning decrement. Epilepsy Res 2008;78:161–70.

131. Köylü B, Walser G, Ischebeck A, et al. Functional imaging of semantic memory predicts postoperative episodic memory functions in chronic temporal lobe epilepsy. Brain Res 2008;1223:73–81.

132. Binder JR, Swanson SJ, Sabsevitz DS, et al. A comparison of two fMRI methods for predicting verbal memory decline after left temporal lobectomy: language lateralization vs. hippocampal activation asymmetry. Epilepsia 2010;51:618–26.

133. Buschke H, Fuld PA. Evaluating storage, retention, and retrieval in disordered memory and learning. Neurology 1974;24:1019–25.

134. Springer JA, Binder JR, Hammeke TA, et al. Language dominance in neurologically normal and epilepsy subjects: a functional MRI study. Brain 1999;122:2033–45.

135. Sabsevitz DS, Swanson SJ, Hammeke TA, et al. Use of preoperative functional neuroimaging to predict language deficits from epilepsy surgery. Neurology 2003;60:1788–92.

136. Baxendale S, Thompson PJ, Duncan JS. The role of the Wada test in the surgical treatment of temporal lobe epilepsy: an international survey (with multi-author commentary). Epilepsia 2008; 49:715–27.

137. Binder JR. Functional MRI is a valid noninvasive alternative to Wada testing. Epilepsy Behav 2010. [Epub ahead of print].

138. Di Gennaro G, Grammaldo LG, Quarato PP, et al. Severe amnesia following bilateral medial temporal lobe damage occurring on two distinct occasions. Neurol Sci 2006;27:129–33.

139. Guerreiro CAM, Jones-Gotman M, Andermann F, et al. Severe amnesia in epilepsy: causes, anatomopsychological considerations, and treatment. Epilepsy Behav 2001;2:224–46.

140. Baxendale S. Amnesia in temporal lobectomy patients: historical perspective and review. Seizure 1998;7:15–24.

141. Kapur N, Prevett M. Unexpected amnesia: are there lessons to be learned from cases of amnesia following unilateral temporal lobe surgery? Brain 2003;126:2573–85.

142. Baxendale SA, Thompson PJ, Duncan JS. A reevaluation of the intracarotid amobarbital procedure (Wada test). Arch Neurol 2008;65: 841–5.

143. Wyllie E, Naugle R, Awad I, et al. Intracarotid amobarbital procedure: I. prediction of decreased modality-specific memory scores after temporal lobectomy. Epilepsia 1991;32:857–64.

144. Medina LS, Aguirre E, Bernal B, et al. Functional MR imaging versus Wada test for evaluation of language lateralization: cost analysis. Radiology 2004;230:49–54.

Transcranial Brain Stimulation: Clinical Applications and Future Directions

Umer Najib, MD[a], Shahid Bashir, PhD[a],
Dylan Edwards, PhD[a,b], Alexander Rotenberg, MD, PhD[a,c],
Alvaro Pascual-Leone, MD, PhD[a,d],*

KEYWORDS

- Transcranial brain stimulation • Brain mapping
- Transcranial magnetic stimulation
- Functional neuroimaging

In human brain mapping, 2 basic strategies are commonly used to obtain information about cortical functional representation: (1) recording brain activity during task performance (the passive approach) and (2) observing the effects of eliciting/extinguishing brain activity (the active approach).[1] Techniques using the passive approach include magnetoencephalography (MEG) and electroencephalography (EEG), which provide direct measures of neuronal activity, and positron emission tomography (PET) and functional magnetic resonance imaging (fMRI), which capture brain hemodynamic and metabolic responses as indirect measures of neuronal activation. For the most part, such approaches fail to provide information about causal relationships between certain cortical regions and behavior or cognition. Furthermore, all these techniques are generally based on changes in brain activity that occur during task performance, and therefore depend on collaboration of the individual and careful behavioral assessments. Resting-state fMRI or EEG measures[2] are valuable, novel approaches to studying brain connectivity and network activity, but their usefulness in cortical output mapping is unclear. On the other hand, the active approach minimizes dependency on the individual's cooperation, because external stimuli are used to elicit or extinguish brain activity, although state-dependent influences on the effects of and responses to brain stimulation need to be considered and controlled for.[3] The active approach investigates whether a specific region of the brain is critical for implementing particular cognitive or behavioral functions and therefore is able to answer questions about causal relationships between brain and function. Noninvasive techniques using such an approach include transcranial electric stimulation (TES) and transcranial magnetic stimulation (TMS).

The noninvasive approach has the advantage of having a greater safety profile and low cost burden for the patients (detailed safety considerations are discussed in later sections). Because of the noninvasiveness of such approaches, they can be repeated as desired, and because

[a] Department of Neurology, Berenson-Allen Center for Noninvasive Brain Stimulation, Beth Israel Deaconess Medical Center, Harvard Medical School, 330 Brookline Avenue, Boston, MA 02215, USA
[b] Non-Invasive Brain Stimulation and the Human Motor Control Laboratory, Burke Medical Research Institute, Inc, 785 Mamaroneck Avenue, White Plains, NY 10605, USA
[c] Division of Epilepsy and Clinical Neurophysiology, Department of Neurology, Children's Hospital, Harvard Medical School, 300 Longwood Avenue, Boston, MA 02115, USA
[d] Institut Guttman de Neurorehabilitació, Institut Universitari, Universitat Autonoma de Barcelona, Camí de Can Ruti s/n, 08916 Badalona, Spain
* Corresponding author. Department of Neurology, Berenson-Allen Center for Noninvasive Brain Stimulation, Beth Israel Deaconess Medical Center, Harvard Medical School, 330 Brookline Avenue, Boston, MA 02215.
E-mail address: apleone@bidmc.harvard.edu

Neurosurg Clin N Am 22 (2011) 233–251
doi:10.1016/j.nec.2011.01.002

stimulation-naive patients get acclimatized to such stimulation techniques quickly, the stress confounders are limited. There is also the added benefit of the lack of medication confounders because most of the noninvasive approaches are based on the underlying activation threshold, thus controlling for the effects of medications on cortical excitability. However, in recent years brain-mapping studies using the passive approach have outnumbered those using the active approach. This situation has been in part because of the problems in correlating the site of stimulation noninvasively to the stimulated cortical region and in part because of the lack of focality of the available noninvasive stimulation devices. The advent of navigated TMS (nTMS) systems has significantly increased the usefulness of TMS in cortical mapping. Such systems can be easily recalibrated after patient movement and, during each stimulation train, the angle and the position of the coil on the scalp can be held constant as verified by real-time visual guidance using the navigation. Using navigation, TMS is able to provide precise information related to the individual's functional anatomy that can be visualized and used during surgical interventions and critically aid in presurgical planning, reducing the need for riskier and more cumbersome intraoperative or invasive mapping procedures. This article reviews the methodological aspects and clinical applications of noninvasive, brain-stimulation-based mapping.

HISTORICAL BACKGROUND

The realization that stimulating/mapping brain areas can guide surgical interventions dates back to Hughlings Jackson, who speculated that the cortex around the central sulcus contained an organized representation of body movements. He suggested that there was a discrete representation of movements of different body parts in this area, and that irritation could produce movements of the corresponding part of the contralateral body. This notion was later confirmed by Fritsch and Hitzig, and then by David Ferrier in the 1870s, who showed that electrical stimulation of the central area in dogs and monkeys could produce movements of the opposite side of the body. Bartholow[4] performed the first stimulation of the human motor cortex a few years later in a patient whose cortex was exposed by a large ulcer on her scalp. This cortical organization was later popularized in the now familiar motor homunculus drawn by Penfield and coworkers (**Fig. 1**).[5,6]

The work of Penfield and colleagues established invasive cortical mapping as a standard tool to

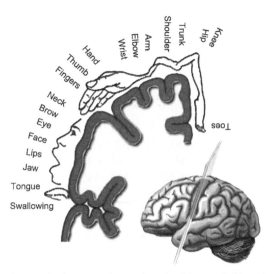

Fig. 1. The homunculus as described by Penfield and Rasmussen. (*Adapted from* Penfield W, Rasmussen T. The cerebral cortex of man. New York: Macmillan; 1950. p. 44, 56, 214–5.)

investigate cortical organization. However, the limited resolution of the early cortical surface stimulation techniques led to the development of better and more advanced stimulation methods such as intracortical microstimulation (ICMS). Nevertheless, all such techniques remained invasive. With the advancement in noninvasive methods of brain stimulation, techniques such as TMS can now be used to leverage the same principle but do so noninvasively, with minimal discomfort to the patients.

Noninvasive brain stimulation provides a valuable tool for interventional neurophysiology applications, modulating brain activity in a specific, distributed, corticosubcortical network so as to induce controlled and controllable manipulations in behavior, as well as for focal neuropharmacology delivery, through the release of neurotransmitters in specific neural networks and the induction of focal gene expression, which may yield a specific behavioral effect. Noninvasive brain stimulation is also a promising treatment of a variety of medical conditions, and the number of applications continues to increase with the large number of ongoing clinical trials in a variety of diseases. Therapeutic usefulness of noninvasive brain stimulation has been claimed in the literature for psychiatric disorders, such as depression, acute mania, bipolar disorders, hallucinations, obsessions, schizophrenia, catatonia, posttraumatic stress disorder, or drug craving; neurologic diseases, such as Parkinson disease (PD), dystonia, tics, stuttering, tinnitus, spasticity, or epilepsy; rehabilitation of aphasia or of hand function after stroke; and pain syndromes, such as those caused by migraine, neuropathies, and low-back pain; or internal visceral diseases, such as chronic pancreatitis or cancer. Although such claims are insufficiently supported by clinical trial data, the potential significance of noninvasive brain stimulation is huge, affecting a large number of patients with debilitating conditions.

In the realm of cortical mapping, the 2 most commonly used techniques for noninvasive brain stimulation are TES and TMS (**Fig. 2**). Such stimulation of the corticobulbar and corticospinal tracts within the brain are used for intraoperative monitoring and for extraoperative diagnostic assessment of central motor pathways. TMS is more useful for extraoperative diagnostic motor-evoked potential (MEP) studies as well as research applications to establish and map causal brain-behavior relations in nonmotor cortical areas. Both TES and TMS depolarize neurons by producing an electrical current within brain parenchyma, although the ways in which these intraparenchymal currents are generated are different. The advantage of TMS is that it does not activate scalp pain fibers as strongly as TES, and it is therefore useful for assessing central motor pathways in conscious individuals. Furthermore, TMS can also be applied to nonmotor regions in the brain convexity. This article focuses on the methodological aspects and clinical application of TMS in cortical mapping.

TMS

TMS mapping of cortical motor areas follows the basic principles of Penfield, and is based on the idea of stimulating different regions of the brain and measuring the modulatory effect (which can be either excitatory or inhibitory). TMS is a noninvasive technique that uses magnetic stimulation to generate electrical current in the cerebral cortex via a device that generates a brief electric current in a coil placed near the patient's head. The electric current in the coil in turn creates a magnetic-field variation of 1.5 to 2 T, which penetrates the skull to about 1.5 to 2.0 cm and reaches the brain. The magnetic field then produces currents changing at rates up to 170 A/μs and induces electric fields in the cortex of up to about 150 V/m. Thus, via electromagnetic induction, TMS painlessly induces ions to flow in the brain without exposing the skull to an electric current.

TMS with a focal figure-of-eight coil can be used to show the gross somatotopy of the motor homunculus. Stimuli are applied at various scalp sites using a latitude/longitude-based coordinate system referenced to the vertex,[7] and the amplitude of MEPs, recorded via electromyography (EMG), evoked in

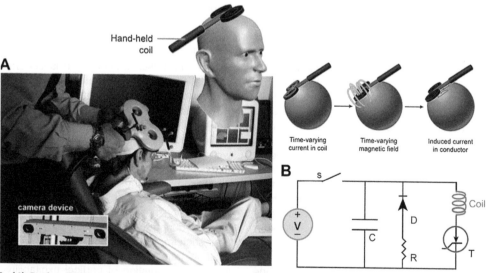

Fig. 2. (A) During TMS, a time-pulsed current is discharged through the TMS coil. The resulting time-varying magnetic field is focused onto underlying neural tissue. The eddying currents, produced in the tissue, can affect the neural activity during and after stimulation. The patient is shown wearing a frameless stereotactic device that can be used to predict the location of stimulation relative to the TMS coil, which is tracked via the camera device (*inset*). (B) A simplified circuit diagram of a single-pulse magnetic stimulator. C, capacitor; D, diode; R, resistor; s, switch; T, thyristor; V, voltage source.

contralateral muscles is measured. This process gives a map of sites on the scalp from which responses can be obtained in each muscle of interest. Specifically, the MEP amplitude data recorded at discrete sites over the motor cortex are transformed to a continuously defined function such that the intermediate values are estimated[7,8] (see article by Thickbroom on mapping elsewhere in this issue for details). The target muscle representation then has a maximum value (optimal site), a center of gravity (CoG) (elements of the representation exceeding 50% of the maximum are used to form a weighted average of their location, in which the weights are given by the normalized value of the element), and a surface area (area where amplitude exceeds 50% of maximum). One of the advantages of this mapping technique is that the optimal site is determined by data from multiple sites, rather than selecting 1 site of largest response. This method has a resolution sufficient to distinguish the optimal site for 2 muscles within the same hand.[8]

Mapping performed with TMS can thus be used to reveal the size of the corticospinal representation of a particular muscle at a given stimulus intensity. As cortical representation increases, the current depolarizes a greater number of cortical cells (in part because of increased current spread), resulting in a steeper curve. Changes in motor cortical maps are also reflected in changes in the slope of stimulus-response curves. Increased excitability of the corticospinal projection is evident from larger MEPs, resulting in a steeper slope of stimulus-response curves and greater area of the representational map.

TMS has developed into a technique that allows the closest noninvasive approximation to electrical cortical stimulation. There have been numerous general reviews of the technique and of the potential for TMS in studies and treatment in neurorehabilitation.[9] Although modeling TMS effects on the brain is an area of active research, the current standard approach is to examine simple maps of responses and determine the CoG and a metric of map size. The CoG is a useful metric because it gives each location stimulated a weight based on the size of the response there. Because the CoG is the result of so many data points, it has a low standard error and high degree of reproducibility. It can be determined with millimeter accuracy, but has no bearing on the spatial extent of the representation. For that purpose, the map volume is often used, which is a sum of the average MEP at each location stimulated, normalized to the average MEP at the location of the largest response. The map volume thus varies from 1, indicating a response at only 1 location, to N, where N is the number of locations in which any response is

measured. Stimulation is generally performed at a fixed percentage of the motor threshold, the stimulus strength that elicits measurable MEP in at least half the stimulations.[10] Map volume can be a confusing term, because it refers to the volume of a contour graph constructed on the scalp surface, but represents the area in which stimulation evokes a response.

The area of the map is more difficult to interpret because the site of stimulation with TMS is considerably less focal than that excited via electrodes placed on the cortical surface. The area of a TMS map is therefore a function of both the area of the underlying corticospinal map and the distance from the coil that corticospinal neurons can be activated. One consequence of this situation is that the higher the intensity of the TMS stimulus, the larger the area of the MEP map. In addition, the higher the excitability of the cortical neurons, the easier it is to stimulate them at a distance from the coil. Again, the apparent area of the MEP map is larger than if excitability is low. Levels of excitability are particularly problematic in mapping studies that are performed in individuals who are at rest. The excitability of the corticospinal system in individuals at rest is ill defined: neurons can be quiescent because they are 1 mV from firing threshold or because they are 10 mV from threshold. In the former case, excitability is higher and the MEP map larger than in the latter. In addition to cortical excitability, the area of MEP maps also depends on the excitability of spinal mechanisms. Mapping of the patient typically takes place with the individual at rest, the coil placed tangentially on the scalp with the handle pointing backward and perpendicular to the central sulcus (**Fig. 3**). After determination of resting motor threshold of the small hand muscles, stimulation is performed at stimulation sites approximately 2 mm apart over an array centered on the central sulcus.

At times, the induced electrical charge after single-pulse TMS is often insufficient to disrupt cortical activity. Instead, repetitive TMS (rTMS) with fast repetition rates is necessary to map these functions. rTMS provides a new window into brain function by creating transient deficits in normal individuals. The higher the stimulation frequency and intensity, the greater is the disruption of cortical function during the train of stimulation. However, after such immediate effects during the TMS train itself, a train of repetitive stimulation can also induce a modulation of cortical excitability. This effect may range from inhibition to facilitation, depending on the stimulation variables (particularly frequency of stimulation).[11] Lower frequencies of rTMS, in the 1-Hz range, can suppress excitability of the motor cortex,[11,12] whereas 20-Hz stimulation

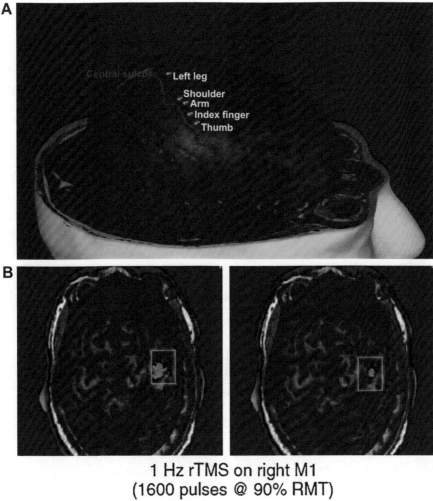

1 Hz rTMS on right M1
(1600 pulses @ 90% RMT)

Fig. 3. (*A*) Head model showing right M1 mapping performed in a healthy individual for upper and lower limb. Each mark represents the hot spot for the muscle mapped. The position of the head of the mark represents the direction of stimulation. The brain is peeled to a depth of 25 mm (ie, the visualized stimulation surface resides at this depth from the scalp). (*B*) Comparison between navigated (*right*) and nonnavigated (*left*) stimulation (1 Hz rTMS) performed in the same individual, on the same target. Note that in the navigated intervention, the dispersion of the stimuli is less and it is more focal than the nonnavigated intervention.

trains seem to lead to a temporary increase in cortical excitability.[12,13]

Advantages of nTMS

Recent advances in image processing have allowed the refinement of current TMS-mapping strategies by combining MRI modalities with TMS using a three-dimensional (3D) digitizer to measure the position of the stimulating coil and map this position onto an MRI data set. A frameless stereotactic system (FSS) that is rigidly fixated to the stimulating coil is used to correlate scalp stimulation sites to the underlying brain anatomy in real time (**Fig. 4**A). The anatomic accuracy as provided by

MRI is combined thereby with the functional motor specificity provided by TMS to introduce stereotactic or nTMS as a new brain-mapping modality. The accuracy of this new technique has been validated by correlating nTMS maps to cortical output maps obtained with direct electrical cortical stimulation (DECS)[14] and to fMRI motor output maps.[15] In addition to the structure-function correlation of nTMS, this technique further allowed for integration of different brain-mapping methodologies by providing a common coordinate system for fMRI and DECS maps.

Coregistration of anatomic MRI data to the sites of stimulation during the TMS session is obtained with the aid of an FSS. This system consists of a

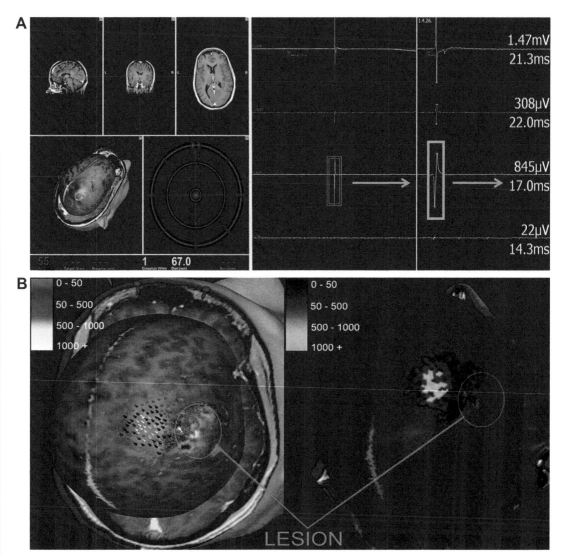

Fig. 4. (*A*) An nTMS system user interface. (*Left panel*) The interface allows the user to identify and select stimulation targets based on the patient's anatomic or functional imaging. It also generates a 3D head model (*bottom left*) for accurate estimation of the target electric field strength. The targeting system (*bottom right*) allows the user to stimulate with enhanced spatial resolution. The position feedback indicator provides real-time feedback surface location, roll, pitch, and yaw of the coil, for consistent and reliable targeting. (*Right panel*) Online EMG recording, along with a modifiable epoch view (*right half*). A single evoked response is measured as peak-to-peak amplitude and onset latency. ADM, abductor digiti minimi; APB, abductor pollicis brevis; ECR, extensor carpi radialis. (*B*) Presurgical cortical maps produced in a patient with right parietal lesion. EMG amplitude-based map on the left side can be viewed only in the navigated brain stimulation system. Amplitude-weighted maps on the right side can be viewed in any third-party imaging system capable of reading DICOM (digital imaging and communications in medicine) images.

jointed mechanical arm, functioning as a stereotactic 3D digitizer, and a computer workstation. Optical encoders in the arm continually measure the angular position of the arm and transmit this information to the computer-graphics workstation, where the spatial position of the tip of the arm is computed in real time and plotted on the MRI data set of the individual's head. The individual's head is spatially coregistered to the MRI by means of fiducial markers that are identified on both the MRI data set after imaging is completed and the head during the TMS session. From those 2 sets of coordinates, a matrix transformation is calculated that allows the computer to display the coordinates of the arm tip on the 3D MRI in real time.[16,17]

Recent studies have highlighted the usefulness of such real-time navigation in identifying cortical motor representation (see **Fig. 4**B). Säisänen and colleagues[18] showed that TMS readily identified the primary motor area when it was impossible to elucidate, from visual inspection alone, where the central region was located. The localization was confirmed via DECS during open brain surgery. The same study showed in another patient in whom both fMRI and nTMS were obtained preoperatively to identify the cortical representation of the tongue muscles, fMRI showed a large cortical region after motor activation of the tongue extending to postcentral areas, whereas nTMS exclusively identified precentral cortical regions. It was hypothesized that the postcentral areas identified by fMRI were caused by sensory coactivation during the performance of the task. This assumption was confirmed during open brain surgery, in which MEPs were elicited only from the precentral cortical areas as previously identified by nTMS.

INTEGRATION OF TMS WITH OTHER BRAIN-MAPPING TECHNIQUES

Neuroimaging techniques, commonly used to acquire functional cortical representation, such as fMRI, PET, EEG, or MEG, have limitations. fMRI and PET provide indirect measures of brain activity with low temporal resolution. EEG and MEG lack in spatial resolution. None of these methods can provide true insights into causal relations between brain activity and behavior. However, combining such neuroimaging and neurophysiologic methods with TMS offers unique advantages: (1) MRI or PET activation can guide where to stimulate and (2) real-time EEG recording can guide when to stimulate.

For example, Sack and colleagues[19] used neuronavigated TMS to quantify the interindividual variance in the exact location of human middle temporal complex (hMT/V5+) and the respective TMS target position on the skull of the study participants. These investigators showed that targets for

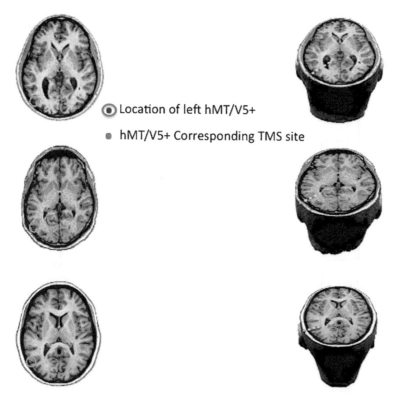

Location of left hMT/V5+

hMT/V5+ Corresponding TMS site

Fig. 5. Axial slices through head reconstructions showing the hMT/V5+ stimulation site (*green sphere*) relative to motion-specific activation, representing the location of hMT/V5+ (*red sphere*; calculated using a motion-mapping paradigm; for details see text). The yellow spheres visualize the orientation of the TMS coil. The imagined line through the spheres corresponds to the normal vector originating from the TMS focus (distance between spheres is 1 cm). (*Data from* Sack AT, Kohler A, Linden DE, et al. The temporal characteristics of motion processing in hMT/V5+: combining fMRI and neuronavigated TMS. Neuroimage 2006;29(4):1326–35.)

TMS application can be reliably selected by individual activation patterns from an fMRI experiment (**Fig. 5**). Area hMT/V5+ was identified in individual participants using a motion-mapping paradigm. Anatomic and fMRI data were coregistered with stereotaxic data from the participants' heads, and TMS was applied to the individually defined stimulation sites. TMS at hMT/V5+ but not at a parietal control site led to a significant reduction of correct motion discriminations in an early (−40 to −30 ms) and a late (130–150 ms) time window. In such paradigms, using individual neuronavigation proves to be an important methodological improvement because, first, the exact location of hMT/V5+ can vary considerably between participants and, second, moving phosphenes, which are used to identify hMT/V5+ functionally, can be produced only in a small percentage of participants.[20] Such a methodological approach enables us to reveal and quantify the interindividual variance in the exact location of the target cortex and the respective TMS target position on the skull of the participants.

Since epileptiform spikes were shown in epileptics by Fisher and Lowenback in 1934, the use of EEG in a clinical setting has grown to include other areas such as sleep disorders, strokes, infectious diseases, brain tumors, mental retardation, severe head injury, drug overdose, and brain death.[21] EEG is especially useful in exploring the virtual lesions caused by TMS (areas where normal operation is disrupted), which are not limited to the stimulated spot but distributed along the neuronal network.[22,23] Furthermore, a growing number of studies indicate that the effects of TMS depend on the state of neuronal activation in the targeted brain region at time of stimulation.[3,22,23] Thus it is conceivable that individual EEG, which is carrying useful information to infer momentary brain state across time and participants, can be used for tailoring TMS effects by fine-tuning the time of stimulation (**Fig. 6**). The notion of EEG-gated TMS to maximize therapeutic efficacy is appealing; however, future studies of TMS coupled with real-time EEG (TMS-EEG) are needed to address this point.

On the other hand, although fMRI has revealed much about the processing in the human brain, it can provide insight only into the brain areas associated with a given behavior, failing to establish a causal relation between brain activity and behavior. To bridge the gap between association and causality it is necessary to disrupt the activity and assess the effect on behavior. fMRI cannot tell the neurosurgeon that lesioning a given brain region, whether it shows activation during a task or not, will cause a postsurgical deficit. The combination of fMRI with TMS can provide such insight.[24]

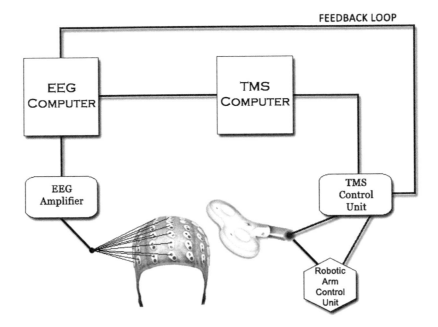

Fig. 6. A combined TMS-EEG system. Note that in addition to triggering TMS using criteria based on online EEG recording (such as a specific event-related potential), TMS triggering can be used to control EEG recording as well (such as momentary stoppage of EEG recording immediately after a TMS pulse to prevent saturation of EEG amplifiers because of excessive voltages induced between the leads because of the magnetic field).

CLINICAL APPLICATIONS OF TMS MAPPING

Over the last 2 decades, several studies have used TMS mapping in a wide range of experimental conditions. In addition to providing insights into the state of cortical representation in healthy individuals, TMS mapping has been used in studying the evolution of various pathologic conditions. Some of the most relevant neurosurgical uses of TMS mapping have been in patients with brain tumors, cerebral palsy, epilepsy, and stroke.

Tumor Mapping

Motor mapping

DECS is considered the gold standard for functional mapping of the motor cortex; however, for the planning of surgical approaches and procedures, preoperative functional maps of the motor cortex are required as well. Furthermore, in some cases the ability to precisely locate functional areas can become a determinant for feasibility of the neurosurgical intervention. Traditionally, most of the perioperative functional analysis has been dependent on recording regional differences in metabolic or electric activity during patient movement by means of fMRI, PET, MEG, and EEG. Although fMRI in particular has found widespread use in the preoperative planning, recent evidence points out the shortcomings of this technique because of the pathologic vessel architecture and the space-consuming effect in the tumor area, which make the interpretation of the fMRI data difficult.[25–27] Moreover, it remains unclear whether or not the activated areas are essential for the function.

More recently nTMS has been used for the functional mapping of the motor cortex in multiple studies[28–31] and has shown analogous functional testing to direct current stimulation (DCS) (**Fig. 7**). Although a spatial resolution of 5 mm is reported with TMS,[29,32] and spatial resolution may be even better with newer navigated systems, doubt regarding the spatioanatomic resolution of TMS remains, mainly because activation of the corticospinal tract is, in part, mediated transsynaptically through cortical interneurons.[33] **Table 1** summarizes the major studies using TMS mapping as a perisurgical functional assessment tool. Data suggest strong correlation between the maps obtained through TMS and DCS (see **Table 1**), by showing that the specification of the position of the tumor in relation to the central sulcus is consistent between the 2 modalities. TMS is found to be useful not only in the preoperative functional mapping of the motor strip but also in the preoperative planning of the operative approach and intraoperative planning of the direction of brain retraction and operative corridor.

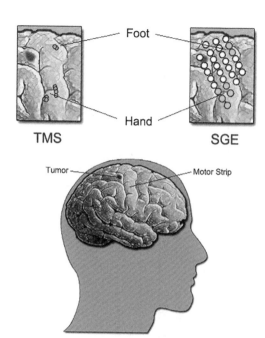

Fig. 7. Head-model recreation of a comparison between navigated brain stimulation (*left*) and direct cortical stimulation (*right*) in a patient with right parietal tumor. Yellow marks on the TMS panel represent the hot spots for hand and lower-limb muscles. Green dots on the SGE grid represent points that resulted in responses from hand and lower limb. SGE, subdural grid electrodes.

Mapping of language areas

Tumors located in the proximity of the language areas represent a special challenge for neurosurgeons. Involvement of the language functions with defined anatomic structures is not enough for the preservation of speech, because of variability of the cortical organization and distortion of the brain convolutions and fibers as a consequence of the mass effect of the tumor, as well as the functional reorganization related to neuroplasticity in the adaptation to the insult.[39–41] Of the various methods used to study language areas, DCS remains the most accurate method but as with other tumor resection procedures, it is associated with prolonged operative time, awake craniotomy, and discomfort for the patients. Conventionally, the intracarotid amobarbital procedure, more commonly known as the Wada test, has been used in the assessment of language lateralization; however, this test has major shortcomings because of its invasiveness, lack of standardization, absence of spatial resolution, and difficulties related to its application and interpretation.[42–44] In addition to the use of TMS in investigations of the motor system, high-frequency rTMS (20 Hz), which can cause transient deficits, has been used in the determination of the lateralization of motor speech

Table 1
Major studies using TMS mapping as a perisurgical functional assessment tool

Studies	Techniques Used for Cortical Mapping	Areas Mapped	n	Diagnoses	Side Effects of Mapping	Surgical Implications and Insights
Focal Lesions						
Krings et al,[29] 1997	nTMS MRI DCS	M1 (tongue and hand area) Left hemisphere	2	1 oligodendroglioma 1 mixed astrocytoma and oligodendroglioma	None reported	TMS mapping helpful in surgical planning One patient had temporary word-finding difficulty for several days Distance between optimal point determined via TMS and DCS = 2.5 mm (average); 0–4.7 mm (range)
Krings et al,[1] 2001	nTMS MRI fMRI	M1	10	–	None reported	TMS mapping helpful in surgical planning No major postoperative complications reported Distance between optimal point determined via TMS and fMRI = 0.6 cm (average); 0–1.2 cm (range)
Picht et al,[30] 2009	nTMS MRI DCS	M1 (hand area) Bilateral	10	3 gliomas 1 meningioma 3 glioblastma 3 metastasis	None reported	TMS mapping helpful in surgical planning No major postoperative complications reported Distance between optimal point determined via TMS and DCS = 3.4 mm (average); 0–7 mm (range)
Juenger et al,[34] 2009	nTMS MRI MEG fMRI DCS SEP	M1 (hand area) Bilateral	1	AVM	None reported	TMS mapping helpful in surgical planning No major postoperative complications reported
Shamov et al,[31] 2010	rTMS MRI CT	Opercular area Left hemisphere	5	5 gliomas	None reported	TMS mapping helpful in surgical planning 3 patients had transient postoperative motor aphasia, which resolved within 1 month Mean operative time reduced from 7 h (without TMS) to 3 h 40 min (for tumors >50 cm^3) with TMS

Study	Methods	Site	n	Pathology	Complications	Comments
Kantelhardt et al,[28] 2010	R-nTMS, MRI, fMRI, DCS	M1 (hand area), Bilateral	5	1 meningioma (grade 1), 1 astrocytoma (grade 2), 1 astrocytoma (grade 3), 2 glioblastomas (grade 4)	Focal seizure in 1 patient: mapping discontinued	TMS mapping helpful in surgical planning. No major postoperative complications reported. Distance between optimal point determined via TMS and DCS <5 mm (1 patient) Preresection DCS not performed in the rest
Epilepsy						
Rutten et al,[35] 2002	nTMS, MRI, fMRI	M1 (hand area), Bilateral	1	Left hemispheric stroke resulting in epilepsy/cortical atrophy	None reported	TMS mapping helpful in surgical planning. No major postoperative complications reported
Kamida et al,[98] 2003	TMS, MRI, DCS, SEPs	M1, Bilateral	5	Intractable epilepsy and hemiplegia	None reported	TMS mapping helpful in surgical planning. No major postoperative complications reported
Vitikainen et al,[36] 2009	nTMS, MRI, fMRI, DCS	M1, Bilateral	2	Intractable epilepsy	None reported	TMS mapping helpful in surgical planning. No major postoperative complications reported
Barba et al,[37] 2010	TMS, fMRI, SEPs	M1, Bilateral	1	Intractable epilepsy and left perisylvian polymicrogyria	None reported	TMS helpful in defining the relationship between epileptogenic zones and somatomotor areas. Surgery not performed because multimodal assessment suggested that removal of the polymicrogyric cortex would have caused severe deficits
Schmidt et al[38] 2010	nTMS, MRI	M1, Bilateral	1	Intractable epilepsy, somatosensory auras, and epilepsia partialis continua	None reported	TMS mapping helpful in surgical planning. No major postoperative complications reported

Abbreviations: AVM, arteriovenous malformation; CT, computed tomography; R-nTMS, robot assisted nTMS; SEP, somatosensory evoked potential.

with high concordance to the Wada test.[45,46] Tokimura and colleagues[47] have suggested an alternative approach to identify the dominant hemisphere with single-pulse TMS to measure the increase in motor-cortical excitability of the dominant (but not of the nondominant) hemisphere during language tasks. In any case, the correlation of TMS results with those of the Wada test is high but not fully satisfactory for a complete presurgical assessment.[46,48] However, Shamov and colleagues[31] have recently reported that using TMS for presurgical planning, the operative time was reduced from an average of 7 hours (using DCS) to an average time of 3 hours and 40 minutes (using TMS) in patients with opercular tumors with a volume more than 50 cm^3. The usefulness of TMS in such cases is augmented by the fact that studies looking at the use of fMRI for functional mapping of the language areas have shown discrepancies between DCS and fMRI results. For example, Giussani and colleagues[49] report the contradictory results when speech zone was mapped using DCS in comparison with fMRI mapping. This data inconsistency could be because DCS suppresses the projection fibers, whereas fMRI depicts the increased deoxygenated hemoglobin in the areas with an increased metabolic activity.

Beyond cortical mapping: promoting presurgical plasticity to optimize surgical outcomes

Repeated surgery of low-grade gliomas with DCS and serial fMRI studies have shown that the cortical location of certain eloquent functions can be displaced as a consequence of the tumor growth.[50,51] This situation occurs when the tumor grows slowly (compared with a quicker onset of symptoms as in high-grade gliomas)[50] and apparently there is not a predictable pattern of reorganization.[52] A great advantage for increasing the extent of tumor resection would occur if we could artificially promote the displacement of eloquent functions in a quicker and more ordered way away from the vicinity of tumors. For example, it can thus be hypothesized that using high-frequency TMS, thetaburst stimulation, it might be possible to promote reorganization by disrupting the activity of the Broca area. Such reorganization might lead to compensatory changes away from the peritumoral area, which could minimize the postoperative deficit. Barcia and colleagues[53] have recently reported a case of 59-year-old woman operated for a left-sided precentral oligodendroglioma, which affected language areas. The patient was submitted to rTMS directed to the Broca area, next to the anterior pole of the tumor, with the aim of provoking a relay of potentially ancillary motor language areas

that could justify a complete tumor removal. Twelve daily sessions of thetaburst rTMS followed by intensive language rehabilitation were performed. Although the initial expectation of anatomic displacement of the Broca area was not met, the experiment data showed modification in the language motor function, especially in repetition and denomination. The investigators concluded that this effect of rTMS could be potentially used to displace the topographic location of language cortical representation. Further studies seem warranted to examine the potential feasibility of such an approach to promote plasticity as a strategy to minimize postsurgical disability and maximize surgical resection.

Epilepsy

Functional mapping before respective epilepsy surgery

Patients with epilepsy who are candidates for resective surgery and whose seizure focus lies close to the eloquent cortex require accurate preoperative functional mapping of the epileptogenic zone and the surrounding area. The standard of care for preoperative functional localization is DCS via subdural electrodes. In this setting, preoperative functional mapping using nTMS can noninvasively localize the sensorimotor cortex and can determine its spatial relationship to the seizure focus.

Detailed preoperative nTMS mapping is particularly well founded when the epileptogenic focus is located near the sensorimotor cortex, and in instances in which cortical malformation might have altered the anatomic organization of the motor representation. In support of this approach, Vitikainen and colleagues[36] used nTMS mapping in epilepsy patients who subsequently underwent a week-long intracranial recording evaluation via subdural electrodes and resective surgery. These investigators showed that nTMS produced spatially more precise mapping of the motor cortical representations than subdural electrode DCS, and proposed that nTMS mapping should be added to the standard preoperative workup. Given that some morbidity and substantial financial cost are associated with any length of time that subdural electrodes are implanted, nTMS preoperative mapping may translate to improved efficiency of the epilepsy workup before respective surgery.

TMS in spike provocation

TMS-EEG has potential as a neurologic stressor to provoke epileptiform activity in a vulnerable cortical region. The usefulness of such TMS application in general may be to identify patients with lowered seizure threshold, but particularly with nTMS, a plausible application may be to enhance seizure focus mapping. Epileptiform discharge provocation by TMS has been shown in patients with epilepsy, but early results suggested that TMS was no more likely than hyperventilation to activate a seizure focus.[54–56] However, more recently, Valentin and colleagues[57] applied single-pulse TMS-EEG to patients with focal epilepsy and to a group of healthy controls. The investigators identified 2 broad categories of electrographic-evoked response: an early (<100 millisecond) slow-wave response and a late (100–1000 millisecond) response, which was either epileptiform in morphology (resembling a sharp wave or spike) or was characterized by rhythmical EEG activity. Although the early responses were present in all patients, the late epileptiform responses were detected only in patients with complex partial seizures. These late discharges often appeared similar to the patients' habitual spikes or sharp waves and were lateralized to the epileptogenic hemisphere in most cases. Moreover, in some instances in which epileptiform abnormalities were triggered by TMS, the interictal scalp EEG was normal.[57] As Valentin and colleagues propose, these data raise the prospects for eventual applications of TMS-EEG to enhance the sensitivity of the scalp EEG in detecting epileptiform abnormalities. Whether and to what extent nTMS can enhance the spatial resolution of seizure focus localization is the work of ongoing experiments. However, if sufficiently sensitive and specific, nTMS seizure focus localization, like nTMS presurgical functional mapping, may translate to a reduced number of subdural electrodes and a shorter invasive recording time, and thus reduced morbidity and economic cost.

Beyond cortical mapping: modulating cortical excitability with therapeutic intent

A further conceivable application of TMS in evaluation of epilepsy is its potential to reduce cortical excitability and by this means raise the seizure threshold. The mechanisms that underlie therapeutic effects of rTMS are not entirely known, but seem to resemble those of long-term depression and long-term potentiation of synaptic strength that result from low- or high-frequency electrical brain stimulation, respectively.[58,59] In epilepsy, the inhibitory effect of low ($\leq$1 Hz) rTMS is most widely used to suppress seizures, with encouraging antiepileptic results in open-label trials.[60–62] Yet, results from placebo-controlled trials are mixed, with 1 trial reporting a reduction in seizures and improvement of the EEG,[63] and 2 others reporting insignificant clinical improvement, or improvement of the EEG without a significant reduction of seizures.[64,65] Similarly, results from open-label rTMS applications in ongoing seizures of epilepsia partialis continua are

mixed with some instances of seizure termination after rTMS, and other instances of continued seizures despite stimulation.[66]

The partial efficacy of rTMS in seizure suppression may relate to suboptimal targeting of the seizure focus. Here, nTMS may be useful in targeting more precisely a radiographically apparent seizure focus such as a tumor or a cortical dysplasia.

Stroke

Functional mapping in poststroke recovery

The molecular and cellular changes after stroke are reflected by a significant reorganization of the postlesion motor cortical map. The pattern of the postlesion map depends on the initial lesion size and on its precise position in the brain. Frost and colleagues[67] showed that the smaller the damage to M1, the less compensatory reorganization was seen in the ventral premotor cortex (PMv). An animal model has shown that destroying 33% of the M1 hand area does not promote observable changes in PMv, as seen with larger lesions.[68] As a consequence of that finding, reorganization of motor cortical maps induced by small M1 lesions is not necessarily easy to detect by custom stimulation/imaging techniques outside the core of the lesion. Nevertheless, many postlesion stimulation studies with ICMS (monkeys, rats) or TMS (humans) have provided insight into motor cortical reorganization. Such insights prove invaluable for surgical planning in patients who have undergone such reorganization after stroke.

TMS mapping provides dual insight in tracking recovery after stroke. In addition to providing information about the processes arising naturally during stroke recovery, it also allows for the investigation of poststroke brain plasticity that may result from therapeutic interventions. For example, studies have shown that the arm- or hand-muscle MEP amplitudes measured soon after a stroke can predict the degree of behavioral recovery weeks to months later.[69–73] Others suggest that stroke alters intracortical excitability[73] (as measured by the paired-pulse TMS paradigms) and successful recovery is associated with normalization of these measures.[74] Moreover, rTMS can be used to determine whether a particular region participates in a recovered function by assessing whether focal stimulation of that region alters behavior.[12,75]

Beyond cortical mapping: modulating cortical excitability with therapeutic intent

TMS can also be used to modulate cortical excitability and corticocortical and corticosubcortical connectivity with therapeutic intent. For example, there is increasing evidence that during voluntary movement generation after stroke, the interhemispheric inhibitory drive from the unaffected to the affected motor cortex is abnormal.[76] Acutely after a stroke, increased inhibitory input from the healthy to the lesioned hemisphere may develop as the neural attempt to control perilesional activity. However, after the acute phase we might expect a shift of interhemispheric interactions from inhibitory to excitatory to maximize the capability of the preserved neurons in the injured tissue to drive behavioral output. Should such a shift fail to take place, the resulting functional outcome may be undesirable, with limited behavioral restoration, in part because of persistent inhibitory inputs from the healthy to the injured hemisphere. Some neuroimaging studies show that long-term, persistent activation of the ipsilateral cortex during motor tasks is associated with poor motor outcomes, whereas a good motor recovery is associated with a decrease in activity of the unaffected motor cortex, and an increase in the affected primary sensorimotor cortex activity.[77,78] Leveraging this information, one can conceive that suppression of the ipsilateral motor cortex through low-frequency (inhibitory) rTMS may enhance motor performance in patients who have stabilized after the acute phase of stroke. Mansur and colleagues[79] showed that in patients 1 to 2 months after a stroke, 0.5 Hz rTMS for 10 minutes to the unaffected hemisphere can suppress cortical activity and release the damaged hemisphere from potentially excessive transcollosal inhibition. Longitudinal studies with larger samples of patients after a stroke and correlation of interhemispheric interactions with functional measures are needed to further explore these avenues.

Other Clinical Applications of TMS Mapping

Chronic pain

The principle of mapping the cortex to gain insight into cortical reorganization can be applied to other clinical conditions as well. In chronic neuropathic pain, studies have shown a reduction of intracortical inhibition in the contralateral hemisphere. This disinhibition has been shown to be more pronounced in patients with moderate/severe pain intensity than in patients with mild pain intensity.[80,81] Krause and colleagues[82] have shown that in patients with complex regional pain syndrome, the cortical representation (size, MEP, and calculated volumes) is significantly larger for the unaffected hand than for the affected hand. Furthermore, in patients with low-back pain, TMS mapping has provided preliminary evidence of reorganization of trunk-muscle representation at

the motor cortex and suggest that this reorganization is associated with deficits in postural control.[83]

The motor cortex has extensive projections to some thalamic nuclei (which along with the somatosensory cortex and the limbic system are considered critical in the pathophysiology of chronic pain).[84] Converging evidence suggests that modulation of the motor cortex may be beneficial in chronic pain.[80] The primary motor cortex might represent a convenient portal for the modulation of deep brain structures with difficult access: the motor cortex stimulation triggers corticothalamic output to brainstem, spinal cord, and also limbic system, exerting an inhibitory effect on these pathways. Several studies, using rTMS and transcranial DCS for therapeutic modulation, have been conducted in this area and significant results have been shown.[85] Moreover, treatment of chronic visceral pain with brain stimulation is also being explored, with promising preliminary results.[86]

PD

TMS-mapping studies of patients with PD have shown altered cortical physiology in basal-ganglia-connected areas such as the supplementary motor area, dorsolateral prefrontal cortex, and primary motor cortex, characterized by excessive corticospinal output at rest and reduced intracortical inhibition.[87,88] Because a given motor task is associated with suppression of competing motor networks, these cortical changes in patients with PD might result in decreased suppression and therefore decrease the performance of the motor system, resulting in symptoms such as tonic contractions and rigidity.[87]

Although the motor symptoms of PD are mainly treated with drugs, the clinical usefulness of these medications tends to become limited over the years, often because of adverse effects such as dyskinesias. Nonpharmacologic approaches, such as deep brain stimulation (DBS), are effective in the treatment of PD motor symptoms in selected patients. Recent developments in DBS have reduced surgical risks and morbidity, but noninvasive approaches are still appealing. rTMS has been used in patients with PD to modulate activity in specific neural networks, using cortical targets as entry ports. Two pathophysiologic mechanisms can be proposed to explain how cortically directed rTMS may improve PD symptoms: either (1) rTMS induces network changes that connect with and positively affect basal-ganglia function[89,90] or (2) rTMS to cortical sites compensates for systematic abnormal changes in cortical function associated with PD.[91–93] Although these mechanisms of action are based on several studies that have attempted to elucidate the pathophysiology of motor disturbance in PD, they remain unproved, and further investigations are required.

SAFETY CONSIDERATIONS FOR TMS MAPPING

Single-pulse stimulation within current guidelines poses low risk of adverse effects in healthy individuals and patients.[94] TMS has been safely used in both children and adults for the explicit purpose of presurgical mapping.[18,28–31] The most severe adverse effect is considered nonintentional seizure after rTMS. From the several thousands of studies that have used TMS, 16 such cases have been reported. Based on the available data, the reported risk of seizures is less than 1 in 1000 for rTMS.[94] Because TMS can have lasting effects on cortical excitability depending on the stimulation parameters (largely frequency and intensity), the seizure risk is related to how the stimulation is applied. High-frequency stimulation can raise cortical excitability and may be unsafe if performed outside the safety guidelines, whereas low-frequency stimulation can reduce cortical excitability.[95] However, the seizure risk is considered minimal with single-pulse stimulation, which is most frequently used for presurgical mapping. The intensity typically use for mapping is 120% of the resting motor threshold, but in some patient groups, in which no response can be elicited at this intensity, up to 100% maximal stimulator output has been reported.[96] Operators should be aware that sedation and anesthesia might raise cortical excitability. With increasingly more powerful coils and stimulators emerging, one should take care to gradually increase the stimulus intensity in a stepwise fashion (see safety guidelines).[94]

In some cases, depending on the stimulus intensity and current spread from TMS, mapping can exceed the anatomic primary motor area and border nonmotor areas; because the stimulus intensity selected remains relative to the motor threshold, stimulating nonmotor areas at this intensity is not considered harmful.[94]

Physiologic monitoring should minimally involve visual inspection that the muscle twitch from TMS remains limited to the associated body part and seems to immediately follow the stimulus. A more quantitative method may be to additionally record EMG from higher threshold or more proximal muscles represented outside the region to be evaluated. If single-pulse TMS over the region of interest begins to elicit responses in this second EMG channel, this would be an indication of increased cortical excitability, and possible spread of intracortical excitation. EEG monitoring is routinely used as a safety feature in intracranial cortical stimulation and could be used during TMS mapping, yet provides equivocal additional benefit.[94]

Based on the ex vivo and in vivo studies, it is suggested that TMS can be safely applied to patients who have implanted stimulators of the central and peripheral nervous system when the TMS coil is not in close proximity to the internal pulse generator system.[94] However, detailed information as to what constitutes a safe distance between the TMS coil and the implanted stimulator is still lacking. Therefore, TMS should only be performed in patients with implanted stimulators if there are medically compelling reasons justifying it.[94] Furthermore, recent data show the absence of adverse events related to titanium (Ti) skull plates in patients undergoing 1-Hz rTMS.[97] These initial data showed that Ti skull plates, even if positioned directly beneath the TMS coil, were minimally heated and unlikely to be displaced by a conventional low-frequency rTMS protocol. However, more data are required to conclude that rTMS in patients with Ti skull plates is definitively minimal risk.

SUMMARY

The notion of remapping has led to significant advances in how we understand the multifactorial process of recovery after injury of the central nervous system. There are experience-dependent processes that likely involve disinhibition of previously inhibited connections as well as stabilization of new synapses. However, the map metaphor has also led to an exaggerated conception of postlesion plasticity. For example, the map expansion found by TMS that seems to be related to therapy may come about through changes in inhibition, excitability, and potentially spinal cord circuitry, and therefore may not represent the same kind of remapping as found in experimental motor cortical lesions. Although such cortical maps need to be reviewed in conjunction with clinical and other diagnostic evidence, they provide us with an important set of electrophysiologic information both for a healthy brain, and for cortical reorganization after lesion.

The presurgical usefulness of nTMS depends mainly on the spatial resolution and the application error of the method by which TMS is used. With the development of newer and more focal nTMS systems, the resolution of the stimulation maps can be further enhanced, by moving the coil in small increments and stimulating just over the threshold with a controlled and monitored level of muscle contraction. Using such meticulous mapping protocols, TMS can prove to be an indispensable tool to study cortical connections in humans noninvasively and painlessly. Moreover, integration of TMS with functional neuroimaging can add to both the spatial and temporal resolution of the mapping strategies.

REFERENCES

1. Krings T, Chiappa KH, Foltys H, et al. Introducing navigated transcranial magnetic stimulation as a refined brain mapping methodology. Neurosurg Rev 2001;24(4):171–9.
2. Raichle ME. A brief history of human brain mapping. Trends Neurosci 2009;32(2):118–26.
3. Silvanto J, Pascual-Leone A. State-dependency of transcranial magnetic stimulation. Brain Topogr 2008;21(1):1–10.
4. Bartholow R. Experimental investigations into the function of the human brain. Am J Med Sci 1874; 134:305–13.
5. Penfield W, Rasmussen T. The cerebral cortex of man. New York: Macmillan; 1950. p. 44, 56, 214–5.
6. Penfield W, Boldrey E. Somatic motor and sensory representation in the cerebral cortex of man as studied by electrical stimulation. Brain 1937;37: 389–443.
7. Thickbroom GW, Byrnes ML, Mastaglia FL. Methodology and application of TMS mapping. Electroencephalogr Clin Neurophysiol Suppl 1999;51:48–54.
8. Wilson SA, Thickbroom GW, Mastaglia FL. Transcranial magnetic stimulation mapping of the motor cortex in normal subjects. The representation of two intrinsic hand muscles. J Neurol Sci 1993;118(2):134–44.
9. Kobayashi M, Pascual-Leone A. Transcranial magnetic stimulation in neurology. Lancet Neurol 2003;2:145–56.
10. Rossini PM, Barker AT, Berardelli A, et al. Non-invasive electrical and magnetic stimulation of the brain, spinal cord and roots: basic principles and procedures for routine clinical application. Report of an IFCN committee. Electroencephalogr Clin Neurophysiol 1994;91:79–92.
11. Pascual-Leone A, Valls-Sole J, Wassermann EM, et al. Responses to rapid-rate transcranial magnetic stimulation of the human motor cortex. Brain 1994; 117:847–58.
12. Pascual-Leone A, Tormos JM, Keenan J, et al. Study and modulation of human cortical excitability with transcranial magnetic stimulation. J Clin Neurophysiol 1998;1(15):333–43.
13. Yozbatiran N, Alonso-Alonso M, See J, et al. Safety and behavioral effects of high-frequency repetitive transcranial magnetic stimulation in stroke. Stroke 2009;40(1):309–12.
14. Tharin S, Golby A. Functional brain mapping and its applications to neurosurgery. Neurosurgery 2007; 60:201–2.
15. Diekhoff S, Uludağ L, Sparing R, et al. Functional localization in the human brain: gradient-echo, spin-echo, and arterial spin-labeling fMRI compared with neuronavigated TMS. Hum Brain Mapp 2010. DOI: 10.1002/hbm.21024.
16. Julkunen P, Säisänen L, Danner N, et al. Comparison of navigated and non-navigated transcranial magnetic stimulation for motor cortex mapping, motor threshold and motor evoked potentials. Neuroimage 2009;44:790–5.
17. Teitti S, Määttä S, Säisänen L, et al. Non-primary motor areas in the human frontal lobe are connected directly to hand muscles. Neuroimage 2008;40: 1243–50.
18. Säisänen L, Könönen M, Julkunen P, et al. Non-invasive preoperative localization of primary motor cortex in epilepsy surgery by navigated transcranial magnetic stimulation. Epilepsy Res 2010;92(2–3): 134–44.
19. Sack AT, Kohler A, Linden DE, et al. The temporal characteristics of motion processing in hMT/V5+: combining fMRI and neuronavigated TMS. Neuroimage 2006;29(4):1326–35.
20. Pascual-Leone A, Walsh V. Fast back projections from the motion to the primary visual area necessary for visual awareness. Science 2001;292:510–2.
21. Nunez PL, Srinivasan R. Electric fields of the brain: the neurophysics of EEG. New York: Oxford University Press; 2006.
22. Thut G, Pascual-Leone A. Integrating TMS with EEG: how and what for? Brain Topogr 2010;22(4):215–8.
23. Thut G, Pascual-Leone A. A review of combined TMS-EEG studies to characterize lasting effects of repetitive TMS and assess their usefulness in cognitive and clinical neuroscience. Brain Topogr 2010; 22(4):219–32.
24. Bestmann S, Ruff CC, Blankenburg F, et al. Mapping causal interregional influences with concurrent TMS-fMRI. Exp Brain Res 2008;191(4):383–402.
25. Hou BL, Bradbury M, Peck KK, et al. Effect of brain tumor neovasculature defined by rCBV on BOLD fMRI activation volume in the primary motor cortex. Neuroimage 2006;32:489–97.
26. Krishnan R, Raabe A, Hattingen E, et al. Functional magnetic resonance imaging-integrated neuronavigation: correlation between lesion-to-motor cortex distance and outcome. Neurosurgery 2004;55: 904–15.
27. Picht T, Wachter D, Mularski S, et al. Functional magnetic resonance imaging and cortical mapping in motor cortex tumor surgery: complementary methods. Zentralbl Neurochir 2008;69:1–6.
28. Kantelhardt SR, Fadini T, Finke M, et al. Robot-assisted image-guided transcranial magnetic stimulation for somatotopic mapping of the motor cortex: a clinical pilot study. Acta Neurochir (Wien) 2010;152(2): 333–43.

29. Krings T, Buchbinder BR, Butler WE, et al. Stereo-tactic transcranial magnetic stimulation: correlation with direct electrical cortical stimulation. Neurosurgery 1997;41:1319–26.

30. Picht T, Mularski S, Kuehn B, et al. Navigated transcranial magnetic stimulation for preoperative functional diagnostics in brain tumor surgery. Neurosurgery 2009;65(6 Suppl):93–8.

31. Shamov T, Spiriev T, Tzvetanov P, et al. The combination of neuronavigation with transcranial magnetic stimulation for treatment of opercular gliomas of the dominant brain hemisphere. Clin Neurol Neurosurg 2010;112(8):672–7.

32. Brasil-Neto JP, McShane LM, Fuhr P, et al. Topographic mapping of the human motor cortex with magnetic stimulation: factors affecting accuracy and reproducibility. Electroencephalogr Clin Neurophysiol 1992;85(1):9–16.

33. Rothwell JC, Thompson PD, Day BL, et al. Stimulation of the human motor cortex through the scalp. Exp Physiol 1991;76(2):159–200.

34. Juenger H, Ressel V, Braun C, et al. Misleading functional magnetic resonance imaging mapping of the cortical hand representation in a 4-year-old boy with an arteriovenous malformation of the central region. J Neurosurg Pediatr 2009;4(4):333–8.

35. Rutten GJ, Ramsey NF, Van Rijen PC, et al. With functional magnetic resonance imaging and transcranial magnetic stimulation interhemispheric reorganization of motor hand function to the primary motor cortex predicted. J Child Neurol 2002;17(4):292–7.

36. Vitikainen AM, Lioumis P, Paetau R, et al. Combined use of non-invasive techniques for improved functional localization for a selected group of epilepsy surgery candidates. Neuroimage 2009;45(2):342–8.

37. Barba C, Montanaro D, Cincotta M, et al. An integrated fMRI, SEPs and MEPs approach for assessing functional organization in the malformed sensorimotor cortex. Epilepsy Res 2010;89(1):66–71.

38. Schmidt S, Holst E, Irlbacher K, et al. A case of pathological excitability located with navigated-TMS: presurgical evaluation of focal neocortical epilepsy. Restor Neurol Neurosci 2010;28(3):379–85.

39. Herholz K, Thiel A, Wienhard K, et al. Individual functional anatomy of verb generation. Neuroimage 1996;3:185–94.

40. Ojemann JG, Miller JW, Silbergeld DL. Preserved function in brain invaded by tumor. Neurosurgery 1996;39:253–8.

41. Wunderlich G, Knorr U, Herzog H, et al. Precentral glioma location determines the displacement of cortical hand representation. Neurosurgery 1998; 42:18–26.

42. Baxendale S, Thompson P, Duncan J, et al. Is it time to replace the Wada test? Neurology 2003;60:354–5.

43. Benbadis SR, Dinner DS, Chelune GJ, et al. Objective criteria for reporting language dominance by intracarotid amobarbital procedure. J Clin Exp Neuropsychol 1995;17:682–90.

44. Meador KJ, Loring DW. The Wada test: controversies, concerns, and insights. Neurology 1999;52:1535–6.

45. Jennum P, Friberg L, Fuglsang-Frederiksen A, et al. Speech localization using repetitive transcranial magnetic stimulation. Neurology 1994;44:269–73.

46. Pascual-Leone A, Gates JR, Dhuna A. Induction of speech arrest and counting errors with rapid-rate transcranial magnetic stimulation. Neurology 1991; 41:697–702.

47. Tokimura H, Tokimura Y, Oliviero A, et al. Speech-induced changes in corticospinal excitability. Ann Neurol 1996;40:628–34.

48. Epstein CM, Jennum P. Language. In: Pascual-Leone A, Davey N, Rothwell J, et al, editors. Handbook of transcranial magnetic stimulation. London: Arnold; 2002. p. 295–302.

49. Giussani C, Roux FE, Ojemann J, et al. Is preoperative functional magnetic resonance imaging reliable for language areas mapping in brain tumor surgery? Review of language functional magnetic resonance imaging and direct cortical stimulation correlation studies. Neurosurgery 2010;66(1):113–20.

50. Duffau H. New concepts in surgery of WHO grade II gliomas: functional brain mapping, connectionism and plasticity–a review. J Neurooncol 2006;79:77–115.

51. Gil Robles S, Gatignol P, Lehéricy S, et al. Long term brain plasticity allowing a multistage surgical approach to World Health Organization Grade II gliomas in eloquent areas. J Neurosurg 2008;109: 615–24.

52. Lee HW, Shin JS, Webber WR, et al. Reorganization of cortical motor and language distribution in human brain. J Neurol Neurosurg Psychiatry 2009;80:285–90.

53. Barcia JA, Sanz A, Gonzalez-Hidalgo M, et al. rTMS stimulation to induce plastic changes at the language motor area in a patient with a left recidivant brain tumor affecting Broca's area. Neurocase 2010, in press.

54. Hufnagel A, Elger CE, Durwen HF, et al. Activation of the epileptic focus by transcranial magnetic stimulation of the human brain. Ann Neurol 1990;27:49–60.

55. Schuler P, Claus D, Stefan H. Hyperventilation and transcranial magnetic stimulation: two methods of activation of epileptiform EEG activity in comparison. J Clin Neurophysiol 1993;10:111–5.

56. Steinhoff BJ, Stodieck SR, Zivcec Z, et al. Transcranial magnetic stimulation (TMS) of the brain in patients with mesiotemporal epileptic foci. Clin Electroencephalogr 1993;24(1):1–5.

57. Valentin A, Arunachalam R, Mesquita-Rodrigues A, et al. Late EEG responses triggered by transcranial magnetic stimulation (TMS) in the evaluation of focal epilepsy. Epilepsia 2008;49(3):470–80.

58. Bliss TV, Lomo T. Long-lasting potentiation of synaptic transmission in the dentate area of the

anaesthetized rabbit following stimulation of the perforant path. J Physiol 1973;232(2):331–56.

59. Dudek SM, Bear MF. Homosynaptic long-term depression in area CA1 of hippocampus and effects of N-methyl-D-aspartate receptor blockade. Proc Natl Acad Sci U S A 1992;89(10):4363–7.

60. Fregni F, Thome-Souza S, Bermpohl F, et al. Antiepileptic effects of repetitive transcranial magnetic stimulation in patients with cortical malformations: an EEG and clinical study. Stereotact Funct Neurosurg 2005;83(2–3):57–62.

61. Santiago-Rodríguez E, Cárdenas-Morales L, Harmony T, et al. Repetitive transcranial magnetic stimulation decreases the number of seizures in patients with focal neocortical epilepsy. Seizure 2008;17(8):677–83.

62. Tergau F, Naumann U, Paulus W, et al. Low-frequency repetitive transcranial magnetic stimulation improves intractable epilepsy. Lancet 1999;353(9171):2209.

63. Fregni F, Otachi PT, Do Valle A, et al. A randomized clinical trial of repetitive transcranial magnetic stimulation in patients with refractory epilepsy. Ann Neurol 2006;60(4):447–55.

64. Cantello R, Rossi S, Varrasi C, et al. Slow repetitive TMS for drug-resistant epilepsy: clinical and EEG findings of a placebo-controlled trial. Epilepsia 2007;48(2):366–74.

65. Theodore WH, Hunter K, Chen R, et al. Transcranial magnetic stimulation for the treatment of seizures: a controlled study. Neurology 2002;59(4):560–2.

66. Rotenberg A, Bae EH, Takeoka M, et al. Repetitive transcranial magnetic stimulation in the treatment of epilepsia partialis continua. Epilepsy Behav 2009;14(1):253–7.

67. Frost SB, Barbay S, Friel KM, et al. Reorganization of remote cortical regions after ischemic brain injury: a potential substrate for stroke recovery. J Neurophysiol 2003;89:3205–14.

68. Dancause N, Barbay S, Frost SB, et al. Effects of small ischemic lesions in the primary motor cortex on neurophysiological organization in ventral premotor cortex. J Neurophysiol 2006;96(6):3506–11.

69. Escudero JV, Sancho J, Bautista D, et al. Prognostic value of motor evoked potential obtained by transcranial magnetic brain stimulation in motor function recovery in patients with acute ischemic stroke. Stroke 1998;29:1854–9.

70. Nascimbeni A, Gaffuri A, Imazio P. Motor evoked potentials: prognostic value in motor recovery after stroke. Funct Neurol 2006;21:199–203.

71. Nascimbeni A, Gaffuri A, Granella L, et al. Prognostic value of motor evoked potentials in stroke motor outcome. Eura Medicophys 2005;41:125–30.

72. Rapisarda G, Bastings E, de Noordhout AM, et al. Can motor recovery in stroke patients be predicted by early transcranial magnetic stimulation? Stroke 1996;27:2191–6.

73. Swayne OB, Rothwell JC, Ward NS, et al. Stages of motor output reorganization after hemispheric stroke suggested by longitudinal studies of cortical physiology. Cereb Cortex 2008;18:1909–22.

74. Manganotti P, Patuzzo S, Cortese F, et al. Motor disinhibition in affected and unaffected hemisphere in the early period of recovery after stroke. Clin Neurophysiol 2002;113:936–43.

75. Maeda F, Keenan JP, Tormos JM, et al. Modulation of corticospinal excitability by repetitive transcranial magnetic stimulation. Clin Neurophysiol 2000; 111(5):800–5.

76. Murase N, Duque J, Mazzocchio R, et al. Influence of interhemispheric interactions on motor function in chronic stroke. Ann Neurol 2004;55(3):400–9.

77. Carey JR, Kimberley TJ, Lewis SM, et al. Analysis of fMRI and finger tracking training in subjects with chronic stroke. Brain 2002;125(Pt 4):773–88.

78. Rossini PM, Dal Forno G. Neuronal post-stroke plasticity in the adult. Restor Neurol Neurosci 2004; 22(3–5):193–206.

79. Mansur CG, Fregni F, Boggio PS, et al. A sham stimulation-controlled trial of rTMS of the unaffected hemisphere in stroke patients. Neurology 2005; 64(10):1802–4.

80. Lefaucheur JP, Drouot X, Menard-Lefaucheur I, et al. Motor cortex rTMS restores defective intracortical inhibition in chronic neuropathic pain. Neurology 2006;67:1568–74.

81. Schwenkreis P, Scherens A, Rönnau AK, et al. Cortical disinhibition occurs in chronic neuropathic, but not in chronic nociceptive pain. BMC Neurosci 2010;11:73.

82. Krause P, Forderreuther S, Straube A. TMS motor cortical brain mapping in patients with complex regional pain syndrome type I. Clin Neurophysiol 2006;117:169–76.

83. Tsao H, Galea MP, Hodges PW. Reorganization of the motor cortex is associated with postural control deficits in recurrent low back pain. Brain 2008; 131(Pt 8):2161–71.

84. Borsook D, Becerra L. Phenotyping central nervous system circuitry in chronic pain using functional MRI: considerations and potential implications in the clinic. Curr Pain Headache Rep 2007;11:201–7.

85. Fregni F, Freedman S, Pascual-Leone A. Recent advances in the treatment of chronic pain with non-invasive brain stimulation techniques. Lancet Neurol 2007;6:188–91.

86. Fregni F, DaSilva D, Potvin K, et al. Treatment of chronic visceral pain with brain stimulation. Ann Neurol 2005;58(6):971–2.

87. Lefaucheur JP. Motor cortex dysfunction revealed by cortical excitability studies in Parkinson's disease: influence of antiparkinsonian treatment and cortical stimulation. Clin Neurophysiol 2005; 116(2):244–53.

88. Vacherot F, Attarian S, Vaugoyeau M, et al. A motor cortex excitability and gait analysis on Parkinsonian patients. Mov Disord 2010;25(16):2747–55.

89. Keck ME, Welt T, Muller MB, et al. Repetitive transcranial magnetic stimulation increases the release of dopamine in the mesolimbic and mesostriatal system. Neuropharmacology 2002;43(1):101–9.

90. Strafella AP, Paus T, Barrett J, et al. Repetitive transcranial magnetic stimulation of the human prefrontal cortex induces dopamine release in the caudate nucleus. J Neurosci 2001;21(15):RC157.

91. de Groot M, Hermann W, Steffen J, et al. [Contralateral and ipsilateral repetitive transcranial magnetic stimulation in Parkinson patients]. Nervenarzt 2001; 72(12):932–8 [in German].

92. Mally J, Stone TW. Improvement in Parkinsonian symptoms after repetitive transcranial magnetic stimulation. J Neurol Sci 1999;162(2):179–84.

93. Siebner HR, Mentschel C, Auer C, et al. Repetitive transcranial magnetic stimulation has a beneficial effect on bradykinesia in Parkinson's disease. Neuroreport 1999;10(3):589–94.

94. Rossi S, Hallett M, Rossini PM, et al. Safety of TMS Consensus Group. Safety, ethical considerations, and application guidelines for the use of transcranial magnetic stimulation in clinical practice and research. Clin Neurophysiol 2009;120(12): 2008–39.

95. Pascual-Leone A, Houser CM, Reese K, et al. Safety of rapid-rate transcranial magnetic stimulation in normal volunteers. Electroencephalogr Clin Neurophysiol 1993;89:120–30.

96. Hallett M. Transcranial magnetic stimulation: a tool for mapping the central nervous system. Electroencephalogr Clin Neurophysiol Suppl 1996;46: 43–51.

97. Rotenberg A, Pascual-Leone A. Safety of 1 Hz repetitive transcranial magnetic stimulation (rTMS) in patients with titanium skull plates. Clin Neurophysiol 2009;120(7):1417.

98. Kamida T, Baba H, Ono K, et al. Usefulness of magnetic motor evoked potentials in the surgical treatment of hemiplegic patients with intractable epilepsy. Seizure 2003;12(6):373–8.

Diffusion Tractography: Methods, Validation and Applications in Patients with Neurosurgical Lesions

Delphine Leclercq, MD[a,b,c,*], Christine Delmaire, MD, PhD[a,d],
Nicolas Menjot de Champfleur, MD[a,e], Jacques Chiras, MD[b],
Stéphane Lehéricy, MD, PhD[a,b,c]

KEYWORDS
- Brain tumor • Diffusion tensor imaging • Fiber tracking
- Tractography • Mapping • Neurosurgery

In patients with surgical lesions in functional areas, the purpose of surgery is to achieve maximal tumor removal while preserving essential brain functions.[1,2] Although intraoperative cortical and subcortical direct electrical stimulations (DESs) remain the gold standard to map the functional boundaries of the resection cavity, the use of DESs can be limited by time constraint. DESs in an awake patient are time consuming and the progressive patient's tiredness explains that only a limited number of tasks can be performed during surgery.[3] In this context, preoperative localization of cortical and subcortical functional areas is crucial. Preoperative evaluation based on anatomic knowledge is insufficient because white matter fiber tracts can be displaced by the tumor and language pathways present high interindividual variability.

Diffusion tensor imaging (DTI) tractography is the only noninvasive technique that permits in vivo dissection of white matter tracts. Tractography can now be easily performed using clinical magnets and therefore is increasingly used to map fiber tracts for surgical planning. Tractography provides a unique anatomic information by reconstructing and visualizing chosen fiber tracts in the 3-dimensional (3D) anatomy of a patient.[4–10] Motor, language, and visual tracts and their relationship with the tumor can then be visualized preoperatively and integrated with a surgical neuronavigation system to guide surgery. Yet, DTI tractography still presents limitations because of the technique and the tumor. This review focuses on the possibilities and limits of DTI imaging in preoperative tumoral mapping and provides an overview of the current knowledge.

The authors have nothing to disclose.
[a] Centre de NeuroImagerie de Recherche—CENIR, Groupe Hospitalier Pitié-Salpêtrière 47-83, Bd de l'Hôpital, 75013 Paris, France
[b] Department of Neuroradiology, Groupe Hospitalier Pitié-Salpêtrière 47-83, Bd de l'Hôpital, 75013 Paris, France
[c] Centre de Recherche de l'Institut du Cerveau et de la Moelle épinière CR-ICM, UPMC—Paris 6/Inserm UMR-S975, CNRS, UMR 7225, 47-83, Bd de l'Hôpital, 75013 Paris, France
[d] Department of Neuroradiology, CHRU Lille, 2, Avenue Oscar Lambret, 59000, Lille, France
[e] Department of Neuroradiology, Gui de Chauliac Hospital, CHU Montpellier, 80, Avenue Augustin Fliche, 34295 Montpellier, France
* Corresponding author. Centre de NeuroImagerie de Recherche – CENIR, Groupe Hospitalier Pitié-Salpêtrière 47-83, Bd de l'Hôpital, 75013 Paris, France.
E-mail address: del.leclercq@gmail.com

Neurosurg Clin N Am 22 (2011) 253–268
doi:10.1016/j.nec.2010.11.004
1042-3680/11/$ – see front matter © 2011 Elsevier Inc. All rights reserved.

POSSIBILITIES AND LIMITS OF DIFFUSION TENSOR BRAIN MAPPING

DTI

Physical basis

Diffusion imaging is based on the self-diffusion of water molecules in tissues.[11]

In a biologic environment, water molecules present with random thermally driven motions that are so-called Brownian motion.[5] When water molecules diffuse equally in all directions, as in the ventricular cerebrospinal fluid (CSF), the diffusion is called isotropic. In brain white matter, the micrometric movements of water molecules are hindered to a greater extent in a direction perpendicular to the fiber orientation than parallel to it. Therefore, diffusion is higher following the direction of fiber bundles. Hindrance is attributed to multiple factors, including myelination, axon density and diameter, and axonal membrane integrity.[5,10,12,13] Diffusion is then not equal in all 3 orthogonal directions, a property called anisotropy. To fully determine the direction of diffusion, a tensor is used, which describes the mobility of water molecules along each direction. Diffusion-weighted images have to be acquired along at least 6 directions along with an image acquired without diffusion weighting. Diffusion anisotropy is subsequently characterized using several indices made of combinations of the terms of the diffusion tensor, that is, the eigenvalues λ_1, λ_2, and λ_3, which characterize the main diffusion directions and associated diffusivities. The most popular measure is fractional anisotropy (FA),[12] which ranges from 0 (isotropy) to 1 (maximum anisotropy). DTI enables to extract the tridimensional orientation of the underlying fibers within each voxel and to quantify the motional anisotropy.

Diffusion tensor color-coded maps and tractography

Diffusion anisotropy can be displayed in several ways. In FA maps, signal intensity codes for the degree of anisotropy (ranging from 0–1). Isotropic

(CSF) or weakly anisotropic voxels (gray matter) usually present an FA less than 0.2, whereas anisotropic white matter presents an FA greater than 0.2. However, FA maps do not provide information on diffusion direction. The white matter tract organization is therefore better represented using ellipsoids or directionally color-coded schematic maps of major diffusion orientation.[14] Ellipsoids are 3D representations of the diffusion distance covered in space by molecules in a given time. In color-coded maps, different colors (red, green, or blue) are attributed to different fiber orientation along the 3 orthogonal spatial axes (**Fig. 1**). Also, the brightness of each color is modulated by the degree of anisotropy.

Fiber tractography enables 3D visualization of fiber bundles. Because water diffusion is preferentially oriented along the direction of fiber tracts, tracts are reconstructed by using this directional property of water diffusion in each voxel. A large number of DTI tractography algorithms have been proposed to reconstruct fiber tracts. The most commonly used algorithm in clinical practice is a deterministic algorithm based on the FACT (fiber assignment by contiguous tracking) algorithm.[15] With this method, tracking is performed on a voxel-by-voxel basis. The entire track is determined from a seed point after the successive orientations associated with adjacent voxels. Tractography necessitates the definition of a seed region of interest (ROI) located on the path of the investigated fiber tract to initiate the fiber tracking procedure.[4,9,15] The termination of line propagation is determined by 2 parameters corresponding to stopping thresholds: (1) when a voxel is less than a predetermined minimum FA value, typically 0.2, or (2) when the maximum angle of the main diffusion orientation between 2 contiguous voxels is reached, typically 30° (**Fig. 2**).

DTI in brain tumors

Reconstructing DTI fiber tracts for tumoral presurgical planning is challenging because in the vicinity

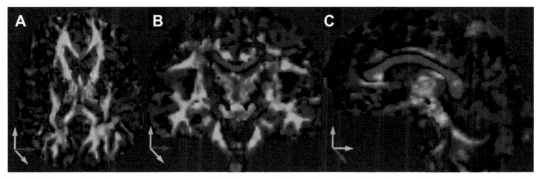

Fig. 1. Color-coded anisotropy maps on axial (*A*), coronal (*B*), and sagittal (*C*) planes. Fibers oriented along the left-to-right direction are seen in red, fibers oriented along the superior-to-inferior direction are seen in blue, and fibers oriented along the anterior-to-posterior direction are seen in green.

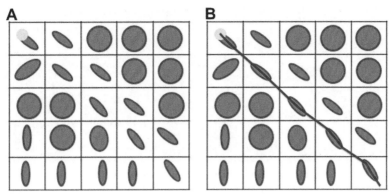

Fig. 2. (*A*) Main diffusion orientation (*ellipses and disks*) in contiguous voxels. Strongly anisotropic voxels are cigar-shaped and isotropic voxels are round. A seeding point is represented in yellow. (*B*) Result of tractography using the yellow ROI as seeding point. The red fiber is propagated voxel by voxel in the orientation of the main diffusion.

of the tumor, fibers can be displaced, infiltrated (by the tumor and/or edema), or destroyed (**Fig. 3**).[16–18] The tumoral cells and the peritumoral edema cause changes in the brain structure. Typically, measurement of diffusion anisotropy in the normal brain parenchyma up to near the tumor demonstrates a decrease in FA values (**Fig. 4**).[19] The reduction in anisotropy can result from fiber depletion (tumor destroys fibers, reducing their absolute numbers), fiber dilution (tumor or

vasogenic edema spreads intact fibers apart, reducing their density), or fiber degradation (fibers themselves become intrinsically less anisotropic, retaining normal numbers and density).[20] Reduced anisotropy explains why DTI tractography can be limited in a tumoral environment (**Fig. 5**).

DTI Artifacts and Limitations

It is important to keep in mind that DTI reconstructed fibers and tracts are not the visualization

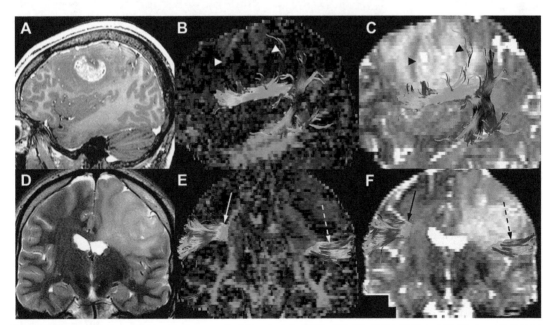

Fig. 3. Tumoral effect on fibers, displacement of the arcuate fasciculus. (*A–C*) Sagittal and (*D–F*) coronal views in a patient with a frontal anaplastic glioma. The tumor is shown in (*A*) a sagittal T1-weighted postgadolinium contrast sequence and (*D*) a T2-weighted image, (*B, E*) color-coded anisotropy maps, and (*C, F*) B0 images acquired without diffusion weighting. In the sagittal plane (*B, C*), the left arcuate fasciculus is in contact with the tumor (*arrow heads*). In the coronal plane (*E, F*), the tract (*dashed arrows*) is displaced downward in comparison with the contralateral tract (*arrows*). Reconstruction was performed using the TrackVis software (www.trackvis.org).

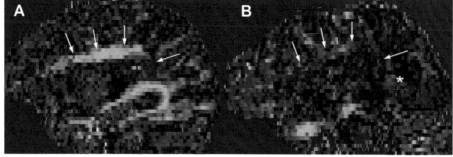

Fig. 4. Tumoral effect on fibers, infiltration and decreased anisotropy. Sagittal views of the right (A) and left (B) arcuate fasciculus in color-coded anisotropy maps in a patient with a left hemispheric low-grade glioma (asterisk). In the healthy hemisphere (A), the anteroposterior and superoinferior fibers (arrows) of the arcuate fasciculus are seen in green and blue, respectively. In the tumoral hemisphere (B), anteroposterior and superoinferior fibers are not evidenced because of the local decrease in anisotropy induced by the tumor.

of an anatomic structure but an estimation of these structures via the diffusion anisotropy. Therefore, there are several limitations inherent to DTI and tractography techniques, which must be known before interpreting the information given by orientation color maps and reconstructed fiber tracts. These limitations have already been described extensively.[21,22]

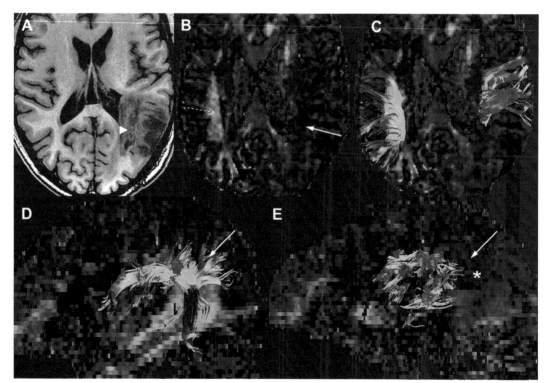

Fig. 5. Tumoral effect on fibers, tumoral infiltration with decreased anisotropy and tractography. (A–C) Axial and (D, E) sagittal images in a patient with a left low-grade glioma (asterisk). (A) The tumor is observed in the left temporoparietal region in the T1-weighted images (arrowhead). (B) In the color-oriented map, the left arcuate fasciculus is visible in green in the normal hemisphere (dashed arrow) and is not visible in the tumoral hemisphere (arrow). DTI tractography using an ROI placed within the tumor showed no fibers (arrow), whereas fibers were reconstructed at the periphery of the tumor. Comparison between the tumoral and the normal contralateral tract is shown in the axial (C) and sagittal planes (D, E) (TrackVis software).

Crossing fibers

In DTI acquisitions, each voxel can contain a large number of fibers. The estimate of orientation of the tensor is therefore an average of the orientations of all the fibers contained within the voxel.[23,24] When the fibers are coherently organized in a parallel fashion, the orientation of the tensor truly reflects the orientation of the underlying fibers. However, when fibers cross within a voxel, the voxel-averaged estimate of orientation cannot accurately summarize the orientation of the underlying fibers.

This explains that DTI tractography fails to reconstruct some existing fibers. For example, the corticospinal tract has a fan-shaped morphology in the centrum semiovale. However, DTI fiber tracking most often reconstructs only fibers originating from the vertex. This reconstruction is attributable to the existence of multiple crossing fibers in the centrum semiovale, which leads to inaccuracy in the estimation of the direction anisotropy in these voxels.[25]

This problem can be overcome with other diffusion techniques, such as the high angular resolution diffusion imaging (HARDI), which has the ability to extract different orientations of fibers in voxels containing multioriented fiber populations.[26] Several algorithms can be used to reconstruct diffusion orientations from HARDI images, the most popular being Q-ball reconstruction.[27] Q-ball can distinguish distinct fiber populations in each voxel and reconstruct portions of tracts that could not be evidenced with DTI.

The main limitation of HARDI in clinical practice is the length of the scan acquisition because it requires a large number of gradient directions and higher b values.

Spurious fibers

Acquisition noise and crossing fibers can induce a corrupted estimate of orientation in a voxel from which a spurious aberrant fiber can be generated.[21] These fibers have the same appearance as the fibers of the expected tract, except that they are anatomically incorrect (**Fig. 6**). Determining whether some fibers are spurious or anatomically coherent can be difficult. Strong a priori knowledge of fiber tract anatomy provides valuable information in this context.

Magnetic susceptibility artifacts

Magnetic susceptibility differences in interfaces among brain tissue (frontal lobe), bone, and air-filled sinuses can induce local image distortions or signal dropout.[21] These artifacts are also observed in calcified structures, after brain hemorrhage because of blood by-products particle deposition as well as after surgery because of the presence of surgical metallic particles.

Tumor infiltration and tumor mass effect

As already described, tumoral infiltration in low-grade gliomas is usually associated with a decrease in anisotropy values. This reduction in anisotropy can be so deep that parts of the tumor are almost isotropic and tractography fails. In this situation, validation studies of DTI tractography with intraoperative subcortical DESs showed that a negative tractography result does not rule out the persistence of a fiber tract, especially when invaded by the tumor.[28–30] Lowering the FA threshold of tractography reconstruction parameters can sometimes help to evidence persistent fibers, which strengthens the fact that when tractography fails, it does not necessarily mean that

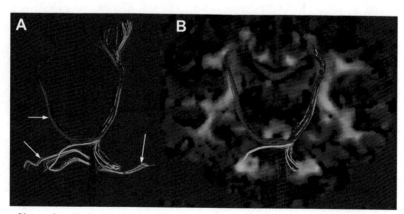

Fig. 6. Spurious fibers. (*A, B*) Coronal representation of DTI fibers resulting from the tractography of the corticospinal tract using a mesencephalic ROI. The tract is superimposed to the color-coded map (*B*). Artifactual cerebellar and contralateral fibers are reconstructed along with the corticospinal tract (*arrows*) (TrackVis software).

the real fiber bundles are interrupted (**Fig. 7**). However, in high-grade gliomas, comparison of DTI tractography with intraoperative subcortical DESs showed a good correspondence between DESs and interrupted fiber tracts, suggesting that the fiber bundles were truly interrupted in these cases.[30]

Tumor mass effect and infiltration can also change the main orientation of diffusion in voxels and lead to fiber crossings (**Fig. 8**) or spurious fibers (**Fig. 9**). Tumor mass effect can result in large modifications of the main diffusion orientation around the tumor and in tractography failure (see **Fig. 8**). As a consequence, presurgical planning should not be done using tractography alone but also with the help of FA color-coded maps.

Selection of the ROIs

Diffusion tractography in presurgical mapping is a user-defined process. Tractography results are dependent on the size and the location of the seed ROIs.[22] Commonly, seed ROIs are traced using anatomic landmarks and positioned on the directionally FA color-coded maps of the patients. The identification of each tract on these color-coded maps is performed by using anatomic atlases and guidelines obtained in healthy individuals.[31,32] ROIs are then placed on the course of the tract (**Fig. 10**). To improve tract delineation, a 2-ROIs approach is usually preferred in patients with tumors. With this approach, only the fibers passing through the 2 ROIs are reconstructed (see **Fig. 10**). The directionally FA color-coded maps enable to locate the different fiber tracts in the anatomy of each patient even if the white matter is deviated from its normal location. However, when tumor infiltration is associated with a reduced anisotropy, the identification of the tract and the selection of the ROIs can be hazardous and highly prone to subjective decisions made by the examiner.[33] In this context, analyzing the relationship of a tract and the tumor with color orientation maps is more robust, although not all tracts are distinguishable on these maps.

To improve tract tracking, studies have attempted to combine DTI with functional magnetic resonance imaging (fMRI) for tracking the corticospinal tract and the arcuate fasciculus.[33–38] Seed ROIs are then defined based on fMRI activation patterns specific to individual patients. Tract tracking using fMRI positioning improved tractography in 6 patients with tumors in language areas and 3 patients with tumors in motor areas as compared with anatomic ROIs.[33] Also, when fiber displacement occurs, fMRI-based selection of seed ROIs may provide more reliable mapping of the fibers path. However, this approach presents limitations. The sensitivity and specificity of cortical sites identified with fMRI also depend on several factors, including the type of tasks used for testing and the thresholds used to display activation maps. Functional images are also subject to magnetic susceptibility artifacts and geometric distortions, and tumor angiogenesis can alter fMRI signal.[39–42]

Reconstruction parameters

The results of tractography depend on the parameters used for tractography,[22] for example, FA and angle thresholds. For example, an increase in the FA threshold reduces the number of detectable

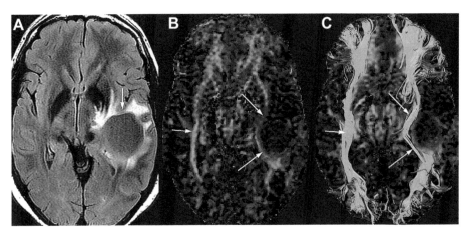

Fig. 7. Importance of reconstruction parameters: angle threshold. (*A*) Patient presenting with a tumoral cyst as seen on a fluid-attenuated inversion recovery image (*arrow*). (*B*) In the axial color-coded orientation image, the left inferior occipitofrontal fasciculus is displaced inwards by the tumor as compared with the contralateral tract (*arrows*). These fibers were not reconstructed with DTI tractography using a 35° threshold angle parameter. With a 45° angle threshold, these fibers were reconstructed (*arrows*) (*C*) (TrackVis software).

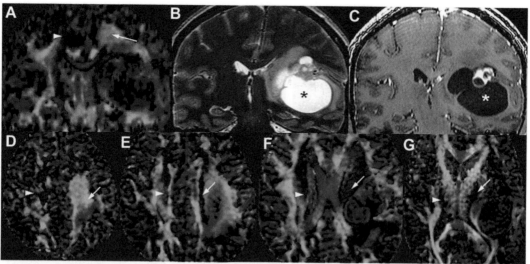

Fig. 8. Tumor mass effect, modification of the diffusion orientation and crossing fibers. Patient presenting a pilocytic astrocytoma with tumor mass effect and peripheral vasogenic edema as seen in (*A*) color-coded FA map and (*B*) (*asterisk*) coronal T2-weighted and (*C*) (*asterisk*) T1-weighted postgadolinium images. In the color-coded anisotropy images in the coronal (*A*) and axial planes (*D–G*), the orientation of anisotropy in the homolateral corticospinal tract was modified. Tumor mass effect induced a modification of the direction of anisotropy at the periphery of the tumor. In the normal hemisphere, the tract was color-coded in blue (*arrowheads in A, D–G*), indicating a superoinferior direction. In the pathologic hemisphere, fibers were seen in green (anteroposterior orientation [*arrows in A, D*]) and red (left-to-right orientation [*arrows in E, F*]). Only the inferior portion of the tract in the internal capsule presented the expected superoinferior orientation (blue, [*A, G, arrow*]). As a result, DTI tractography failed to reconstruct the corticospinal tract in the regions where the directional anisotropy was altered even if the tract was not invaded by the lesion. In this situation, the identification of the tract was performed using the color-coded maps.

fiber bundles and increases the distance between the reconstructed fiber bundles and the tumor.[43] In patients with tumor infiltration and low local FA, lowering the FA threshold can allow proper reconstruction of the tract when no tract is evidenced with the usual threshold.[28,30] The same situation exists with the angle threshold and mass effect (see **Fig. 7**). One has also to keep in mind that DTI fasciculus is not a representation of the actual size of the fiber tracts.[25] The field strength is also important because higher field strength increases the signal to noise ratio and improves fiber tracking.[44]

Brain shifting and coregistration pitfalls

Intraoperative brain shift caused by gravity, loss of CSF, and tumor resection with reexpansion of the formerly compressed brain is a well-known

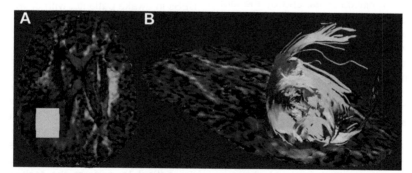

Fig. 9. Tumor effect, modification of the diffusion orientation and spurious fibers. Patient presenting an anaplastic glioma associated with a modification of the directional anisotropy. DTI tractography within the tumor using the ROI in green (*A*) resulted in the reconstruction of multiple spurious fibers as seen in the oblique view (*B*); (TrackVis software). In this case, the interpretation of the tracts inside the tumor is impossible.

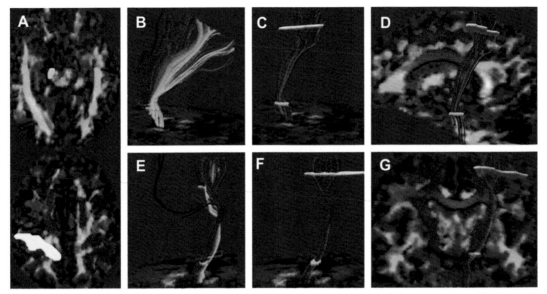

Fig. 10. Reconstruction of the corticospinal tract using 1 (*B, E*) or 2 ROIs (*C, D, F, G*). (*A*) ROI in the midbrain and in the precentral gyrus. (*B–D*) Oblique sagittal and (*E–G*) coronal views showing the tractography results using the midbrain ROI only (*B, E*) and both the midbrain and the precentral ROIs (*C–D* and *F–G*). Tracts are superimposed on the color-coded maps (*D, G*).

phenomenon.[45–48] Intraoperative white matter tract shifting was reported ranging from an inward shift of 8 mm to an outward shift of 15 mm.[47] This inevitable shift significantly reduces the reliability of preoperative images and neuronavigation during surgery. Several investigators have reported the combination of cortical and subcortical stimulation and tractography integrated in a neuronavigation system.[25,30,49–52] Although this integration is very promising, the interpretation of the topography of the tracts into the operation room has to integrate a possible gap between the reconstructed tract and the stimulation site. This gap is multifactorial and can be explained by brain shifting, by registration inaccuracies, and by the fact that DTI fiber tracking can underestimate the size of fiber bundles.[25] As a consequence, subcortical DESs usefully complements DTI fiber tracking during removal of tumors located within 1 cm from the pyramidal tracts.[52]

MAIN FIBER TRACTS, VALIDATION STUDIES, OVERVIEW, AND CURRENT STATE

The main purpose of brain tumor surgery is to achieve maximal tumor resection while preserving essential brain functions, which can be challenging in tumors located in functional areas. In this context, the preservation of motor, language, and visual functions is essential.

Methods of Validation of DTI Fiber Tracks

Postmortem studies
Results of fiber tracking have been correlated with postmortem dissection studies, showing close correspondence for the arcuate fasciculus,[53] the inferior occipitofrontal fasciculus,[53,54] the corticospinal tract,[53] the cingulum,[53] the uncinate fasciculus,[53,54] the cerebellar pathways,[53] and the Meyer loop.[54]

DESs studies
Methods An increasing number of studies have compared the results of motor and language DTI fiber tracks with intraoperative direct subcortical DESs in awake patients, with or without neuronavigation system and also with intraoperative magnetic resonance imaging.[28–30,50,52,55–58]

Limitations of DESs studies Validation of DTI-reconstructed tracts with DESs has some limitations. The correlations are limited by brain shifting, and the testing depends on patient cooperation and fatigue. If the attention level of the patient decreases, erroneous interpretation may result, increasing the number of false positives.[59] Also, DESs interfere directly by blocking the ability of the patient to perform the task. It is assumed that DESs map critical areas only, although it is possible that a tract carries not only critical but also nonessential functions. An example of this situation is the inferior longitudinal fasciculus (ILF) that is suspected to be implicated in the semantic components of speech while its stimulation and resection induce no language deficit and are probably compensated.[60] Another limitation is technical, the testing performed during DESs is time limited and includes only simple tasks. The testing paradigm is then limited to some aspects of language processing,[59] for example, picture naming involves attention, visual perception, visual-conceptual integration, semantic comprehension, motor initiation, phonological expression, and articulation but not semantic processing of sentences or syntax.[61–63]

Specific DTI Fiber Tracks, Reconstruction Methods, and Validation

The following paragraphs present the main fiber tracts implicated in motor, language, and visual functions. Methods to reconstruct the fiber tracts and ROI placement are described in the figure legends.

Corticospinal tract

The anatomy of the corticospinal (pyramidal) tract is well known. This tract contains motor as well as premotor fibers.[64] The corticospinal tract is usually traced using a 2-ROIs approach (see **Fig. 10**). Eloquent cortical areas revealed by intraoperative stimulations were also used as seeding points for fiber tracking, delineating pathways between functional regions.[49,65]

A good correspondence was reported between DTI-reconstructed tracks and positive functional subcortical DESs site, in 92% to 95%.[30,56] As for the reconstructed fiber tracts, the topography of the tract inside or at the boundaries of the tumor

was confirmed by DESs.[30,66] As mentioned previously, HARDI images with Q-ball tractography allow reconstructing the superior-medial and lateral portions of the tract in good agreement with cortical and subcortical DESs.[26,67]

Language tracts

Current theories on brain organization suggest that cognitive functions, such as language, are organized in widespread, segregated, and overlapping networks.[68] Recently, Hickok and Poeppel[69] proposed a dual-stream model for auditory language processing. This model includes a dorsal pathway involved in mapping sound to articulation, mediating sublexical repetition of speech, and a ventral pathway mediating comprehension. Although the dorsal pathway is suspected to include the arcuate fasciculus, the constitution of the ventral pathway is still a matter of debate. Some investigators[70] and subcortical DESs studies[71] suggest that the ventral pathway is composed by the inferior fronto-occipital fasciculus (IFOF), uncinate fasciculus, and ILF, whereas a recent study combining fMRI and tractography suggested the implication of a pathway coursing along the extreme capsule between the insular cortex and the claustrum.[72] Studies combining DESs and tractography reported that DESs-positive subcortical sites corresponded with DTI fiber tracts in 81% to 97%.[28,30] In contrast, DTI fails to evidence insular fibers responsible for speech arrest when stimulated because their anatomy remains unknown.[28]

Arcuate fasciculus The arcuate fasciculus is a large lateral associative bundle composed of long and short fibers connecting the perisylvian cortex of the frontal, parietal, and temporal lobes (**Fig. 11**).[31]

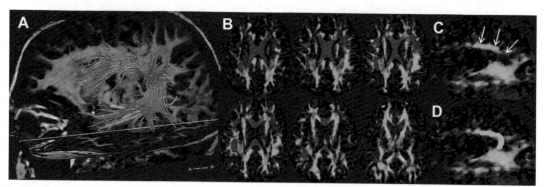

Fig. 11. Reconstruction of the arcuate fasciculus. (*A*) Visualization of the arcuate fasciculus superimposed to the multiplanar anatomy of a patient. ROIs for tractography can be placed on the color-coded maps either on the axial ([*B*], ROI in red) or the sagittal images ([*C, D*], ROI in blue in [*D*]). In the sagittal plane (*C*), the arcuate fasciculus is visualized as a perisylvian bundle with an anteroposterior segment (*green*) and a vertical segment (*blue*) (*arrows*).

The dense part of the fasciculus can be easily visualized as periventricular anteroposterior fibers on an axial plane or on the sagittal plane as C-shaped perisylvian fibers (see **Fig. 11**). In the left dominant hemisphere, stimulations of the arcuate fasciculus suggest that it conveys the phonological components of language. Negative DESs results in areas where DTI showed the presence of the arcuate fasciculus may also indicate that arcuate fibers may not be all functionally relevant for language.[30] In the right hemisphere, the arcuate fasciculus may be involved in visuospatial processing[73,74] and some aspects of language, such as prosody and semantic.[70]

Inferior fronto-occipital fasciculus The IFOF connects the ventral occipital lobe with the orbitofrontal cortex via the external capsule. IFOF fibers are visualized as anteroposterior occipitotemporal fibers in the color-coded orientation maps (**Fig. 12**). Without tractography, IFOF fibers cannot be distinguished from other adjacent anteroposterior tracts, such as the ILF or the optic radiations. Its implication in language and semantic processes is strongly supported by intraoperative DESs studies, which always reported semantic paraphasias[28,55] consecutive to its stimulation. The occipitofrontal fasciculus has also been reported to participate in reading,[73,75] attention, and visual processing.[76,77]

Inferior longitudinal fasciculus The ILF is a fiber bundle linking occipital areas and the temporal lobe (**Fig. 13**).[78] The ILF is likely to play an important role in visual object recognition, in reading,[75] and in linking object representations to their lexical labels.[79] The ILF may not be indispensable for language because it can be compensated both during stimulation and after resection.[60] However, tumoral invasion of the ILF may induce language deficits when the occipitofrontal fasciculus is already disrupted.[80]

Uncinate fasciculus The uncinate fasciculus is a fiber bundle connecting the anterior part of the temporal lobe and the orbitofrontal area (**Figs. 14 and 15**).[24] The functions of this bundle are poorly understood.[31] Uncinate fasciculus is considered to belong to the limbic system and could be involved in emotion processing and memory.[81] It may also play an important role in lexical retrieval, semantic associations, and aspects of naming that require connections from temporal to frontal components of the language network (eg, the naming of actions).[70] Likewise the ILF, a subcortical electrical stimulation study also suggested that uncinate fasciculus is not essential for language.[82]

Optic radiations
The optic radiations originate from the lateral geniculate nucleus and divide into 2 bundles, a ventral temporal loop, also called the Meyer loop, and a dorsal optic radiation. The fibers of the dorsal optic radiations convey the information of the inferior contralateral visual field of both eyes. The fibers bend posteriorly toward the occipital pole and terminate in the upper calcarine lip (see **Fig. 15**).[78,83] The ventral temporal loop bundle passes below the dorsal optic radiation fibers and projects forward and laterally toward the temporal pole. After a short run, the temporal loop describes a sharp arc around the temporal

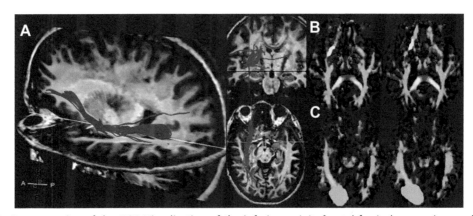

Fig. 12. Reconstruction of the IFOF. Visualization of the inferior occipitofrontal fasciculus superimposed to the multiplanar T1-weighted anatomy of a patient. (*A*). The IFOF is reconstructed with a 2-ROIs approach using an ROI in the anterior and inferior part of the external capsule (yellow in the axial color-coded maps [*B*]) and an ROI in the temporo-occipital white matter, including the lingual (O5) and fusiform (T4) gyri (green on the axial color-coded maps [*C*]).

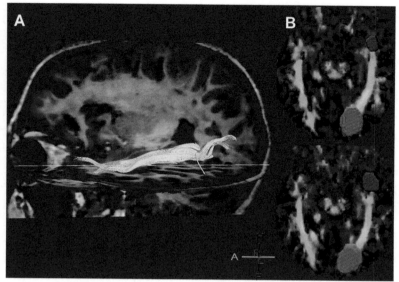

Fig. 13. Reconstruction of the ILF. Visualization of the ILF superimposed to the multiplanar T1-weighted anatomy of a patient (A). The ILF reconstructed with a 2-ROI approach using an ROI in the white matter of the anterior part of the temporal pole (purple on the axial color-coded maps [B]) and the same temporo-occipital ROI used for the tractography of the IFOF (blue on the axial color-coded maps [B]).

horn of the lateral ventricle and continues backward toward the occipital pole where it terminates in the lower calcarine lip. This ventral loop (Meyer loop) transmits visual information from the contralateral superior field of both eyes. Damage to its fibers causes a bilateral homonymous superior quadrantanopia.[84] The anterior extent of this loop presents with a high interindividual variability[6,85–87] and has the particularity to be difficult to reconstruct with tractography.[88] Visual field defects are usually not tested by DESs in the operating room. Two recent studies correlated the results of DTI tracking and postoperative visual field defects after temporal lobectomy.[58,86] Although the Meyer loop is a thin bundle, its evaluation with tractography seems to be feasible,[89] and

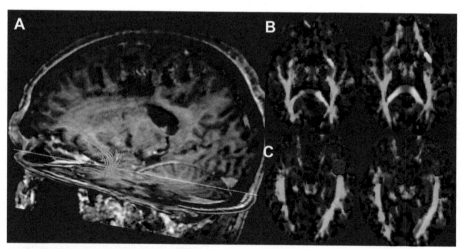

Fig. 14. Reconstruction of the uncinate fasciculus. Visualization of the uncinate fasciculus superimposed to the multiplanar T1-weighted anatomy of a patient (A). The uncinate fasciculus is reconstructed with a 2-ROIs approach using an ROI in the anterior and inferior part of the external capsule as in the reconstruction of the IFOF (yellow on the axial color-coded maps [B]) and the same anterior temporal ROI used for the tractography of the ILF (purple on the axial color-coded maps [C]).

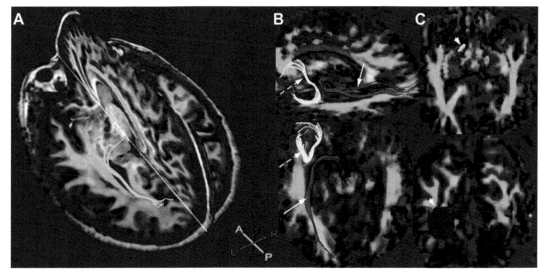

Fig. 15. Reconstruction of the optic radiations. Visualization of the optic radiations in the multiplanar anatomy of the patient (blue in A and red in B, indicated with *arrows*). The optic radiations are reconstructed with a 2-ROIs approach using an ROI positioned on the optic tract and the lateral geniculate body (yellow on the axial color-coded maps [*arrowhead, C*]) and an ROI in the occipital white matter (blue on the axial color-coded maps [*arrowhead, C*]). The uncinate fasciculus is represented in yellow (*dashed arrow* [B]) (TrackVis software).

the confidence in the validity of the anterior limit this loop can be increased by reconstructing the uncinate fasciculus as a reference for its anterior limit.[54,89] In both studies, the distance from the tip of the Meyer loop to the temporal pole and the size of resection were significant predictors of the postoperative visual field defect.

Effect on Patient Care

DTI tractography for presurgical mapping is thus feasible, and there is a good concordance between tractography results and DESs, even if limitations exist. DTI tractography improves patient's care. A lower rate of postoperative deficit and dependency and a higher median survival rate were reported in 118 patients operated with DTI-integrated neuronavigation as compared with 120 patients operated with anatomic imaging and neuronavigation.[57]

Moreover, the combination of DTI fiber tracking and intraoperative DESs decreases the duration of surgery, patient fatigue, and intraoperative seizures.[30] Similarly, combined tractography and subcortical motor evoked potentials resulted in better surgical outcome in the preservation of motor function than outcomes repeated after motor evoked potentials monitoring alone or fiber tracking alone.[52]

However, intraoperative DESs still remain the gold standard to map the functional boundaries of the resection and have significantly improved the survival rate of patients undergoing low-

grade glioma resections.[90] The role of preoperative mapping of the tracks using DTI is then to speed up radical resections by indicating which borders of a resection cavity deserve extensive stimulation.[26]

Therefore, combined DTI preoperative mapping and intraoperative DESs have the potential to improve the overall patient care.

SUMMARY

DTI and tractography is a powerful tool for preoperative and intraoperative subcortical mapping in functional areas. The orientation color maps and 3D fiber tracts provided by this technique present pitfalls, which must be known before using the images in the operation room. Tractography is a user-defined method and can be falsely negative in regions with tumor infiltration and tumor mass effect. Therefore, negative tractography results do not exclude the persistence of functional fibers, and DTI tractography should not be interpreted without color maps of diffusion orientation and strong a priori knowledge of the normal white matter anatomy. Another limitation is a possible gap between the DTI-reconstructed tract and the anatomic tract.

Despite these limitations, concordance between the DTI tracts and subcortical mapping is high, and DTI fiber tracking has proven useful to guide stimulations and resections to improve overall patient care.

REFERENCES

1. Berger MS. Minimalism through intraoperative functional mapping. Clin Neurosurg 1996;43:324–37.

2. Black PM. Brain tumors. Part 1. N Engl J Med 1991; 324(21):1471–6.

3. Duffau H. New concepts in surgery of WHO grade II gliomas: functional brain mapping, connectionism and plasticity—a review. J Neurooncol 2006;79(1): 77–115.

4. Basser PJ, Pajevic S, Pierpaoli C, et al. In vivo fiber tractography using DT-MRI data. Magn Reson Med 2000;44(4):625–32.

5. Beaulieu C. The basis of anisotropic water diffusion in the nervous system - a technical review. NMR Biomed 2002;15(7–8):435–55.

6. Burgel U, Schormann T, Schleicher A, et al. Mapping of histologically identified long fiber tracts in human cerebral hemispheres to the MRI volume of a reference brain: position and spatial variability of the optic radiation. Neuroimage 1999;10(5):489–99.

7. Mori S, Frederiksen K, van Zijl PC, et al. Brain white matter anatomy of tumor patients evaluated with diffusion tensor imaging. Ann Neurol 2002;51(3): 377–80.

8. Mori S, van Zijl PC. Fiber tracking: principles and strategies - a technical review. NMR Biomed 2002; 15(7–8):468–80.

9. Conturo TE, Lori NF, Cull TS, et al. Tracking neuronal fiber pathways in the living human brain. Proc Natl Acad Sci U S A 1999;96(18):10422–7.

10. Pierpaoli C, Jezzard P, Basser PJ, et al. Diffusion tensor MR imaging of the human brain. Radiology 1996;201(3):637–48.

11. Le Bihan D, Breton E, Lallemand D, et al. MR imaging of intravoxel incoherent motions: application to diffusion and perfusion in neurologic disorders. Radiology 1986;161(2):401–7.

12. Basser PJ, Pierpaoli C. A simplified method to measure the diffusion tensor from seven MR images. Magn Reson Med 1998;39(6):928–34.

13. Le Bihan D. The 'wet mind': water and functional neuroimaging. Phys Med Biol 2007;52(7):R57–90.

14. Pajevic S, Pierpaoli C. Color schemes to represent the orientation of anisotropic tissues from diffusion tensor data: application to white matter fiber tract mapping in the human brain. Magn Reson Med 1999;42(3):526–40.

15. Mori S, Crain BJ, Chacko VP, et al. Three-dimensional tracking of axonal projections in the brain by magnetic resonance imaging. Ann Neurol 1999; 45(2):265–9.

16. Field AS, Alexander AL, Wu YC, et al. Diffusion tensor eigenvector directional color imaging patterns in the evaluation of cerebral white matter tracts altered by tumor. J Magn Reson Imaging 2004;20(4):555–62.

17. Witwer BP, Moftakhar R, Hasan KM, et al. Diffusion-tensor imaging of white matter tracts in patients with cerebral neoplasm. J Neurosurg 2002;97(3):568–75.

18. Jellison BJ, Field AS, Medow J, et al. Diffusion tensor imaging of cerebral white matter: a pictorial review of physics, fiber tract anatomy, and tumor imaging patterns. AJNR Am J Neuroradiol 2004;25(3):356–69.

19. Cruz LC Jr, Sorensen AG. Diffusion tensor magnetic resonance imaging of brain tumors. Magn Reson Imaging Clin N Am 2006;14(2):183–202.

20. Field AS. Diffusion tensor imaging at the crossroads: fiber tracking meets tissue characterization in brain tumors. AJNR Am J Neuroradiol 2005;26(9):2168–9.

21. Le Bihan D, Poupon C, Amadon A, et al. Artifacts and pitfalls in diffusion MRI. J Magn Reson Imaging 2006;24(3):478–88.

22. Clark CA, Barrick TR, Murphy MM, et al. White matter fiber tracking in patients with space-occupying lesions of the brain: a new technique for neurosurgical planning? Neuroimage 2003; 20(3):1601–8.

23. Virta A, Barnett A, Pierpaoli C. Visualizing and characterizing white matter fiber structure and architecture in the human pyramidal tract using diffusion tensor MRI. Magn Reson Imaging 1999;17(8): 1121–33.

24. Catani M, Howard RJ, Pajevic S, et al. Virtual in vivo interactive dissection of white matter fasciculi in the human brain. Neuroimage 2002;17(1):77–94.

25. Kinoshita M, Yamada K, Hashimoto N, et al. Fiber-tracking does not accurately estimate size of fiber bundle in pathological condition: initial neurosurgical experience using neuronavigation and subcortical white matter stimulation. Neuroimage 2005; 25(2):424–9.

26. Berman J. Diffusion MR tractography as a tool for surgical planning. Magn Reson Imaging Clin N Am 2009;17(2):205–14.

27. Tuch DS. Q-ball imaging. Magn Reson Med 2004; 52(6):1358–72.

28. Leclercq D, Duffau H, Delmaire C, et al. Comparison of diffusion tensor imaging tractography of language tracts and intraoperative subcortical stimulations. J Neurosurg 2010;112(3):503–11.

29. Spena G, Nava A, Cassini F, et al. Preoperative and intraoperative brain mapping for the resection of eloquent-area tumors. A prospective analysis of methodology, correlation, and usefulness based on clinical outcomes. Acta Neurochir (Wien) 2010; 152(11):1835–46.

30. Bello L, Gambini A, Castellano A, et al. Motor and language DTI Fiber Tracking combined with intraoperative subcortical mapping for surgical removal of gliomas. Neuroimage 2008;39(1):369–82.

31. Catani M, Thiebaut de Schotten M. A diffusion tensor imaging tractography atlas for virtual in vivo dissections. Cortex 2008;44(8):1105–32.

32. Thiebaut de Schotten M, Ffytche DH, Bizzi A, et al. Atlasing location, asymmetry and inter-subject variability of white matter tracts in the human brain with MR diffusion tractography. Neuroimage 2011; 54(1):49–59.

33. Schonberg T, Pianka P, Hendler T, et al. Characterization of displaced white matter by brain tumors using combined DTI and fMRI. Neuroimage 2006; 30(4):1100–11.

34. Kleiser R, Staempfli P, Valavanis A, et al. Impact of fMRI-guided advanced DTI fiber tracking techniques on their clinical applications in patients with brain tumors. Neuroradiology 2010;52(1):37–46.

35. Guye M, Parker GJ, Symms M, et al. Combined functional MRI and tractography to demonstrate the connectivity of the human primary motor cortex in vivo. Neuroimage 2003;19(4):1349–60.

36. Hendler T, Pianka P, Sigal M, et al. Delineating gray and white matter involvement in brain lesions: three-dimensional alignment of functional magnetic resonance and diffusion-tensor imaging. J Neurosurg 2003;99(6):1018–27.

37. Watts R, Liston C, Niogi S, et al. Fiber tracking using magnetic resonance diffusion tensor imaging and its applications to human brain development. Ment Retard Dev Disabil Res Rev 2003;9(3):168–77.

38. Staempfli P, Reischauer C, Jaermann T, et al. Combining fMRI and DTI: a framework for exploring the limits of fMRI-guided DTI fiber tracking and for verifying DTI-based fiber tractography results. Neuroimage 2008;39(1):119–26.

39. Roux FE, Ibarrola D, Tremoulet M, et al. Methodological and technical issues for integrating functional magnetic resonance imaging data in a neuronavigational system. Neurosurgery 2001;49(5):1145–56 [discussion: 1156–7].

40. Schiffbauer H, Ferrari P, Rowley HA, et al. Functional activity within brain tumors: a magnetic source imaging study. Neurosurgery 2001;49(6):1313–20 [discussion: 1320–1].

41. Bogomolny DL, Petrovich NM, Hou BL, et al. Functional MRI in the brain tumor patient. Top Magn Reson Imaging 2004;15(5):325–35.

42. Lehericy S, Duffau H, Cornu P, et al. Correspondence between functional magnetic resonance imaging somatotopy and individual brain anatomy of the central region: comparison with intraoperative stimulation in patients with brain tumors. J Neurosurg 2000;92(4):589–98.

43. Stadlbauer A, Nimsky C, Buslei R, et al. Diffusion tensor imaging and optimized fiber tracking in glioma patients: histopathologic evaluation of tumor-invaded white matter structures. Neuroimage 2007;34(3):949–56.

44. Okada T, Miki Y, Fushimi Y, et al. Diffusion-tensor fiber tractography: intraindividual comparison of 3.0-T and 1.5-T MR imaging. Radiology 2006; 238(2):668–78.

45. Nimsky C, Ganslandt O, Cerny S, et al. Quantification of, visualization of, and compensation for brain shift using intraoperative magnetic resonance imaging. Neurosurgery 2000;47(5):1070–9 [discussion: 1079–80].

46. Nimsky C, Ganslandt O, Hastreiter P, et al. Preoperative and intraoperative diffusion tensor imaging-based fiber tracking in glioma surgery. Neurosurgery 2005;56(1):130–7 [discussion: 138].

47. Nimsky C, Ganslandt O, Hastreiter P, et al. Intraoperative diffusion-tensor MR imaging: shifting of white matter tracts during neurosurgical procedures—initial experience. Radiology 2005;234(1):218–25.

48. Reinges MH, Nguyen HH, Krings T, et al. Course of brain shift during microsurgical resection of supratentorial cerebral lesions: limits of conventional neuronavigation. Acta Neurochir (Wien) 2004;146(4): 369–77 [discussion: 377].

49. Berman JI, Berger MS, Mukherjee P, et al. Diffusion-tensor imaging-guided tracking of fibers of the pyramidal tract combined with intraoperative cortical stimulation mapping in patients with gliomas. J Neurosurg 2004;101(1):66–72.

50. Kamada K, Todo T, Masutani Y, et al. Combined use of tractography-integrated functional neuronavigation and direct fiber stimulation. J Neurosurg 2005; 102(4):664–72.

51. Okada T, Mikuni N, Miki Y, et al. Corticospinal tract localization: integration of diffusion-tensor tractography at 3-T MR imaging with intraoperative white matter stimulation mapping—preliminary results. Radiology 2006;240(3):849–57.

52. Mikuni N, Okada T, Enatsu R, et al. Clinical impact of integrated functional neuronavigation and subcortical electrical stimulation to preserve motor function during resection of brain tumors. J Neurosurg 2007; 106(4):593–8.

53. Lawes IN, Barrick TR, Murugam V, et al. Atlas-based segmentation of white matter tracts of the human brain using diffusion tensor tractography and comparison with classical dissection. Neuroimage 2008;39(1):62–79.

54. Kier EL, Staib LH, Davis LM, et al. MR imaging of the temporal stem: anatomic dissection tractography of the uncinate fasciculus, inferior occipitofrontal fasciculus, and Meyer's loop of the optic radiation. AJNR Am J Neuroradiol 2004;25(5):677–91.

55. Bello L, Gallucci M, Fava M, et al. Intraoperative subcortical language tract mapping guides surgical removal of gliomas involving speech areas. Neurosurgery 2007;60(1):67–80 [discussion: 80–2].

56. Coenen VA, Krings T, Axer H, et al. Intraoperative three-dimensional visualization of the pyramidal tract in a neuronavigation system (PTV) reliably

predicts true position of principal motor pathways. Surg Neurol 2003;60(5):381–90 [discussion: 390].

57. Wu JS, Zhou LF, Tang WJ, et al. Clinical evaluation and follow-up outcome of diffusion tensor imaging-based functional neuronavigation: a prospective, controlled study in patients with gliomas involving pyramidal tracts. Neurosurgery 2007;61(5):935–48 [discussion: 948–9].

58. Chen X, Weigel D, Ganslandt O, et al. Prediction of visual field deficits by diffusion tensor imaging in temporal lobe epilepsy surgery. Neuroimage 2009; 45(2):286–97.

59. De Witt Hamer PC, Moritz-Gasser S, Gatignol P, et al. Is the human left middle longitudinal fascicle essential for language? A brain electrostimulation study. Hum Brain Mapp 2010. [Epub ahead of print].

60. Mandonnet E, Nouet A, Gatignol P, et al. Does the left inferior longitudinal fasciculus play a role in language? A brain stimulation study. Brain 2007; 130(Pt 3):623–9.

61. DeLeon J, Gottesman RF, Kleinman JT, et al. Neural regions essential for distinct cognitive processes underlying picture naming. Brain 2007;130(Pt 5): 1408–22.

62. Glaser WR. Picture naming. Cognition 1992;42(1–3): 61–105.

63. Johnson CJ, Paivio A, Clark JM. Cognitive components of picture naming. Psychol Bull 1996;120(1): 113–39.

64. Newton JM, Ward NS, Parker GJ, et al. Non-invasive mapping of corticofugal fibres from multiple motor areas—relevance to stroke recovery. Brain 2006; 129(Pt 7):1844–58.

65. Henry RG, Berman JI, Nagarajan SS, et al. Subcortical pathways serving cortical language sites: initial experience with diffusion tensor imaging fiber tracking combined with intraoperative language mapping. Neuroimage 2004;21(2):616–22.

66. Bello L, Castellano A, Fava E, et al. Intraoperative use of diffusion tensor imaging fiber tractography and subcortical mapping for resection of gliomas: technical considerations. Neurosurg Focus 2010; 28(2):E6.

67. Berman JI, Clark DJ, Berger MS, et al. Improved diffusion MR fiber tracking for neurosurgical application ISMRM Toronto, Oral Presentation. 2008.

68. Mesulam MM. Large-scale neurocognitive networks and distributed processing for attention, language, and memory. Ann Neurol 1990;28(5):597–613.

69. Hickok G, Poeppel D. Dorsal and ventral streams: a framework for understanding aspects of the functional anatomy of language. Cognition 2004;92(1–2): 67–99.

70. Catani M, Mesulam M. The arcuate fasciculus and the disconnection theme in language and aphasia: history and current state. Cortex 2008;44(8):953–61.

71. Duffau H, Gatignol P, Mandonnet E, et al. New insights into the anatomo-functional connectivity of the semantic system: a study using cortico-subcortical electrostimulations. Brain 2005;128 (Pt 4):797–810.

72. Saur D, Kreher BW, Schnell S, et al. Ventral and dorsal pathways for language. Proc Natl Acad Sci U S A 2008;105(46):18035–40.

73. Doricchi F, Thiebaut de Schotten M, Tomaiuolo F, et al. White matter (dis)connections and gray matter (dys)functions in visual neglect: gaining insights into the brain networks of spatial awareness. Cortex 2008;44(8):983–95.

74. Thiebaut de Schotten M, Kinkingnehun S, Delmaire C, et al. Visualization of disconnection syndromes in humans. Cortex 2008;44(8):1097–103.

75. Epelbaum S, Pinel P, Gaillard R, et al. Pure alexia as a disconnection syndrome: new diffusion imaging evidence for an old concept. Cortex 2008;44(8): 962–74.

76. Fox CJ, Iaria G, Barton JJ. Disconnection in prosopagnosia and face processing. Cortex 2008;44(8): 996–1009.

77. Rudrauf D, Mehta S, Grabowski TJ. Disconnection's renaissance takes shape: formal incorporation in group-level lesion studies. Cortex 2008;44(8): 1084–96.

78. Catani M, Jones DK, Donato R, et al. Occipito-temporal connections in the human brain. Brain 2003;126(Pt 9):2093–107.

79. Mummery CJ, Patterson K, Wise RJ, et al. Disrupted temporal lobe connections in semantic dementia. Brain 1999;122(Pt 1):61–73.

80. Shinoura N, Suzuki Y, Tsukada M, et al. Deficits in the left inferior longitudinal fasciculus results in impairments in object naming. Neurocase 2010; 16(2):135–9.

81. Gaffan D, Wilson CR. Medial temporal and prefrontal function: recent behavioural disconnection studies in the macaque monkey. Cortex 2008;44(8):928–35.

82. Duffau H, Gatignol P, Moritz-Gasser S, et al. Is the left uncinate fasciculus essential for language? A cerebral stimulation study. J Neurol 2009;256(3): 382–9.

83. Choi C, Rubino PA, Fernandez-Miranda JC, et al. Meyer's loop and the optic radiations in the transsylvian approach to the mediobasal temporal lobe. Neurosurgery 2006;59(4 Suppl 2):ONS228–35 [discussion: ONS235–6].

84. Jacobson DM. The localizing value of a quadrantanopia. Arch Neurol 1997;54(4):401–4.

85. Ebeling U, Reulen HJ. Neurosurgical topography of the optic radiation in the temporal lobe. Acta Neurochir (Wien) 1988;92(1–4):29–36.

86. Yogarajah M, Focke NK, Bonelli S, et al. Defining Meyer's loop-temporal lobe resections, visual field

deficits and diffusion tensor tractography. Brain 2009;132(Pt 6):1656–68.

87. Nilsson D, Starck G, Ljungberg M, et al. Intersubject variability in the anterior extent of the optic radiation assessed by tractography. Epilepsy Res 2007;77(1): 11–6.

88. Yamamoto A, Miki Y, Urayama S, et al. Diffusion tensor fiber tractography of the optic radiation: analysis with 6-, 12-, 40-, and 81-directional motion-probing gradients, a preliminary study. AJNR Am J Neuroradiol 2007;28(1):92–6.

89. Taoka T, Sakamoto M, Nakagawa H, et al. Diffusion tensor tractography of the Meyer loop in cases of temporal lobe resection for temporal lobe epilepsy: correlation between postsurgical visual field defect and anterior limit of Meyer loop on tractography. AJNR Am J Neuroradiol 2008;29(7):1329–34.

90. Duffau H. Lessons from brain mapping in surgery for low-grade glioma: insights into associations between tumour and brain plasticity. Lancet Neurol 2005;4(8):476–86.

Intraoperative Acquisition of fMRI and DTI

Christopher Nimsky, MD, PhD

KEYWORDS

- Brain shift • Functional navigation • Multimodal navigation
- Intraoperative functional magnetic resonance
- Intraoperative diffusion tensor imaging

FUNCTIONAL NAVIGATION

The integration of functional data from functional MRI (fMRI) and magnetoencephalography (MEG) identifying eloquent cortical brain areas into standard 3-dimensional (D) anatomic datasets is known as functional navigation.[1–3] Eloquent functional structures, such as the motor strip or language-related areas can be identified during surgery by visualizing their position using the microscope-based heads-up display technology. Functional navigation allows resection of tumors close to eloquent brain areas with low postoperative deficits, whereas intraoperative imaging ensures that the maximum extent of a resection can be achieved.

Especially in surgery of high-grade tumors, it is of no benefit to maximize the extent of a resection to potentially increase the survival time by only some weeks when risking permanent neurologic deficits right after surgery. It is absolutely mandatory to combine the goal of maximum resection with the goal of preservation of function. Intraoperative imaging helps to maximize the extent of resection, and in combination with functional multimodal navigation it helps to minimize postoperative neurologic deficits.[4,5] With the advances in surgical techniques and perioperative technology, it is now possible to maximally resect malignant intrinsic glial neoplasms, even close to functionally critical areas, without increased morbidity. Studies have demonstrated a survival advantage in these lesions with a resection extent of 98% or greater, particularly in younger patients with good Karnofsky scores.[6]

To achieve this advantage, functional navigation, that is, integrating functional data into anatomic navigational datasets, is an important add-on to intraoperative MRI because it prevents too extensive resections, which would otherwise result in new neurologic deficits. Meanwhile, data from MEG and fMRI are routinely integrated in functional navigation, allowing identification of eloquent brain areas, such as the motor area and speech-related areas.[1,2]

In a retrospective study, the author's group investigated how the decision to resect a glioma was influenced by MEG.[1,7] Altogether, 191 patients were examined, 119 of them harbored supratentorial gliomas. About every forth patient (26.8%) yielded a severe possible danger of postoperative neurologic morbidity according to MEG and thus was not considered to be a good candidate for surgery. This result corresponds to published data in which 12 of 40 investigated patients (30%) with tumors and vascular malformations underwent nonsurgical therapy based on the MEG results.[8] When functional data were used in combination with frameless stereotactic devices the postoperative morbidity was as low as 2.3%. However, the overall morbidity was 6.8%. These data reflect the beneficial effects of functional navigation in comparison to data of other studies with morbidity rates varying from 6% to 31.7%.[9–13] These figures can also be interpreted as a result of a more careful patient

This work was supported by DFG grant SFB603/C9 & NI568/3–1.
The author is a scientific consultant regarding intraoperative magnetic resonance imaging for Brainlab.
Department of Neurosurgery, University Marburg, Baldingerstrasse, Marburg 35033, Germany
E-mail address: nimsky@med.uni-marburg.de

selection based on preoperative brain mapping. Preoperative identification of eloquent brain areas has an effect in the risk evaluation in glioma surgery, and functional navigation reduces the risk for postoperative neurologic deficits. Besides identification of the motor strip, the localization of language areas has a great clinical effect.[14,15]

The concept of functional navigation was expanded by the integration of further data leading to the so-called multimodal navigation. To prevent postoperative neurologic deficits, it is also mandatory to preserve major white matter tracts, such as the pyramidal tract for the motor system, that are connected to eloquent cortical brain areas, which are localized by fMRI and MEG.

As a first attempt to integrate information about major white matter tracts into a multimodal navigation setup, diffusion data with limited directional information were used for a rough estimation of the course of the pyramidal tract and applied for intraoperative guidance during brain tumor resection.[16,17] These methods often required time-consuming preoperative manual data processing, such as the segmentation of the assumed major white matter tract in single slices and subsequent image registration. The reliability of the reconstructed white matter tract depended mainly on the experience of the individual person processing the data.

Diffusion tensor imaging (DTI) is based on measuring multiple diffusion-weighted images in different gradient directions to resolve the orientation of the white matter tracts. DTI can resolve the dominant fiber orientation in each voxel element. The direction of greatest diffusion measured by DTI parallels the dominant orientation of the tissue structure in each voxel, representing the mean longitudinal direction of axons in the major white matter tracts. DTI provides information about the normal course, the displacement, or interruption of white matter tracts around a tumor, and the widening of fiber bundles due to edema or tumor infiltration can be detected.[18–26]

To integrate DTI data into navigational datasets, the first step was to register fractional anisotropy (FA) maps with the standard anatomic 3D images.[27–29] In contrast to using diffusion-weighted images for the delineation of major white matter tracts, the manual segmentation in color-coded FA maps was more reliable and less user dependent. However, still it was a time-consuming process, which allowed, especially close to a lesion, only a rough and quite unreliable estimation of the course of the pyramidal tract.

Fiber tracking is probably the most clinically appealing and understandable technique for representing major white matter tracts. Various tracking algorithms that compare local tensor field orientations measured by DTI from voxel to voxel have been developed, allowing a noninvasive tracing of large fiber tract bundles in the human brain (**Fig. 1**).

Initially, most approaches did not satisfy the needs of neurosurgical planning. For clinical intraoperative use, the actual border of a major white matter tract is of interest. A line representation such as the visualization in standard fiber tracking lacks the ability to provide a border, so the user has to interpret the visualization as a model for the tract. The generation of hulls is a possibility to overcome this drawback. A surface wrapping a particular subset of previously computed

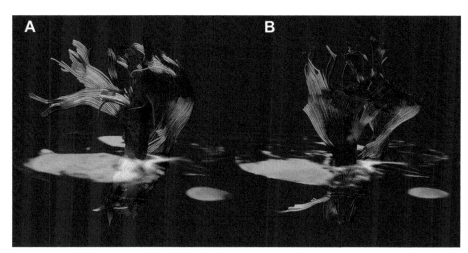

Fig. 1. Fiber tracking. Right temporal World Health Organization grade III astrocytoma in a 29-year-old man. Displayed is the fiber tracking of the pyramidal tract and an axial slice of the B0 diffusion images preoperatively (*A*) and postoperatively (*B*) depicting the clear outward shifting of the pyramidal tract on the right side after tumor removal.

streamlines represents a certain fiber tract bundle. This representation results in an intuitive visualization with flexible tubes, which is closely related to the expected appearance of a major white matter bundle or a complete 3D object representing the major white matter tract of interest. The combination with volume rendering of anatomic magnetic resonance (MR) data provides a good spatial orientation. Alternatively to this wrapping approach, volume-growing techniques can also generate 3D objects representing major white matter tracts.

Integration of tractography data into a stereotactic coordinate system was the next major step in the development of major white matter tract navigation. Most of these applications and approaches, however, were stand-alone applications developed for individual clinical sites.[27,29–31] A broad application for routine clinical use was not possible with the various prototype applications, and the missing standardization did not allow comparing the different approaches.

The implementation of a fiber tracking algorithm into a standard navigation system, allowing routine usage and broad availability, solved these restrictions.[32] Registration with standard anatomic image data greatly facilitated the generation and selection of the fibers of interest as well as eased the delineation of the relationship of the tracked fibers to certain anatomic structures because the seed regions for the tracking algorithms could be defined in high-resolution 3D anatomic images. The implemented approach allowed a straightforward definition of volumes of interest for selecting the fiber tracts of interest. Only 2 parameters, the FA threshold and the minimum length of the fibers that will be computed, have to be selected by the user. The total generation of the fiber tracts, including image transfer, registration of the diffusion data with the standard anatomic image data, tensor calculation, fiber tracking, and the final generation of a 3D object, needs less than 10 minutes, depending to some extent on the strategy by which the different seed volumes of interest during initiation of the tracking algorithm are selected.

The intraoperative visualization of the course of the pyramidal tract by microscope-based navigation during the resection of supratentorial gliomas has resulted in reduced neurologic deficits, which may serve as a proof of the concept per se. This concept is also supported by studies comparing preoperative and postoperative reconstructions of major white matter structures in the brain stem well correlating to clinical deficits.[33] Visual field deficits in temporal lobe surgery for pharmacoresistant epilepsy provide an ideal model to analyze the clinical validity of changes in fiber tracking by correlating the extent of visual field defects with the changes in preoperative and intraoperative DTI-based reconstruction of the optic radiation. The significant correlation between postoperative visual field deficits and the extent of alterations of the optic radiation also proved that reconstruction of major white matter tracts can be reliably used in a clinical setting.[34]

All these data clearly support the concept of functional navigation, that is, adding functional information to 3D anatomic datasets to reduce postoperative morbidity when operating on lesions close to eloquent brain structures. Of course, intraoperative knowledge of the exact position of the pyramidal tract does not prevent neurologic deficits per se; intraoperative events, such as the necessity to coagulate small vessels close to the pyramidal tract, may result in an injury of the pyramidal tract leading to neurologic deficits. The closest distance to which a reconstructed major white matter tract can be approached is not yet clearly defined. Analyzing the DTI-based navigation data with regard to the distance between tumor and pyramidal tract revealed that a distance of 5 mm seems to be a critical distance, which should be taken into account as safety margin.[35] This value corresponds well to an identical critical distance of about 5 mm when approaching functionally eloquent cortical brain areas delineated by fMRI or MEG data.[36]

Additional hulls around the reconstructed 3D objects representing major white matter tracts make visualization of these safety margins possible. Ideally, these encompassing hulls would vary in thickness with respect to the quality and reliability of the reconstructed fiber bundle.[37] In case of noisy unreliable data a thick hull would be added, whereas in highly reliable data the hull would be thinner. The technical and clinical definition of the extent of these safety margins has still to be established.

The major question is whether the tracking results actually reflect reality. First attempts correlating the DTI findings to intraoperative electrophysiological measurements showed quite some discrepancies,[31,38] which are probably mainly attributable to a distinct shifting of major white matter tracts during a neurosurgical procedure, which could be demonstrated by comparing preoperative and intraoperative fiber tracking, acquired by high-field MRI applied during surgery.

INTRAOPERATIVE IMAGING

Navigation systems have a decreasing accuracy during the course of a surgical procedure because these systems are normally based on preoperative data only. This decreasing accuracy is because of brain shift, that is, the intraoperative deformation of the brain, which is caused by tumor removal, brain swelling, the use of brain retractors, and cerebrospinal fluid drainage.[39,40] Intraoperative imaging offers a possibility to compensate for the effects of brain shift. It depicts a virtual reproduction of the actual intraoperative physical reality, on how the brain is deformed and on the extent of tumor removal.[39,41–43] The ability to objectively determine the extent of tumor removal during surgery is of great value. If a resection is incomplete, tumor residues that were initially missed can be further removed during the same operation. Intraoperative imaging allows an objective evaluation of the actual intraoperative situation, thus serving as quality control during surgery.[41,44–48]

Intraoperative high-field MRI is the most sophisticated possibility for intraoperative imaging compared with the alternatives such as intraoperative computed tomography and intraoperative ultrasonography.[49] Combining high-field MRI and microscope-based navigation enables an intraoperative possibility to compensate for the effects of brain shift by intraoperatively updating the image information.[41] For the update, the intraoperative images have to be registered either by a calibrated registration matrix that is attached to the upper part of the imaging coil and tracked by the navigation system[50] or by a direct registration of preoperative and intraoperative images, assuming that there is no positional shift, that is, that the initial patient registration was correct, so that the coordinate system of the initial patient registration can also be applied for the intraoperative images. Updated navigation with intraoperative image data allows a reliable identification of tumor remnants. Microscope-based heads-up displays with the direct visualization of the segmented tumor remnant in the surgical field play a crucial role in the precise localization and orientation in the resection cavity.

However, these updates typically are updates of anatomic data, so that the initially integrated preoperative functional data are lost. On the other hand, intraoperative high-field MRI not only allows for standard anatomic imaging such as T1- and T2-weighted sequences but also makes intraoperative fMRI and, more important clinically, intraoperative DTI feasible. Intraoperative MR spectroscopy (MRS) still has its limitations because of the brain-air interface. So there remains some distinct challenges for updating also the MRS information intraoperatively.

INTRAOPERATIVE FMRI

To implement intraoperative fMRI a passive stimulation paradigm with shielded electrical peripheral nerve stimulation of the median and tibial nerves was applied. For electric stimulation, an electromagnetically shielded coaxial lead was developed, while shielding was achieved by connecting the conductor's shielding mesh to the MRI cage. The impulse generator was located outside the radiofrequency-shielded cabin, and the conductor was threaded through a waveguide array into the actual operating theater. After induction of anesthesia and patient positioning, the stimulation electrodes were attached and the motor threshold was defined. After an initial anatomic and functional MR scan, 2 further data sets were acquired during and at the end of the surgical procedure. The block design stimulation paradigm alternated 4 rest and 4 activation periods of 33 seconds each. For functional imaging, slices parallel to the anterior-posterior commissural plane were acquired as T2*-weighted echo planar imaging sequences (echo time 60 milliseconds, repetition time 3300 milliseconds, flip angle 90°, slice thickness 3 mm, field of view 220 mm, matrix 64 × 64) with data acquisition covering the whole cerebrum. The fMRI data were analyzed during acquisition by an online statistical evaluation package installed in the MR scanner console (**Fig. 2**). In addition, phase reversal of somatosensory evoked potentials was used for verification of intraoperative fMRI. In 4 anesthetized patients with lesions in the vicinity of the central region, a total of 11 fMRI measurements were successfully acquired and analyzed online. Activation was found in the somatosensory cortex, which could be confirmed by intraoperative phase reversal for each measurement. Furthermore, statistical parametric mapping was used for an extensive offline data analysis. No neurologic deteriorations or complications caused by the stimulation technique were observed. Thus, intraoperative fMRI is technically feasible, allowing a real-time identification of eloquent brain areas despite brain shift.[51] In a recent investigation by Gasser and colleagues[52] it was shown that similar results are also possible applying a sophisticated setup with a low-field (0.3 T) scanner.

Nevertheless, the clinical necessity for intraoperative fMRI is debatable because the position of eloquent cortical brain areas can be identified and marked after dural opening when applying preoperative data–based functional navigation. Shifting of the eloquent cortical areas during a procedure can be observed by the surgeon without much guesswork, so a time-consuming

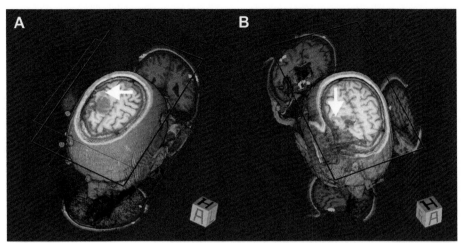

Fig. 2. Intraoperative fMRI. Right precentral World Health Organization grade II astrocytoma in a 28-year-old woman patient, 3D representation of the immediate fMRI analysis on the MR console applying a passive stimulation paradigm with shielded electric peripheral nerve stimulation of the median and tibial nerve. (*A*) Preoperative fMRI with the head already fixed in the MR-compatible headholder-coil combination under anesthesia (*white arrow* depicts the activation delineating the motor strip). (*B*) Intraoperative fMRI after subtotal tumor removal (*white arrow* depicts the fMRI activity in the motor strip. Note the tumor remnant directly adjacent to the motor strip).

fMRI update procedure might be of interest only in selected cases, whereby the updated fMRI information is used as seed region for fiber tracking algorithms to intraoperatively reconstruct the arcuate fasciculus, applying intraoperative DTI to update reconstructed language fibers.

Alternatively, mathematical models simulating the brain shift behavior[53,54] can be used to coregister preoperative functional data with intraoperative anatomic images.[55] However, these models are still too time consuming and not yet reliable enough to be applied during surgery. On the other hand, comparing predicted functional localizations by these models with the real intraoperative fMRI measurements are a possibility to validate the mathematical models.

INTRAOPERATIVE DTI

In contrast to the fMRI and MEG data, brain shift clinically affects the DTI data much more. The intraoperative shifting of cortical areas during surgery can be well detected by the naked eye; however, changes in the depth of a resection cavity, close to major white matter tracts, are nearly undetectable for the neurosurgeon during tumor resection. Thus, it was of great interest to implement intraoperative DTI.

Preoperative and intraoperative DTI for tractography of major white matter tracts in glioma surgery was established using a 1.5-T MR scanner, which is placed in an operating theater.[49,56–58] Intraoperative fiber tract visualization using a software solution that was running on the MR scanner platform needed less than 1 minute, so the whole evaluation could be performed during surgery (**Fig. 3**). The interactive 3D display with coregistered diffusion images gave a quick and intuitive overview of the position of major white matter tracts. It could be shown that fiber tracking is a method not only for preoperative neurosurgical visualization but also for further intraoperative planning. Only in 2.7% of patients in a study with intraoperative DTI a neurologic aggravation was observed. The measured extent of shifting of the major white matter tracts in glioma surgery (+2.7 ± 6.0 mm) corresponded well to previous data on brain shift of the so-called deep tumor margin, which was reported to be in the range of +4.4 ± 6.8 mm or +5.1 mm.[59,60] Furthermore, the individually unpredictable direction and great interindividual variability of white matter tract shifting confirmed these previous data.[39,59,61] The absolute amount of shifting correlated with the tumor volume; that is, in larger tumors greater deformations were likely to occur. However, the direction of white matter tract shifting, whether in the outward or inward direction with respect to the craniotomy opening, seemed to be unpredictable. Even the opening of the ventricular system was no reliable parameter to predict inward shifting caused by the loss of cerebrospinal fluid.

The knowledge of the actual position of major white matter tracts during glioma resection helps

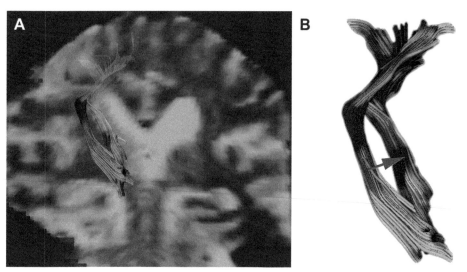

Fig. 3. Intraoperative DTI. Right temporal World Health Organization grade III astrocytoma in a 66-year-old man. (*A*) Coregistration of the coronal preoperative and intraoperative B0 images with the tracked right pyramidal tract. (*B*) The overlay of the preoperative and intraoperative pyramidal tracts depicts the distinct inward shifting after tumor removal (*gray arrow*).

to prevent too extensive resections that could potentially damage major white matter tracts and subsequently result in postoperative neurologic deficits. When data from fiber tracking are integrated into a navigational setup, preferably with the simultaneous application of fMRI, serving as seed regions for DTI fiber tracking algorithms, it is essential that the effects of brain shift, which clearly affect the spatial position of major white matter tracts, are compensated for. In contrast to mathematical models, which still have great restrictions simulating the brain shift behavior for deep brain structures, intraoperative DTI is a reliable possibility to obtain actual data for fiber tracking representing the intraoperative situation after substantial parts of a glioma are removed and when further guidance is needed.

The implementation of a DTI-tracking algorithm in the navigation software allows to perform an intraoperative update of the navigation system with the intraoperative DTI data in less than 5 to 10 minutes, thus compensating for the effects of brain shift not only for standard 3D anatomic data but also for the position of major white matter tracts. This update possibility delineating the course of major white matter tracts based on intraoperative data is a prerequisite for a real electrophysiological validation of the white matter tract data. Reports on comparisons between subcortical electric stimulations and preoperative DTI data showed some inconsistencies, which were probably caused by the effects of brain shift.[31,38]

Maximal safety may require combining electrophysiological brain mapping with functional navigation that integrates fMRI/MEG data and DTI-based fiber tracking acquired before or during surgery. Because eloquent cortical brain areas can be identified by intraoperative electrophysiological mapping subcortical electric stimulation helps to identify major white matter tracts intraoperatively. Recent studies emphasize that functional navigation and subcortical stimulation are complementary methods that may facilitate the preservation of pyramidal tracts.

Future research will have to be in quantification and reduction of spatial inaccuracies of the raw DTI data[62] and to improve sequence design, tracking parameters, and algorithms. Besides progress in sequence development with reduced image distortion, denoising, increased number of diffusion directions, and higher resolution of the raw data, further progress will also relate to a more accurate reconstruction of neural connectivity patterns. Correct identification of areas of fiber crossings is not possible by standard DTI because of its inability to resolve more than a single axon direction within each imaging voxel. Techniques that can resolve multiple axon directions within a single voxel may solve the problem of white matter fiber crossings as well as white matter insertions into the cortex.

Further challenges relate to the effects of edema surrounding a tumor, whereby fiber tracking is performed. Effects of edema, the resection cavity, and tumor remnants may directly impede the correct tracking so that either existing fibers are not visualized at all or are tracked erroneously.

SUMMARY

Multimodal functional navigation enables removing a tumor close to eloquent brain areas with low postoperative deficits, whereas additional intraoperative imaging ensures that the maximum extent of the resection can be achieved and updates the image data compensating for the effects of brain shift. Intraoperative imaging beyond standard anatomic imaging, that is, intraoperative fMRI and especially intraoperative DTI, add further safety for complex tumor resections.

REFERENCES

1. Nimsky C, Ganslandt O, Kober H, et al. Integration of functional magnetic resonance imaging supported by magnetoencephalography in functional neuronavigation. Neurosurgery 1999;44:1249–56.
2. Ganslandt O, Fahlbusch R, Nimsky C, et al. Functional neuronavigation with magnetoencephalography: outcome in 50 patients with lesions around the motor cortex. J Neurosurg 1999;91(1):73–9.
3. Kober H, Nimsky C, Möller M, et al. Correlation of sensorimotor activation with functional magnetic resonance imaging and magnetoencephalography in presurgical functional imaging: a spatial analysis. Neuroimage 2001;14:1214–28.
4. Nimsky C, Ganslandt O, Fahlbusch R. Functional neuronavigation and intraoperative MRI. Adv Tech Stand Neurosurg 2004;29:229–63.
5. Nimsky C, Ganslandt O, Fahlbusch R. 1.5 T: intraoperative imaging beyond standard anatomic imaging. Neurosurg Clin N Am 2005;16(1):185–200, vii.
6. Hentschel SJ, Sawaya R. Optimizing outcomes with maximal surgical resection of malignant gliomas. Cancer Control 2003;10(2):109–14.
7. Ganslandt O, Buchfelder M, Hastreiter P, et al. Magnetic source imaging supports clinical decision making in glioma patients. Clin Neurol Neurosurg 2004;107(1):20–6.
8. Hund M, Rezai AR, Kronberg E, et al. Magnetoencephalographic mapping: basic of a new functional risk profile in the selection of patients with cortical brain lesions. Neurosurgery 1997;40(5):936–43.
9. Ammirati M, Galicich JH, Arbit E, et al. Reoperation in the treatment of recurrent intracranial malignant gliomas. Neurosurgery 1987;21(5):607–14.
10. Black PM. Surgery for cerebral gliomas: past, present and future. In: Howard MA III, Elliott JP, Haglund MM, et al, editors, In: Clinical neurosurgery, vol. 47. Boston: Lippincott Williams & Wilkins; 1999. p. 21–45.
11. Cabantog AM, Bernstein M. Complications of first craniotomy for intra-axial brain tumour. Can J Neurol Sci 1994;21(3):213–8.
12. Ciric I, Ammirati M, Vick N, et al. Supratentorial gliomas: surgical considerations and immediate postoperative results. Gross total resection versus partial resection. Neurosurgery 1987;21(1):21–6.
13. Fadul C, Wood J, Thaler H, et al. Morbidity and mortality of craniotomy for excision of supratentorial gliomas. Neurology 1988;38(9):1374–9.
14. Grummich P, Nimsky C, Pauli E, et al. Combining fMRI and MEG increases the reliability of presurgical language localization: a clinical study on the difference between and congruence of both modalities. Neuroimage 2006;32(4):1793–803.
15. Kober H, Moller M, Nimsky C, et al. New approach to localize speech relevant brain areas and hemispheric dominance using spatially filtered magnetoencephalography. Hum Brain Mapp 2001;14(4):236–50.
16. Coenen VA, Krings T, Mayfrank L, et al. Three-dimensional visualization of the pyramidal tract in a neuronavigation system during brain tumor surgery: first experiences and technical note. Neurosurgery 2001;49(1):86–93.
17. Kamada K, Houkin K, Takeuchi F, et al. Visualization of the eloquent motor system by integration of MEG, functional, and anisotropic diffusion-weighted MRI in functional neuronavigation. Surg Neurol 2003;59(5):352–62.
18. Beppu T, Inoue T, Shibata Y, et al. Measurement of fractional anisotropy using diffusion tensor MRI in supratentorial astrocytic tumors. J Neurooncol 2003;63:109–16.
19. Clark CA, Barrick TR, Murphy MM, et al. White matter fiber tracking in patients with space-occupying lesions of the brain: a new technique for neurosurgical planning? Neuroimage 2003;20(3):1601–8.
20. Hendler T, Pianka P, Sigal M, et al. Delineating gray and white matter involvement in brain lesions: three-dimensional alignment of functional magnetic resonance and diffusion-tensor imaging. J Neurosurg 2003;99(6):1018–27.
21. Lu S, Ahn D, Johnson G, et al. Peritumoral diffusion tensor imaging of high-grade gliomas and metastatic brain tumors. AJNR Am J Neuroradiol 2003;24(5):937–41.
22. Price S, Burnet N, Donovan T, et al. Diffusion tensor imaging of brain tumours at 3T: a potential tool for assessing white matter tract invasion? Clin Radiol 2003;58(6):455–62.
23. Tummala RP, Chu RM, Liu H, et al. Application of diffusion tensor imaging to magnetic-resonance-guided brain tumor resection. Pediatr Neurosurg 2003;39:39–43.
24. Wieshmann UC, Clark CA, Symms MR, et al. Reduced anisotropy of water diffusion in structural cerebral abnormalities demonstrated with diffusion tensor imaging. Magn Reson Imaging 1999;17(9):1269–74.
25. Witwer BP, Moftakhar R, Hasan KM, et al. Diffusion-tensor imaging of white matter tracts in patients with cerebral neoplasm. J Neurosurg 2002;97(3):568–75.

26. Yamada K, Kizu O, Mori S, et al. Brain fiber tracking with clinically feasible diffusion-tensor MR imaging: initial experience. Radiology 2003;227(1):295–301.

27. Talos I, O'Donnell L, Westin CF, et al. Diffusion tensor and functional MRI fusion with anatomical MRI for image-guided neurosurgery. Heidelberg (Germany). In: Ellis R, Peters T, editors. MICCAI 2003. Berlin: Springer-Verlag; 2003. p. 407–15.

28. Nimsky C, Grummich P, Sorensen AG, et al. Visualization of the pyramidal tract in glioma surgery by integrating diffusion tensor imaging in functional neuronavigation. Zentralbl Neurochir 2005;66(3): 133–41.

29. Wu JS, Zhou LF, Hong XN, et al. [Role of diffusion tensor imaging in neuronavigation surgery of brain tumors involving pyramidal tracts]. Zhonghua Wai Ke Za Zhi 2003;41(9):662–6 [in Chinese].

30. Kamada K, Sawamura Y, Takeuchi F, et al. Functional identification of the primary motor area by corticospinal tractography. Neurosurgery 2005; 56(Suppl 1):98–109.

31. Kinoshita M, Yamada K, Hashimoto N, et al. Fiber-tracking does not accurately estimate size of fiber bundle in pathological condition: initial neurosurgical experience using neuronavigation and subcortical white matter stimulation. Neuroimage 2005; 25(2):424–9.

32. Nimsky C, Ganslandt O, Fahlbusch R. Implementation of fiber tract navigation. Neurosurgery 2006; 58(4 Suppl 2):ONS-292–304.

33. Chen X, Weigel D, Ganslandt O, et al. Diffusion tensor imaging and white matter tractography in patients with brainstem lesions. Acta Neurochir (Wien) 2007;149(11):1117–31 [discussion: 1131].

34. Chen X, Weigel D, Ganslandt O, et al. Prediction of visual field deficits by diffusion tensor imaging in temporal lobe epilepsy surgery. Neuroimage 2009; 45(2):286–97.

35. Nimsky C, Ganslandt O, Weigel D, et al. Intraoperative tractography and neuronavigation of the pyramidal tract. Jpn J Neurosurg 2008;17:21–6.

36. Krishnan R, Raabe A, Hattingen E, et al. Functional magnetic resonance imaging-integrated neuronavigation: correlation between lesion-to-motor cortex distance and outcome. Neurosurgery 2004;55(4): 904–14 [discussion: 914–5].

37. Merhof D, Meister M, Bingol E, et al. Isosurface-based generation of hulls encompassing neuronal pathways. Stereotact Funct Neurosurg 2009;87(1): 50–60.

38. Kamada K, Todo T, Masutani Y, et al. Combined use of tractography-integrated functional neuronavigation and direct fiber stimulation. J Neurosurg 2005; 102(4):664–72.

39. Nabavi A, Black PM, Gering DT, et al. Serial intraoperative magnetic resonance imaging of brain shift. Neurosurgery 2001;48(4):787–98.

40. Hastreiter P, Rezk-Salama C, Nimsky C, et al. Registration techniques for the analysis of the brain shift in neurosurgery. Comput Graph 2000;24(3):385–9.

41. Hastreiter P, Rezk-Salama C, Soza G, et al. Strategies for brain shift evaluation. Med Image Anal 2004;8(4):447–64.

42. Nimsky C, Ganslandt O, Hastreiter P, et al. Intraoperative compensation for brain shift. Surg Neurol 2001; 56(6):357–65.

43. Wirtz CR, Bonsanto MM, Knauth M, et al. Intraoperative magnetic resonance imaging to update interactive navigation in neurosurgery: method and preliminary experience. Comput Aided Surg 1997;2:172–9.

44. Black PM, Moriarty T, Alexander E III, et al. Development and implementation of intraoperative magnetic resonance imaging and its neurosurgical applications. Neurosurgery 1997;41(4):831–45.

45. Hall WA, Kowalik K, Liu H, et al. Costs and benefits of intraoperative MR-guided brain tumor resection. Acta Neurochir Suppl 2003;85:137–42.

46. Hall WA, Liu H, Martin AJ, et al. Safety, efficacy, and functionality of high-field strength interventional magnetic resonance imaging for neurosurgery. Neurosurgery 2000;46(3):632–42.

47. Nimsky C, Ganslandt O, Fahlbusch R. Comparing 0.2 Tesla with 1.5 Tesla intraoperative magnetic resonance imaging analysis of setup, workflow, and efficiency. Acad Radiol 2005;12(9):1065–79.

48. Sutherland GR, Kaibara T, Louw D, et al. A mobile high-field magnetic resonance system for neurosurgery. J Neurosurg 1999;91(5):804–13.

49. Nimsky C, Ganslandt O, von Keller B, et al. Intraoperative high-field strength MR imaging: implementation and experience in 200 patients. Radiology 2004;233(1):67–78.

50. Rachinger J, von Keller B, Ganslandt O, et al. Application accuracy of automatic registration in frameless stereotaxy. Stereotact Funct Neurosurg 2006; 84(2–3):109–17.

51. Gasser T, Ganslandt O, Sandalcioglu E, et al. Intraoperative functional MRI: implementation and preliminary experience. Neuroimage 2005;26(3):685–93.

52. Gasser T, Szelenyi A, Senft C, et al. Intraoperative MRI and functional mapping. Acta Neurochir Suppl (Wien) 2010;109:61–5.

53. Ferrant M, Nabavi A, Macq B, et al. Registration of 3-D intraoperative MR images of the brain using a finite-element biomechanical model. IEEE Trans Med Imaging 2001;20(12):1384–97.

54. Platenik LA, Miga MI, Roberts DW, et al. In vivo quantification of retraction deformation modeling for updated image-guidance during neurosurgery. IEEE Trans Biomed Eng 2002;49(8):823–35.

55. Wolf M, Vogel T, Weierich P, et al. Automatic transfer of preoperative fMRI markers into intraoperative MR-images for updating functional neuronavigation. IEICE Transactions Inf Syst 2001;E84-D(12):1698–704.

56. Nimsky C, Ganslandt O, Hastreiter P, et al. Intraoperative diffusion tensor imaging: shifting of white matter tracts during neurosurgical procedures-initial experience. Radiology 2005;234(1):218–25.

57. Nimsky C, Ganslandt O, Hastreiter P, et al. Preoperative and intraoperative diffusion tensor imaging-based fiber tracking in glioma surgery. Neurosurgery 2005;56(1):130–8.

58. Nimsky C, Ganslandt O, Merhof D, et al. Intraoperative visualization of the pyramidal tract by diffusion-tensor-imaging-based fiber tracking. Neuroimage 2006;30(4):1219–29.

59. Nimsky C, Ganslandt O, Cerny S, et al. Quantification of, visualization of, and compensation for brain shift using intraoperative magnetic resonance imaging. Neurosurgery 2000;47(5):1070–80.

60. Dorward NL, Alberti O, Velani B, et al. Postimaging brain distortion: magnitude, correlates, and impact on neuronavigation. J Neurosurg 1998; 88(4):656–62.

61. Keles GE, Lamborn KR, Berger MS. Coregistration accuracy and detection of brain shift using intraoperative sononavigation during resection of hemispheric tumors. Neurosurgery 2003;53(3):556–64.

62. Merhof D, Soza G, Stadlbauer A, et al. Correction of susceptibility artifacts in diffusion tensor data using non-linear registration. Med Image Anal 2007; 11(6):588–603.

Identification of Neural Targets for the Treatment of Psychiatric Disorders: The Role of Functional Neuroimaging

David R. Vago, PhD[a],*, Jane Epstein, MD[a],
Eva Catenaccio, BA[a], Emily Stern, MD[b]

KEYWORDS
- Neuroimaging • Neurocircuitry • Psychiatric disorders
- Depression

Neurosurgical treatment of psychiatric disorders has a long history, influenced by evolving neurobiological models of symptom generation. In recent years, the advent of functional neuroimaging, along with advances in the cognitive and affective neurosciences, has revolutionized understanding of the functional neuroanatomy of psychiatric disease. The investigational use of techniques such as positron emission tomography (PET) and functional magnetic resonance imaging (fMRI), combined with advanced statistical methods, has led to the development of complex neurocircuitry-based models of an array of psychiatric disorders.

In addition to increasing our understanding of the pathophysiology of neuropsychiatric illness, functional neuroimaging studies are being used for detection, localization, and characterization of final common pathways of major psychiatric disease expression as a foundation for clinical advances. They are also playing a major role in the prediction of response to treatment; identification of biomarkers for risk/resilience; and guiding the development, monitoring, and assessment of targeted biologic therapies, including neurosurgical treatments, for several psychiatric disorders.

HISTORICAL BACKGROUND
Bodily Humors, Mental Faculties, and the Brain

Symptom localization in psychiatric illness has its historical roots in the fifth century BCE, a time at which bodily fluids called humors were believed to be the crucial elements of health and disease. Although it may have its origins in ancient Egypt, it was Hippocrates who systematized the humoral doctrine in a medical theory of mood and behavior based on the balance of the 4 humors: yellow and

The authors have nothing to disclose.

[a] Department of Psychiatry, Functional Neuroimaging Laboratory, Brigham & Womens Hospital/Harvard Medical School, 824 Boylston Street, Chestnut Hill, MA 02143, USA
[b] Department of Radiology, fMRI Service, Functional and Molecular Neuroimaging, Brigham & Women's Hospital/Harvard Medical School, 824 Boylston Street, Chestnut Hill, MA 02143, USA
* Corresponding author.
E-mail address: vago.dave@gmail.com

Neurosurg Clin N Am 22 (2011) 279–305
doi:10.1016/j.nec.2011.01.003
1042-3680/11/$ – see front matter © 2011 Elsevier Inc. All rights reserved.

black bile, phlegm, and blood. The theory was later perpetuated by the Roman physician, Galen of Pergamon, who proposed in the first and second century CE that each bodily humor is related to particular mental faculties of perception, reason, or memory and their corresponding conditions of temperature and moisture. Mental illness was determined to be caused by a loss of 1 or more mental faculties and was treated by balancing the humors through the influence of the temperature/moisture along with the common practice of bloodletting.[1] In melancholia, it was presumed that the faculty of perception was impaired, whereas the faculty of reason was still intact. Black bile from the abdominal cavity was believed to darken the anterior section of the brain, clouding the faculty of perception and leading to long-lasting fear and sadness. It was believed that, with increasing severity, the illness spread to the other faculties.

Within that framework, a few influential pathologists began to associate particular mental faculties with certain parts of the brain. For example, the faculty of reason was believed to reside in the medial aspects of the brain, and memory was believed to be located in the cerebellum.[1–3] Similar classifications were made in cases of mania, in which the faculty of reason was most affected. Although the localization of mental disease remained largely unknown, Galen[4] emphasized both genetic/innate and external factors in his treatise *On the Affected Parts*:

Black bile arises in some people in large quantity either because of their original humoural constitution or by their customary diet ... Like the thick phlegm, this heavy atrabilious blood obstructs the passage through the middle or posterior cavity of the brain and sometimes causes epilepsy. When its excess pervades the brain matter itself, it causes melancholy ...[4]

Avicenna, an Arabic physician and philosopher from the late tenth century, expanded on Galen's perspectives on mental illness and wrote extensively on the topic of melancholy, referring to the melancholy humor (black bile), melancholia the disease, and the melancholic disposition. He was also a pioneer in the association of physiology with emotion. His vast medical and scientific perspectives were published in *The Book of Healing* and fourteen-volume *Canon of Medicine* (1025), texts that influenced medicine into the eighteenth century throughout Europe.

Empirical investigation into the underlying factors influencing mental illness did not resurface until the sixteenth century, when detailed neuroanatomic illustrations were provided by Andreas Vesalius, now considered one of the founders of modern medicine. Vesalius used dissections of cadavers as the primary teaching tool, significantly advancing the understanding of brain and body anatomy through the method of direct observation. By the seventeenth century, the brain was established as the seat of most mental disease, and its association with black bile or melancholic humor was diminishing. Thomas Willis, a pioneer in research into the anatomy of the brain and nervous system, coined the term neurology in his influential medical texts, and proposed alternate chemical theories for the pathogenesis of melancholia. By the eighteenth century, knowledge of the central nervous system, along with detailed classifications of mental illness, had considerably increased in breadth and detail.

The Debate About Localization and the Emergence of Connectionist Models

The work of Willis and the advances made in understanding and describing neuroanatomy set the stage for the work of Franz Joseph Gall and the phrenologists, whose theories of cerebral surface localization in the late 1700s and early 1800s preceded the modern conceptions of cortical localization.[5] In the early 1800s, Gall and his collaborator J.C. Spurzheim developed a model of brain/mind relations in which specific functions were localized within areas of the cortex, with the size of the cortical region reflecting the development and activity of the corresponding function (**Fig. 1**).[6] They posited that the prominence of individual cortical areas could be assessed by measuring the prominence of the overlying skull.[6] After examining the skulls of a variety of subjects ranging from criminals and the mentally ill to prominent figures such as politicians, artists, and intellectuals, including Voltaire and Descartes, Gall described the localization of 27 different faculties in the cerebral cortex, including wisdom, passion, courage, love of offspring, cleverness, and murderous tendencies.[6–8] Gall's theory, ultimately known as phrenology, gained general popularity, but was ultimately vigorously attacked within the scientific community. Although well deserved on methodological grounds, the attack may also have been motivated by entrenched scientific perspectives and religious beliefs regarding the unity of soul and mind.[7,9] The most prominent detractor of phrenology was Pierre Flourens, a leading brain physiologist, who posited that all parts of the cortex are capable of performing all functions.[8]

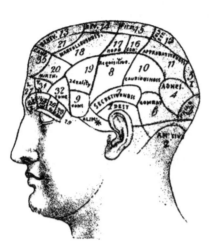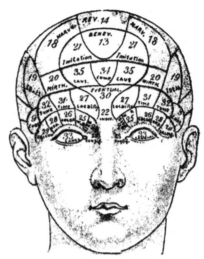

Fig. 1. Phrenological diagram from Spurzheim (1832). Gall and Spurzheim described the localization of 27 different faculties in the cerebral cortex including wisdom, passion, courage, love of offspring, cleverness, and murderous tendencies. (*Reproduced from* Buchanan's Journal of Man, November 1887.)

Although this antilocalizationist view, known as the theory of equipotentiality, gained ascendancy in the early nineteenth century, the question of cortical localization remained a topic of heated debate, kept active by numerous reports of speech dysfunction associated with frontal lesions (a localization suggested by Gall).[7] The French physician Jean-Baptiste Bouillaud, in particular, presented more than 100 cases in support of this association, famously wagering 500 francs, in 1848, that no one could find an example of a deep lesion in the anterior lobes in which speech was not affected.[9,10] Bouillaud's son-in-law, Simon Alexandre Ernest Aubertin, who was also a fierce proponent of localization, threw down a similar challenge, stating that he would renounce all his convictions about localization if 1 case could be shown in which speech was preserved despite massive lesions to both anterior lobes.[11]

A turning point in the debate occurred in 1861, 8 days after Aubertin's challenge, when Paul Broca, a well-respected neurologist who had not previously been active in the debate, delivered a report to the French Societe de'Anthropologie describing the case of a recently deceased patient who had suffered from right hemiplegia, loss of speech, and seizures. Following the patient's death, autopsy revealed a fluid-filled cavity the size of an egg in the left frontal lobe, providing dramatic support for the proposed localization of speech.[11] In the years that followed, Carl Wernicke published a monograph describing various types of aphasia related to lesions in differing brain regions and developed a model, known as associationism or connectionism, which explained

disorders of language or cognition in terms of lesions to different combinations of specialized brain regions and/or the connections between them.[9,12] This model was quickly extended by neurologists such as Lichtheim, Liepmann, and Dejerine to explain syndromes such as pure word deafness, ideomotor apraxia, and alexia without agraphia.[12]

Application of Localization and Connectionist Models to Disorders of Emotion, Motivation, and Social Comportment

In the later years of the nineteenth century, several investigators used lesion or stimulation studies in animals, and autopsy findings in humans, to localize cortical functions. Although early efforts focused on motor areas, attention eventually turned toward localization of emotional, behavioral, and other mental functions. In the mid-1870s, David Ferrier described monkeys with frontal lobe damage who showed deficits in attention, appeared listless and dull, and proposed that thinking was inhibition of action. Eduard Hitzig, a German neuropsychiatrist, suggested that the capacity for abstract thought was affected by frontal lobe damage. Leonardo Bianchi, an Italian neurologist, described deficits involving social interaction, self-perception, and executive functions such as planning and decision making in monkeys with frontal lobe damage.[13] Supplementing these observations and theories was evidence drawn from the case of Phineas Gage, a railroad worker injured in 1848 when an explosion caused a tamping rod to enter his left cheek, shoot through his frontal lobes, and exit through the midline of his skull near the junction of the coronal and sagittal sutures.[14,15] Alterations in Gage's behavioral disposition involving changes in emotional expression and regulation, as well as social decision making, provided further insight into frontal lobe functions, supporting the observations and investigations of Ferrier and others.[11]

Another development promoting investigation of the neural substrates of emotional processing and behavior was the adoption of evolutionary perspectives following the publication of Darwin's *Origin of Species* in 1859 and *Descent of Man* in 1871. In this context, Hughlings Jackson developed a hierarchal model of the brain in which functions are represented at multiple levels of organization acquired through the course of evolution. In this model, lower-level functions, which are simple, stereotyped, and automatic, are controlled by higher-level functions, which are more complex, flexible, and voluntary. Mental alterations produced by lesions in higher-level cortical structures result in impairment of associated cortical function but also reflect ongoing, but distorted, activity in the rest of the brain, including lower-level functions now released from inhibitory control.[16,17]

An evolutionary perspective can also be seen in the writings of James Papez, an American neuroanatomist, who in 1937 delineated a complex system of extensively interconnected brain structures mediating emotion.[18,19] The limbic circuit described by Papez[19] incorporates the phylogenetically primitive and morphologically simple structures surrounding the brainstem, including the cingulate and parahippocampal gyri, hippocampal formation, mamillary bodies, anterior thalamus, and hypothalamus. Papez viewed the cingulate as the "seat of dynamic vigilance by which environmental experiences are endowed with an emotional consciousness," and postulated that projections from the cingulate to other areas of cortex "add emotional coloring."[19] In accordance with theories originally postulated by Walter Cannon (1927, 1931), the functions of this limbic circuit could account for the striking autonomic and behavioral changes associated with bitemporal damage in the Kluver-Bucy syndrome, spontaneous laughter and crying produced by stimulation of the anterior thalamus, and sham rage seen in animals following removal of inhibitory cortex and accompanying increases in diencephalic activity.[20]

Paul MacLean further extended the limbic circuit delineated by Papez[19] to include the amygdala and septal nuclei. He developed an evolutionary model of the tripartite brain, in which the mammalian limbic network provides a variety of emotional and viscerosomatic reactions as it facilitates communication between the hypothalamus and frontal lobes.[18,19] In 1948, Ivan Yakovlev added the orbitofrontal cortex, precuneus, and insula to the limbic system. As discussed later, Papez, MacLean, and Yakovlev were correct in many of their assumptions regarding emotional expression and control.

With the advent of histochemical, immunocytochemical, and autoradiographic methods for tract tracing in the 1960s and 1970s, it became possible to identify the cortical-limbic circuit with more precision. Multiple research teams used these methods in postmortem human tissue and animal models to identify paths of atrophy caused by experimental lesions, guide future ablation techniques, and clarify cytoarchitectonic pathways.[21–23] Projections were identified from the amygdala to orbital and medial prefrontal, insular, and temporal regions (perirhinal cortex, lateral entorhinal cortex, piriform cortex, and hippocampus), mediodorsal thalamus, medial and lateral hypothalamus, periaqueductal gray, and other brainstem nuclei that are involved in visceral control and autonomic function.[21,23–27] More recent studies have been able to show that the bulk of incoming cortical projections terminate within the basolateral amygdaloid nuclei and reciprocally project back on cortical areas in a highly topographic manner.[22,28] The basolateral nuclei of the amygdala project to orbital and medial prefrontal regions, whereas central and medial nuclei have descending projections to the hypothalamus and brainstem that are largely inhibitory.[29]

The Emergence of Neuropsychiatry

In the late twentieth century, advances in several brain-related disciplines and methodologies laid the groundwork for the emergence of neuropsychiatry, a psychiatric subspecialty devoted to understanding emotional, behavioral, cognitive, and perceptual symptoms in terms of their functional neuroanatomy, whether in the context of neurologic or primary psychiatric conditions. One of these advances occurred in 1956, when a Symposium on Information Theory was held at the Massachusetts Institute of Technology. Participants were drawn from fields including artificial intelligence, cognitive psychology, and linguistics. Their interaction gave rise to the multidisciplinary field of cognitive science, which has at its core an attempt to understand mental functions in terms of information processing or computation.[30,31] Cognitive science has delineated ways in which the mind and brain seem to function in accord with computational constructs, developing promising models of brain/mind function such as parallel processing and neural networks, and incorporating data and perspectives from philosophy and the neurosciences.

Another major advance occurred in 1965, when Norman Geschwind published *Disconnection Syndromes in Animals and Man*, establishing behavioral neurology.[32–34] Geschwind and his students revived and built on the nineteenth century connectionist tradition, elucidating the neural substrates of phenomena such as memory, attention, knowledge, and awareness. This neurologic subspecialty developed in conjunction with neuropsychology, a branch of psychology that arose in the wake of World War II in response to a need to characterize the effects of traumatic brain injury. In the following decades, the body of knowledge derived from these clinically based approaches was complemented by animal studies, most often in rats and nonhuman primates. These studies,[35–40] combined with contributions from ethology[41] and evolutionary psychology,[42] were particularly useful in the investigation of the social, motivational, and emotional functions that had been neglected by cognitive science, behavioral neurology, and neuropsychology.

In time, these disciplines (behavioral neurology, neuropsychology, cognitive science, animal studies of brain and behavior, evolutionary psychology, philosophy of mind, ethology, and developmental psychobiology, among others) grew increasingly intertwined and synergistic, to the extent that they are frequently referred to collectively as the cognitive and affective neurosciences. This interdisciplinary understanding of brain/mind functioning was adopted by the nascent field of neuropsychiatry, and applied to the investigation of the neural underpinnings of psychiatric disorders; an application made possible by the development of functional neuroimaging technologies (**Fig. 2**).

THE ROLE OF NEUROIMAGING IN THE DEVELOPMENT OF NEUROCIRCUITRY-BASED MODELS OF PSYCHIATRIC DISORDERS: THE EXAMPLE OF DEPRESSION

In 1980, Jacoby and Levi[43] published the first computed tomography (CT) study of patients with mood disorders; in 1983, Rangel-Guerra and colleagues[44] published the first MRI study of a similar population. These studies were followed, in subsequent years, by a plethora of structural and functional neuroimaging studies of patients with major depressive disorder (MDD) and bipolar disorder (BPD), as well as those experiencing depressive symptoms in the context of primary neurologic disorders or other medical illness. Current neuroimaging research uses analyses based on measurement of regional cerebral blood flow (CBF) or glucose metabolism (GLC); morphologic or volumetric abnormalities using voxel-based morphometry (VBM), cortical thickness, or diffusion weighted imaging (eg, diffusion tensor imaging); and multivariate statistical models to identify critical neurocircuitry, and quantify dysregulation in effective and functional connectivity.[45] Despite considerable variation in study design and methodology, as well as heterogeneity of study populations, significant progress has been made in the last 30 years in delineating the circuitry underlying major depression. This article reviews

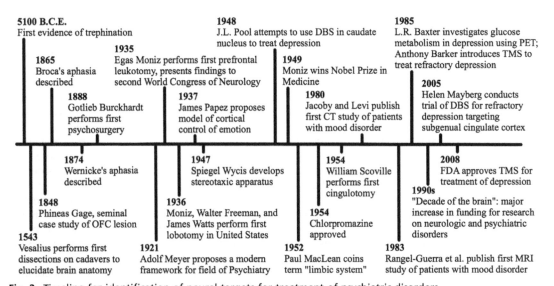

Fig. 2. Timeline for identification of neural targets for treatment of psychiatric disorders.

findings from the last 3 decades and provides evidence for emerging neurocircuitry models of mood disorders, focusing on critical circuits of cognition and emotion, particularly those brain networks regulating the evaluative, expressive, and experiential aspects of emotion.[46–48]

Morphologic and Volumetric Studies

Early studies

Early neuroradiological investigations, based on findings from pneumoencephalography (PEG; a method in which some cerebrospinal fluid is drained and replaced with air, oxygen, or helium to allow the structure of the brain to show up more clearly on a radiograph), indicated morphologic brain changes in patients with affective disorders undergoing subcaudate tractotomy.[49] The earliest CT studies of mood disorders from the early 1980s focused on sulcal and cerebral volume, along with gross structural differences in patients with mood disorders compared with healthy control subjects (see Refs.[50,51] for review). Although results were mixed, significantly increased ventricular size was the most consistent finding across most studies that used manual tracing to measure ventricular/brain ratio (VBR). This crude finding, also reported in conditions such as schizophrenia and alcohol abuse, is clearly nonspecific.[51]

A few studies reported that subcortical atrophy preceding neurologic insult or onset of neurodegenerative disease increases the likelihood of later onset of depression,[52,53] and evidence continues to accumulate that neurologic diseases involving subcortical abnormalities are associated with higher rates of depression.[50] There is also evidence for potential mediators of structural changes related to depression, including genetic predisposition, stress reactivity, and behavioral factors for risk and resiliency.[53,54] There are large volumes of research showing that exposure to increased levels of glucocorticoids can accelerate hippocampal neuron loss and lead to cognitive and affective impairments.[55] Some animal research suggests that maternal grooming early in life leads to increases in density of glucocorticoid receptors in both hippocampus and prefrontal cortex (PFC), which likely play an important role in developing resilience to stress later in life.[56,57] Although the evidence for effects of stress on structure and function is incomplete as it relates to depression, maladaptive stress responses have been shown to correlate positively with increased plasma cortisol levels, degree of hippocampal atrophy, decreased immune response, and decreases in neurogenesis and/or brain-derived neurotrophic factor.[58,59] Ineffective management of chronic stress (physical or psychogenic) is associated with blunted behavioral expression in the presence of stressors and impaired recovery of parasympathetic tone after a stressor is experienced.[53,60] Psychosocial stressors are also associated with the onset,[61,62] symptom severity,[63] and course of MDD.[60]

Investigations of regionally specific structural abnormalities in the 1990s were hampered by the paucity of standards for demarcating complex anatomic regions. Nonetheless, some studies found decreased width of PFC, and virtually all suggested that PFC is a key region in the neuroanatomic model of mood regulation.[50] Findings related to temporal and parietal regions were mixed. The advent of MRI volumetric studies brought improved resolution in distinguishing gray from white matter, allowing for gross morphologic characterizations of density of fiber tracts associated with myelination, anatomic connectivity, and neuronal degeneration. A few early controlled MRI studies found decreased total white matter volume and decreased frontal volumes in MDD and BPD, and a relative increase in gray matter specific to BPD,[64] whereas most studies found nonspecific global atrophy.[51] Several CT and MRI studies have also found increased rates of subcortical white matter or periventricular hyperintensities suggestive of cerebrovascular disease in patients with MDD and BPD, particularly in elderly patients.[50,64,65]

In general, the early structural imaging studies showed that white matter lesions throughout the frontal-striatal-thalamic circuitry are associated with depression. Volumetric abnormalities were most often found in the frontal lobes, but not consistently in any other region.[50,66]

Prefrontal cortices

More recent studies of patients with mood disorders have shown consistent abnormalities in morphometry of several specific medial prefrontal areas, anterior cingulate, and limbic regions.[50,67–70] Anatomic specificity has improved and allowed for more accurate functional localization to lateralized subdivisions of PFC. Based on cytoarchitectonic and functional considerations, the primate PFC has most often been delineated into subdivisions including the dorsolateral PFC (DLPFC), dorsomedial PFC (dmPFC), ventromedial PFC (vmPFC), and orbitofrontal cortex (OFC) sectors.[48,71,72] In addition, there seem to be important functional differences between the left and right sides within each of these subdivisions. In studies of naturally occurring lesions secondary to stroke or trauma, patients with damage to the left hemisphere, specifically the left PFC, were found to be more likely to develop depressive symptoms compared with patients having homologous lesions in the right hemisphere.[72–74] This is consistent with studies of healthy subjects showing that positive mood and affect are associated with left DLPFC function,[72,73,75] whereas negative affect is associated with activation of right anterior PFC in the intact brain.[72] Although a few studies have reported that right hemisphere lesions have been associated with manic symptoms, mania has been less frequent than depression following stroke or brain injury.[72,74,76,77] The more recent literature has largely supported these lateralized observations across methodologies and in various contexts.[78–80]

Volumetric reductions have been observed with less consistency in OFC (BA 11/47) in both MDD and BPD, and in ventrolateral PFC (VLPFC) (BA 45) and DLPFC (BA 9/10) in BPD.[81–84] Some discrepancies may be related to the use of variable subregional specifications as targeted regions of interest (ROIs). In contrast with ROI-based structural studies, the use of VBM allows for voxel-by-voxel comparisons in regions that are difficult to define anatomically, by normalizing individual structural MRI scans to a standard template.[85] However, the VBM method poses risk for type II errors, such that small differences in volume located in other gray matter areas might be missed.

Using VBM methodology, a few studies have reported bilateral reductions in OFC volumes in patients with MDD compared with control subjects.[86,87] Reductions in cortical thickness have also been reported in patients with MDD.[88] Recently, VBM analyses in patients with BPD have revealed a strong correlation between decreased gray matter volume in left DLPFC and number of manic episodes,[89] consistent with the cognitive deficits observed in this population. Neither lifetime number of depressive episodes nor years of illness has been found to correlate with changes in gray matter volume, although voxel-based structural deficits in the left DLPFC were found to characterize a subgroup of people with recurrent MDD who respond poorly to antidepressants.[90]

Anterior cingulate cortex

The most prominent abnormality reported to date in MDD and BPD has been a marked (19%–48%) reduction in gray matter in left subgenual anterior cingulate cortex (sgACC, BA 25) (**Fig. 3**C).[48,85,91–100] This occurs early in the progression of the illness, as well as in young adults at high familial risk for MDD.[48,95] This finding

has been shown to be stable over time. Botteron and colleagues[95] showed that patients with first onset depression had the same degree of volumetric reduction as did patients who had experienced recurrent episodes. Drevets and colleagues[100] showed no change in volume when patients were rescanned after a 3-month interval, regardless of whether their symptoms had resolved. A postmortem study by Ongur and colleagues[101,102] suggested a loss of glial cells as a potential cause. In comparison with unaffected control subjects, patients with MDD and BPD were found to have reduced density and number of glial cells in this region, a finding that was particularly robust in those subjects with a family history of depressive illness.[102,103] Some evidence suggests that left sgACC gray matter reduction may predate illness onset, and act as a biologic marker for familial risk of MDD or BPD.[48,66] Similarly, McDonald and colleagues (2004) showed an association between reduced volumes in right pregenual anterior cingulate cortex (pgACC) and sgACC and genetic risk for BPD.

Hippocampus

Studies examining volumetric changes of the hippocampus in depressed subjects have had mixed results, with findings influenced by a wide array of variables including duration of illness, severity of illness, age of onset, responsiveness to treatment, untreated days of illness, history of childhood abuse, and level of anxiety.[46,53,58,67,76,104–109] However, a recent meta-analysis of 36 studies (more than 2000 subjects) showed that depressed patients overall had significantly lower hippocampal volumes than healthy controls, most prominently in the left hippocampus,[104,106] consistent with studies showing an association between depression and abnormalities of context-dependent memory.[48] Hippocampal atrophy was seen only in those patients with a duration of illness greater than 2 years, or more than 1 depressive episode.[104] In addition, this effect was limited to children and middle-aged or older adults, and appeared to persist during symptom remission.[110] Young adults with MDD had hippocampal volumes equivalent to those seen in healthy controls, a result that has been postulated to reflect a reduced burden of illness in this population.[104]

A positive correlation has also been shown between hippocampal atrophy and extent of depressive symptoms, consistent with hippocampal sensitivity to stress-induced suppression of neurogenesis, and decreases in hippocampal volume associated with chronically increased glucocorticoids.[55,111] Shape analysis methodology

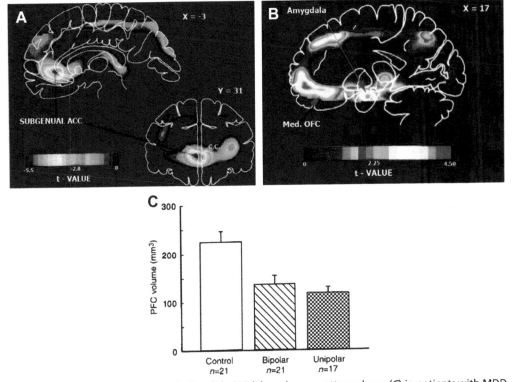

Fig. 3. Areas of abnormal glucose metabolism (*A*), CBF (*B*), and gray matter volume (*C*) in patients with MDD. (*A*) Decreased GLC in sgACC. (*B*) Increased amygdalar CBF. Abnormalities of CBF have also commonly been observed in rostral ACC, with normalization following pharmacologic and cognitive behavioral treatments.[92,131,144,239] (*C*) Reductions in sgACC gray matter volume in bipolar disorder and unipolar depression.[97] Significant reductions are observed irrespective of mood state and after covarying for age, gender, and whole brain volume.[100] (Fig. 3A: *Modified from* Drevets WC, Price JL, Simpson JR Jr, et al. Subgenual prefrontal cortex abnormalities in mood disorders. Nature 1997;386(6627):826; with permission. Fig. 3B: *Modified from* Price JL, Carmichael ST, Drevets WC. Networks related to the orbital and medial prefrontal cortex; a substrate for emotional behavior? Prog Brain Res 1996;107:533; with permission. Fig. 3C: *Reproduced from* Drevets WC, Price JL, Simpson JR Jr, et al. Subgenual prefrontal cortex abnormalities in mood disorders. Nature 1997;386(6627):826; with permission.)

used by Cole and colleagues[107] has localized subregional deformations to the CA1 subregion and the subiculum, the main output regions of the hippocampus. These specific deficits were limited to patients with 2 or fewer episodes of major depression. Although most studies reveal no differences in hippocampal volumes between male and female subjects with depression, a few report gender differences, with men showing a correlation between decreased left hippocampal volume (compared with controls) and length of depression, and women showing no such finding.[58,109,112] Within a group of female subjects, Vakili and colleagues[109] showed greater right hippocampal volume in those women who responded to medication than in those who did not.

Amygdala

Amygdalar volume in MDD or BPD (compared with healthy controls) has been reported to be increased in some studies and decreased in others[46,84,99,105,112–115]; higher volumes have been shown more often in patients with BPD,[84,106] whereas decreased volumes are more often found in cases of depression that are chronic or intermittent.[46] In keeping with these findings, Bowley and colleagues[116] reported substantially lower glial density in the amygdala in patients with MDD, and a recent metaregression analysis of patients with BPD found that those taking lithium were more likely to have increased gray matter volume in the amygdala.[84] Few studies have investigated gender differences; Hastings and colleagues[99] showed significantly smaller volumes in bilateral amygdalae of female depressed patients compared with depressed men.

Basal ganglia

Although morphometric studies of the basal ganglia have been mixed, most studies have found caudate, putamen, and nucleus accumbens to be smaller in depressed subjects than in healthy controls.[64,117–122] Postmortem analysis has similarly shown volume decreases of up to 32%.[118] Lesions of the striatum and pallidum caused by/ gliosis or calcifications are associated with depression, whereas mania has been observed after brain injury or stroke resulting in damage to the head of the right caudate nucleus.[77,123,124] In contrast, increases in striatal volume independent of illness duration have more often been shown in patients with BPD, as well as in their nonaffected twin siblings.[64] Aylward and colleagues (1996) reported increased caudate volumes in male, but not female, patients with BPD compared with controls.

Overall, structural imaging studies have been useful in identifying possible neuroanatomic substrates for depression; however, most results have been mixed, and this approach is clearly limited compared with methods that provide direct measures of energy metabolism, neurophysiologic abnormalities, or functional hemodynamic abnormalities. However, structural differences must be taken into account in the interpretation of functional findings.[102,125]

Functional Studies

Global findings

In an early functional neuroimaging study of MDD and BPD, Baxter and colleaguers[126] used fluorodeoxyglucose PET (FDG-PET) to scan patients in different mood states. Cerebral glucose metabolic rates were found to be globally reduced in bipolar patients in both depressed and mixed states in comparison with bipolar patients in manic states, patients with MDD, and normal controls. For subjects with BPD, whole brain metabolic rates were lowest in the depressed group, intermediate in the euthymic group, and greatest in the manic group, suggesting a state- specific, rather than trait-specific, finding.[126]

Frontal lobes

Functional abnormalities of PFC have been among the most robust findings in depression. Initial single-photon emission computed tomography (SPECT) and PET findings were variable, but most studies suggested maximal CBF reductions in left frontal cortex that normalize with treatment and form an inverse relationship with depression severity.[51,126–128] In 1993, Bench and colleagues[94,129] showed decreased CBF in the left DLPFC, left anterior cingulate cortex (ACC), and left angular gyrus using PET. Subsequent PET and SPECT studies confirmed these findings, supporting an inverse relationship between

depression severity and frontal activity.[56] More recent studies have confirmed the presence of frontal abnormalities, but the direction of findings has been mixed (see Refs.[46,76,80,100,160] for comprehensive review), although some may be confounded by local reductions in gray matter volume, particularly on the left, as described earlier. The most consistent findings have been hypoactivity in dorsal portions of PFC and ACC, and hyperactivity in ventral and medial regions of PFC, including vmPFC, OFC, VLPFC, and anterior insula.[46,48,130] Normalization of this hyperactivity has been seen after treatment with pharmacotherapy,[92] cognitive behavioral therapy (CBT),[131] or deep brain stimulation of the ventral striatum.[132] Hypermetabolism in the frontal lobes has also been reported, but only in patients with pure familial MDD.[125] More often, hypermetabolism is found to be localized to the OFC region along with increased metabolism of the anterior insula during a major depressive episode.[69,125]

There seems to be a pattern of inverse activity in vmPFC and DLPFC, in which vmPFC is hyperactive in depressed patients at rest and healthy subjects during experimentally induced fear/ anxiety, and decreases in activity during remission of symptoms, whereas DLPFC and dorsal cingulate are hypoactive at rest, and increase in activity during remission of symptoms.[59] In contrast, mania has been associated with decreased ventral and increased dorsal activity in PFC and ACC, perhaps resulting in inappropriate behavioral responses to changing inner drive and external environmental contexts.[133,134] Hypoactivation in dorsal PFC regions in depression may underlie alterations in psychomotor function, impairment of initiation and maintenance of goal-directed behavior, and difficulty suppressing automatic responses to emotion-related stimuli, resulting in perseveration of negative affect and decreased inhibitory control.

Anterior cingulate cortex

The ACC has been described as a "point of integration for visceral, attentional and affective information that is critical for self-regulation and adaptability."[135] The ACC has extensive anatomic and functional connections with both dorsal and ventral aspects of frontal lobe networks. The ventral ACC connects with limbic and paralimbic regions such as the amygdala, nucleus accumbens, anterior insula, and autonomic brainstem motor nuclei (periaqueductal gray and parabrachial nucleus), and is assumed to be involved in regulating somatic, visceral, and autonomic responses to stressful events, emotional expression, and social behavior.[80,136] The dorsal ACC connects with DLPFC (BA 46/9), posterior cingulate cortex (PCC), parietal cortex (BA 7), supplementary motor area, and spinal cord, and plays an important role in response selection and processing of cognitively demanding information.[80,136]

Imaging studies of depression in both MDD and BPD have shown abnormalities in ventral, rostral, and dorsal ACC metabolism and hemodynamic activity during a variety of emotion-induction tasks.[48,53,80,97,130,136–138] Abnormalities have been found most consistently in sgACC, supporting prominent structural abnormalities found in this region (see **Fig. 3**A, C).[46] Decreased sgACC metabolism and CBF has been shown in both medicated and unmedicated patients with depression using SPECT,[139] PET,[129,138,140,141] and fMRI.[100,137,142] These regional decreases have been reported to predate the onset of clinical symptoms[143] and predict recovery.[144] Decreases in dorsal regions of ACC (BA 24a/b/32) have also been reported.[80]

In contrast, there have also been reports of increased ACC, GLC, and CBF in the depressed versus remitted state, most often in dorsal and rostral aspects of ACC, including the subgenual and pregenual ACC,[130,145,146] a finding supported by activation in healthy subjects during experimentally induced sadness.[147–149] Metabolism in rostral ACC has been shown to correlate positively with severity of depression[150]; to decrease during remission induced by antidepressant drugs,[151] electroconvulsive therapy,[152] deep brain stimulation (DBS),[153] and placebo[154]; and to increase during relapse.

The inconsistent directionality of these findings may be caused by differential reductions in gray matter volume within heterogeneous study populations, and failure to account for partial volume effects in functional brain images with poor spatial resolution. When this volumetric deficit has been taken into account by correcting for partial volume effects and corresponding gray matter reduction, sgACC metabolism seems to be increased in unmedicated patients in the depressed state, and normal in medicated patients in remission.[48,76] Directional discrepancies may also reflect an inverse relationship between dorsal and ventral ACC similar to that seen in other dorsal and ventral frontal regions.

Along with studies showing strong modulatory connections to the lateral hypothalamus, these imaging studies suggest that sgACC activity may serve as an effective regulator of autonomic responsivity and, in conjunction with rostral and dorsal ACC, a predictor of treatment response.

Mayberg[92] found that depressed patients who showed increased pretreatment resting state metabolism in rostral ACC (BA 24a/b) were more likely to respond to pharmacotherapy, whereas those in whom it was decreased remained significantly depressed after 6 weeks of treatment (**Fig. 4**A). In a pretreatment activation study involving negative emotional stimuli, Siegle and colleagues[144] showed that lower reactivity in sgACC, and higher pretreatment reactivity in the amygdale, were associated with improved response to CBT (see **Fig. 4**B). Studies suggest that rostral ACC may also have the capacity to facilitate restoration of dynamic equilibrium between the hypoactive dorsal and hyperactive ventral prefrontal circuitry through inhibitory modulation,[48] consistent with Thayer and Lane's[135] observation that rostral ACC is ideally positioned to modulate both dorsal and ventral prefrontal circuitry. Future studies will need to clarify the functional differences between dorsal and ventral ACC in relation to depressive subtypes.

Amygdala

Increases in resting amygdalar CBF and GLC metabolism have been consistently reported in individuals with mood disorders during both symptomatic and asymptomatic states, although this has not been reported in all depressive subtypes.[48,76,114,119] Increases correlate with severity of depression,[114] whereas decreases are seen with effective pharmacologic treatment, and correlate with clinical improvement.[114] Increased metabolism in the left amygdala has also been shown to correlate with plasma cortisol concentrations measured in stressful conditions in patients with MDD and BPD.[114]

Increases in left amygdalar CBF are also typically seen in healthy individuals during exposure to fear-related stimuli, a response that is present, but blunted, in both depressed adolescents and adults, perhaps because of increased regional resting metabolism.[114,155] Although healthy subjects display habituation of hemodynamic response to fear-related stimuli, prolonged blood oxygen level–dependent (BOLD) increases in bilateral amygdalae have been observed in patients with MDD and BPD,[156] suggesting dysfunctional fear conditioning mechanisms related to extinction. Current data suggest that the prolonged response to threat-related stimuli may be associated with right amygdalar dysfunction, whereas negative biases observed in mood and anxiety disorders may be associated with dysfunction of the left amygdala.[69]

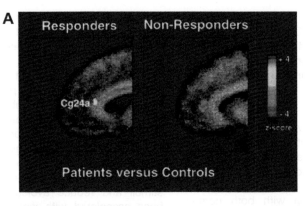

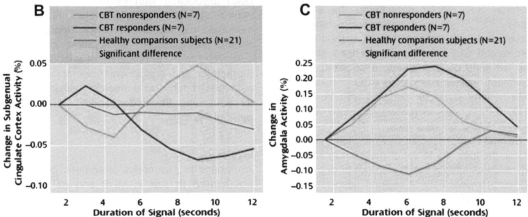

Fig. 4. Pretreatment CBF abnormalities in anterior cingulate cortex (ACC) and amygdala. (*A*) Depressed patients with high pretreatment resting metabolism in rostral ACC showed greater response to antidepressant medication; those with lower regional metabolism remained significantly depressed after 6 weeks of treatment. (*B, C*) Pretreatment changes in cingulate cortex (*B*) and amygdala (*C*) activity in response to negative emotional words in depressed versus healthy subjects. Positive response to CBT was associated with lower pretreatment reactivity in subgenual cingulate cortex (*B*) and higher pretreatment reactivity in amygdala (*C*). Shaded regions depict significant pretreatment differences in subgenual ACC responsivity between CBT responders and nonresponders (*B*), and in amygdalar responsitivity between depressed patients and healthy subjects (*C*). (Fig. 4A: *Reproduced from* Mayberg HS. Limbic-cortical dysregulation: a proposed model of depression. J Neuropsychiatry Clin Neurosci 1997;9(3):476; with permission. Fig. 4B, C: *Reproduced from* Siegle GJ, Carter CS, Thase ME. Use of FMRI to predict recovery from unipolar depression with cognitive behavior therapy. Am J Psychiatr 2006;163(4):736; with permission.)

Hippocampus

Although structural and histopathologic assessments of the hippocampus in depressed individuals have revealed significant abnormalities, functional abnormalities are rarely observed, with the exception that bilateral hippocampal hypoactivation has consistently been reported in studies of geriatric depression,[108] a condition commonly associated with memory impairment. Although there is a general lack of evidence for functional abnormalities in MDD or BPD, alterations in hippocampal neurogenesis have been associated with MDD, and some antidepressants have been shown to promote hippocampal neurogenesis.[106,157] Rather than an overall increase or decrease in hippocampal activation, dysregulation during context-dependent conditioning is more likely in MDD. Davidson and colleagues[80] suggest that there may be a link between inappropriate context-dependent affective responding and hippocampal atrophy, a suggestion that is consistent with the role of the hippocampus in context-specific memory formation and retrieval.

Mediodorsal thalamus

The mediodorsal thalamic nucleus has extensive connections with the amygdala and with ventral regions, as well as other PFC regions including OFC, VLPFC, and sgACC.[48,158] Depressed patients with MDD and BPD have shown consistent increases in GLC and CBF in the left mediodorsal nucleus (MD),[67,119] implicating a limbic-thalamocortical circuit involving amygdala, MD, and medial PFC in depression.

Basal ganglia
Early PET studies showed state-dependent changes in CBF throughout the basal ganglia in both BPD and unipolar depression.[118,126,159] A significantly lower metabolic rate within the caudate nucleus has been observed in depressed patients in comparison with both normal controls and bipolar patients in the euthymic state,[125,126,146] although manic states have been associated with increased right compared with left striatal CBF,[133,160] and increased activity in the left head of the caudate associated with an ipsilateral increase in dorsal ACC.[133] Compared with healthy subjects, patients with both MDD and BPD show increased caudate CBF in response to aversive stimuli.[161,162]

Several recent studies have focused on anhedonia, the loss of interest or pleasure in activities, which constitutes a core symptom of depression, showing hypoactivity of regions associated with the processing of reward and positive stimuli in patients with depression. In depressed subjects and those with trait anhedonia, this symptom has been associated with decreased activity in ventral striatum (particularly nucleus accumbens) **(Fig. 5)** and dmPFC, a region associated with the processing of self-related stimuli,[161,163] as well as increases in vmPFC in response to positive stimuli and monetary reward. Anticipation of reward has been associated with abnormal activity in caudate and dorsal striatum.[67,161] Reduced volume

of nucleus accumbens and anterior caudate, and decreased functional resting activity in rostral ACC, have also been associated with anhedonia.[164]

These data are consistent with the reduction in effortful and sustained positively motivated behavior seen across all subtypes of depressive disorder,[165] and suggest that inability to experience interest or pleasure in activities is associated with dysfunction of mesolimbic dopamine reward and prefrontal-striatal pathways. Psychotherapies designed to increase engagement with rewarding stimuli and reduce avoidance behaviors have been associated with increased metabolism in ventral striatum during monetary reward, and increased metabolism in dorsal striatum during reward anticipation.[166] In addition, it has been suggested that the presence of anhedonia could represent an endophenotype for particular subtypes of depressive disorder, with implications for advancing the understanding of depressive pathophysiology.[162]

Insula
Alterations in awareness of somatic characteristics related to self in MDD and BPD may be reflected in various somatovegetative symptoms associated with depression, along with an apparent hypervigilance to bodily changes, and exaggerated negative self-image.[167] The insula has been referred to as the interoceptive cortex, and shown to contain somatotopic representations of distinct feelings from the body (eg, pain, temperature, thirst, hunger, and other visceral sensations).[168] The posterior-to-anterior progression of neural processing through the insula provides a foundation for the sequential

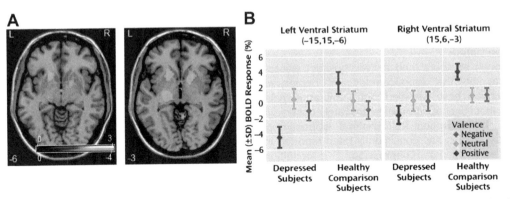

Fig. 5. Axial brain images (A) and graphs (B) showing significant bilateral ventral striatal decreases in activation to positive stimuli in depressed versus healthy subjects. The ventral striatum, particularly the nucleus accumbens, is associated with processing of reward and positive stimuli. Decreased activation was associated with anhedonia, or the inability to experience interest and pleasure. (Data from Epstein J, Pan H, Kocsis JH, et al. Lack of ventral striatal response to positive stimuli in depressed versus normal subjects. Am J Psychiatr 2006;163(10):1784–90.)

integration of the primary homeostatic condition of the body with salient features of the sensory environment, and then with motivational, hedonic, and social conditions represented in interconnected brain regions.[169] Studies in normal subjects have shown insular activation during anticipation of aversive stimuli, and in experimentally induced sadness,[141] suggesting a role for this structure in conveying aversive (or potentially aversive) visceral information to the amygdala. The insula has also been implicated in numerous studies involving the manipulation of emotion, and has been postulated to mediate self-awareness of behavioral patterns related to emotional expression, emotional control, and interpersonal relations.[170]

Evidence is accumulating for dysfunctional interoception in depression and anxiety, a finding integrated increasingly into neurocognitive models of depression.[47,141,171,172] Both early PET and more recent fMRI studies of patients with MDD have shown abnormal insular activity following interoceptive awareness tasks, or during experimentally induced sad autobiographical memories or negative self-relevant affective expression.[141,171,173,174] This altered insular activation, along with abnormal metabolism in medial PFC, may reflect an inability to shift the focus of perception/awareness from one's own body to the environment, consistent with the phenomenology of depression.[172] In keeping with this hypothesis, Wiebking and colleagues[172] showed a hypersensitive bodily awareness in patients with MDD compared with healthy controls that correlated positively with sustained activity in left anterior insula and severity of depression. Decreased activation of insular cortex in response to negative stimuli has also been reported in depressed patients, and observed to normalize following 2 weeks of treatment with venlafaxine, with correlation between symptom reduction and signal change in the left insular cortex.[175]

Connectivity studies

In recent years, functional neuroimaging research has focused increasingly on interregional neural interactions, most often via functional connectivity analyses that identify temporal correlations of low-frequency (0.01–0.1 Hz) BOLD fluctuations between spatially remote regions presumed to function as a network in the execution of a given task. Multivariate analyses have also identified spontaneous intrinsic activity in the resting brain that is anticorrelated with activity related to any particular attention-demanding task, and seems to be consistent across time and with anatomic connectivity.[176–180] This intrinsic activity is referred to as the default mode network (DMN).[176,177,181,182]

The DMN increases in activity during passive states, in which individuals are left to themselves to think, and during spontaneous and experimentally induced stimulus-independent thought or the state of a wandering mind.[183,184]

The DMN involves 2 subsystems that interact with a common core, and overlap with circuitry associated with self-reflective thought.[181,182,185] Core areas of the DMN are the anterior medial prefrontal cortex (aMPFC) and PCC. The dorsal medial prefrontal cortex (dMPFC) subsystem includes the dMPFC, temporoparietal junction (TPJ), lateral temporal cortex (LTC), and temporal pole (TempP); the medial temporal lobe (MTL) subsystem includes the vmPFC, posterior inferior parietal lobe (pIPL), retrosplenial cortex (Rsp), parahippocampal cortex (PHC), and hippocampal formation (HF+).[181] The dMPFC subsystem preferentially engages when participants make self-referential judgments about their present situation or mental states, whereas the MTL subsystem preferentially engages during episodic judgments about the personal future.[181]

Several studies of depressed subjects have shown abnormalities in functional connectivity within the network of structures described earlier (see Broyd and colleagues[189] for review).[142,186–189] Depressed subjects at rest displayed increased DMN connectivity with sgACC, correlating positively with length of current depressive episode.[186,190] Increased connectivity between the DMN, the sgACC, and the thalamus has also been observed, suggesting increased incorporation of emotional processing at the expense of executive functions.[186] Grimm and colleagues[187] also found abnormalities in connectivity between vmPFC and PCC, in addition to sgACC.

In depressed individuals, attentional resources are disproportionately allocated from the external environment to internal experiences such as negative cognitions and sadness, manifested clinically as rumination.[165] Berman and colleagues[190] showed that resting state correlation between PCC and sgACC in depressed subjects correlates positively with self-reflective rumination. Anticorrelations or negative BOLD responses in the DMN, typical during emotional stimulation in healthy individuals, have been absent in patients with MDD, suggesting increased self-reflective processing.[187] Recently, Epstein and colleagues observed a failure to segregate emotional processing from cognitive and sensorimotor processing in depressed subjects viewing positive stimuli. In BPD patients, functional connectivity analyses have identified abnormal correlations between left ventral PFC, amygdala, and right ventral striatum, along with weak inverse correlations between ventral PFC and dorsal PFC, providing support for behavioral observations of dysregulated affect and reward processing.[191] Although characterization using functional and effective connectivity methodology is in its infancy, existing data suggest that excessive activation of functional resting state networks in depressed subjects is associated with increases in ruminative thought, and with perseveration on negative, self-referential thoughts.[186,190]

Neurochemical Studies

Magnetic resonance spectroscopy (MRS) investigations into MDD and BPD have revealed a variety of abnormalities in brain chemistry. Decreased levels of γ-aminobutyric acid (GABA) have been observed in dmPFC and DLPFC,[192] consistent with postmortem studies showing reduced glial cell density in these regions. Glutamatergic abnormalities, as measured by the Glx peak, reflecting combined concentrations of glutamate plus glutamine, have also been observed in depressed subjects, and found to be linearly correlated with resting state functional connectivity between pgACC and anterior insula, a correlation not seen in healthy controls.[193] The most consistent finding has been abnormalities in the Cho signal, which is believed to reflect concentrations of choline-containing compounds, membrane turnover, and changes in synaptic plasticity.[194]

Choline abnormalities have also been reported in BPD. Several studies have shown increased choline concentrations in striatum and cingulate cortex that are independent of mood state or treatment with lithium.[160,195] One study of patients with BPD (compared with healthy controls) found lateralized differences in the cingulate: on the left, choline concentrations correlated positively with ratings of depression, whereas, on the right, choline was increased regardless of the presence of depressive symptoms.[160] Changes in N-acetyl aspartate (NAA), a marker for functional and structural neuronal integrity, have also been shown in BPD, with decreases reported in DLPFC and hippocampus of adolescents and adults with the disorder.[160] These data suggest a subcortical basis for the expression of bipolar symptoms, and impaired neural signaling during depressed states, especially in PFC and hippocampus.

Overall, the most common functional metabolic findings in patients with MDD and BPD, irrespective of mood state, are abnormalities in the amygdala and rostral ACC, including the subgenual and pregenual regions (see Fig. 3A, B). Some of these findings seem to normalize with pharmacologic or psychotherapeutic treatment and/or serve as predictors of treatment response (see Fig. 4).[56,130,131,144,145,152]

REFINING NEUROCIRCUITRY MODELS FOR MOOD DISORDERS: CURRENT PERSPECTIVES

The brain regions consistently implicated in the production of depressive signs and symptoms via neuroimaging, neuropsychological, and histopathologic methods are shown in Fig. 6 within a schematic model of corticolimbic-insular-striatal-pallidal-thalamic circuitry (CLIPST).[46,48,50,53,69,119] Consistent with the wide variety of symptoms that comprise depression, the model includes structures involved in the processing of fear, reward, attention, motivation, memory, stress, social cognition, and somatic functions.[48,80,130] Depression may arise in the context of dysfunction of 1 or more of these regions, or because of a failure of coordinated interactions within or between the broader circuits. It is likely that different subtypes of depression are mediated by disorders localized to different brain areas, and respond accordingly to different treatments.

Prevailing models for mood disorders have focused on critical dissociations between the highly integrated dorsal and ventral circuits of the frontal lobe and their respective interactions with elements of the limbic system (amygdala, hippocampus, thalamus), basal ganglia, insula, and hypothalamic-pituitary-adrenal (HPA) axis.[68,76,97,129,130,139,142,196–198] Tract-tracing methods in animals have further subdivided ventral regions into orbital and medial prefrontal networks.[48,199] Recently, graph analytical and hierarchical clustering analysis of low-frequency, intrinsic functional BOLD connectivity in the resting brain has revealed distinct dorsomedial and ventromedial subsystems that interact with a common midline core (orbitomedial PFC [OMPFC] and PCC).[181] The dorsal circuit includes portions of the middle and superior frontal gyri on the lateral surface of the frontal lobe (BA 9/46/44); has dense interconnections with premotor areas; and projects to the dorsal cingulate (BA 24b/32), posterior cingulate (PCC, BA 29/30/31), inferior parietal cortex (BA 39/40), head of the caudate, and putamen.[46,69,130,200] The ventral circuit includes the medial and ventrolateral aspects of orbitofrontal cortex (BA 10/11/47/12) and has reciprocal projections with the adjacent anterior agranular insular cortex (AIC, BA 13), pgACC and sgACC (BA 24a/25/32), amygdala and hippocampus, ventromedial striatum, midline thalamic nuclei (PVT), and hypothalamus.[46,48,50,68] Behavioral observations of experimental lesions in animals[1,93,201,202] and naturally occurring

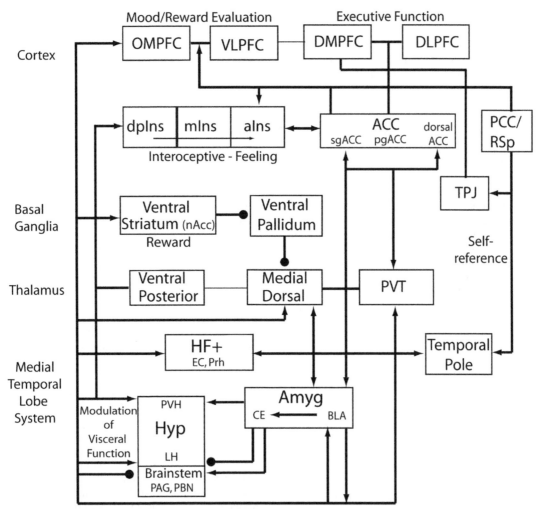

Fig. 6. Neuroanatomic model of circuitry implicated in depression by neuroimaging and neuropathological studies of mood disorders. Solid lines, anatomic connections; arrows, excitatory projections; terminal endings, strong inhibitory projections. ACC, anterior cingulate cortex; aIns, anterior insula; Amyg, amygdala; BLA, basolateral nucleus of the amygdale; CE, central nucleus of the amygdala; DLPFC, dorsolateral prefrontal cortex; dpIns, dorsal-posterior insula; EC, entorhinal cortex; HF+, hippocampal formation; LH, lateral hypothalamus; mIns, medial insula; nAcc, nucleus accumbens; OMPFC, orbitomedial prefrontal cortex; PAG, periacqueductal gray; PBN, peribrachial nucleus; Prh, perirhinal cortex; PVH, periventricular hypothalamus; PVT, periventricular thalamus; RSp, retrosplenial cortex; VLPFC, ventrolateral prefrontal cortex.

disorders in humans[14,149,203] provide ample evidence for the role of CLIPST circuitry in the pathophysiology of depression. Late-onset depression is associated with cerebrovascular disease and white matter changes within this network.[67,120,163,204,205] Traumatic brain injury to regions within the circuit is associated with hyperactivity, agitation, mood swings, irritability, excitation, impulsivity, hostility, and impaired affective evaluation.[174,203,206] The application of imaging techniques to the skull of Phineas Gage, the well-known exemplar of behavioral changes secondary to frontal lobe injury, suggests that

the lesion affected left anterior OFC (BA 11/12), polar and anterior medial frontal cortices (BA 8/9/10/32), and possibly vmPFC and ACC (BA 24).[14,15] Specific abnormalities in CLIPST circuitry may also serve as biomarkers either for resilience to stress, or for risk of subsequent development of mood disorders.[55,207] There are data to suggest that structural and functional abnormalities caused by genetic endowment or early traumatic experience may initiate a pathologic process that remains presymptomatic through adolescence, but subsequently manifests at clinical levels after exposure to a significant stressor toward which cognitive and emotional processing is maladaptive.[46,165,207]

In the model delineated earlier, lesions in any part of the circuitry could lead to a constellation of symptoms related to depression, but specific to the precise functional location. Dorsal circuitry is characterized as regulating executive functions (forming, maintaining, switching set), sensory discrimination, and cognitive forms of apprais-al.[50,130,156,171,208] Lesions in dorsolateral circuitry lead to broadly defined deficits in executive function and working memory, whereas those in dorsomedial circuitry lead to deficits in reason and emotional expression.[149,208] Ventral circuitry is characterized as regulating affective, motivational, evaluative, and self-relevant process-ing.[93,125,174,203] Symptoms arising from ventral circuitry lesions may reflect dysregulated attempts to interrupt unreinforced aversive thoughts and emotions, raising the possibility that disturbed synaptic interactions between these regions and the amygdala, striatum, hypothalamus, or periaqueductal gray may impair the ability to inhibit unreinforced or maladaptive emotional, cognitive, and behavioral responses.

Generally, the functional neuroimaging studies described earlier show that sadness and depressive symptoms are associated with decreases in dorsal, and relative increases in ventral, circuit activity.[48,68,80,129,142,156,209,210] In response to a real or imagined threat, abnormalities in metabolism or function within the dorsal circuit may disinhibit the autonomic and emotional expression regulated by ventral circuitry. With successful pharmacologic or behavioral treatment, reversal of these findings is observed.[48,119,174] Current models of emotion regulation propose that depressive remission occurs when there is inhibition of the hyperactive ventral regions and activation of the previously hypofunctioning dorsal areas.[130,174,211] Based on the overwhelming evidence for abnormal functioning of the rostral ACC in depression, its strong reciprocal connections with both dorsal and ventral circuitry, and evidence that pretreatment metabolism in the BA 24a region uniquely predicts treatment response, the region is postulated to play a major regulatory role and to be necessary for adaptive behavioral change.[130] Disruption of the rostral cingulate is likely to have a significant effect on the CLIPST network, particularly those circuits regulating mood, cognition, and autonomic response.

Data from neuroimaging studies are consistent with cognitive models of psychopathology such that depressive episodes are caused, in part, by heightened limbic reactivity to emotionally significant events, followed by a form of cognitive

reactivity that includes deployment of increased attentional resources to such events (ie, rumination) and results in negative attentional bias and recall.[165] The cognitive control of emotional appraisal in this context of real or imagined threat is significantly attenuated, and thus reappraisal of negative interpretations is limited. Cognitive models further propose that a negatively biased information processing system translates into stable dysfunctional attitudes with distorted negative interpretations (eg, selective abstraction, overgeneralization) of benign emotional experiences. Thus, depressive symptoms emerge from a continuous feedback loop of negative interpretations and attentional biases, with subjective and behavioral symptoms reinforcing one another.

CIRCUITRY-BASED NEUROTHERAPEUTICS

Neurosurgical treatment of psychiatric disease has a long and controversial history (**Box 1**). This approach is currently reserved for a select patient population characterized by severe and refractory symptoms, or strongly adverse side effects. Although neurosurgical treatments are most widely used for obsessive-compulsive disorder, various procedures have also been used for severe forms of refractory depression. The circuitry-based model described earlier provides insight into the physiologic mechanisms of the neurosurgical, DBS, and rapid transcranial magnetic stimulation (rTMS) treatments for refractory depression that have been reported in the literature.[92,212–215] In addition to their role in delineating this model, neuroimaging methods have also been instrumental in preoperative localization of targets and postoperative confirmation of lesion extent.

Stereotactic Ablation

The most effective surgical procedure for the treatment of refractory depression has been the subcaudate tractotomy, a procedure that involves interrupting white matter tracts that link various structures including vmPFC, basal forebrain, amygdale, and hypothalamus (**Fig. 8**).[200,215,219,220] In general, procedures that induce damage to vmPFC and/or its white matter connections have been reported to be efficacious in alleviating depression.[220] In a retrospective study of patients who had suffered severe mood or obsessive-compulsive disorders before surgery between 1979 and 1991, 84 of 249 (34%) had significantly reduced symptoms 1 year after subcaudate tractotomy.[221] Other procedures have included anterior cingulotomy, limbic leukotomy, anterior capsulotomy, bilateral amygdalotomy,

---

Box 1
History of psychosurgery

The earliest evidence of surgical methods targeting psychiatric illness comes from an archaeological site in France where skulls carbon dated to 5100 BCE were observed to contain carefully drilled holes rounded off by growth of new bony tissue, suggesting healing around the opening. Similar finds from subsequent eras suggest that the holes resulted from a surgical intervention called trephination, an opening of the cranium to relieve depressive symptoms along with headaches, seizures, or other spiritual or psychiatric disturbances.[215,216]

In the nineteenth century, neurobiologic models of mental dysfunction began to emerge, providing the groundwork for the development of somatic treatments. By the end of the century, increasing excitement surrounding connectionist models of mental function set the stage for the first psychosurgical intervention, a topectomy performed by Gottlieb Burckhardt, a Swiss psychiatrist. In 1888, Burckhardt removed cortical tissue from multiple foci in frontal, parietal, and temporal lobes in 6 patients characterized as aggressive and demented, with limited success.[215,216]

It was not until the 1930s that psychosurgery (now firmly focused on frontal incisions) gained prominence. Given the pressures of overcrowded psychiatric institutions and the limited success of other somatic therapies including convulsive, insulin shock, and hydrotherapy, the use of psychosurgery began to peak following World War II. More than 5000 outpatient lobotomies were performed in 1949 alone, and more than 15,000 more by the time the practice declined in the 1950s.[215–217]

The term psychosurgery was coined by Egas Moniz, a Portuguese neurologist credited as the first to target smaller areas of the frontal lobes, using either ethyl alcohol or a leucotome, for treatment of melancholy, anxiety, and delusions.[200,215–217] Along with a neurosurgical colleague, Almeida Lima, Moniz performed frontal leucotomies, targeting fibers that connect anterior frontal cortex with thalamic and cortical regions, with the intention of disrupting abnormally stabilized neural connections believed to be responsible for the fixed ideas that constitute mental illness.[202,216] Variations of the method were later used throughout the world to treat symptoms of psychosis.

In North America, James Watts, a neurosurgeon, and Walter Freeman, a neuropsychiatrist, refined the location and extent of the surgical lesion based on clinical responsiveness, and renamed the procedure frontal lobotomy, with minimal, standard, radical, and transorbital modifications (**Fig. 7**).[216,218] In 1942, Freeman and Watts reported that, of the first 200 patients to undergo frontal lobotomy, 63% manifested an improvement in symptoms, and noted that postmortem examination of some patients who had undergone the procedure confirmed retrograde degeneration in specific areas of the thalamus.[216] Transorbital lobotomies became the most common procedure for treating mental illness until the practice declined in the 1950s with the introduction of the antipsychotic drug, chlorpromazine, a safer, cheaper, more effective, and reversible treatment.

Despite the gains provided by the subsequent proliferation of pharmacologic treatments, it gradually became apparent that a surgical alternative might be useful for a select patient population characterized by severe and refractory symptoms, or strongly adverse side effects. In 1976, the National Commission for the Protection of Human Subjects of Biomedical and Behavioral Research addressed this issue, creating guidelines for the ethical use and regulation of neurosurgical procedures for psychiatric disease.

---

bimedial leukotomy, orbital gyrus undercutting, thalomotomy, and hypothalamotomy.[200,219,222,223]

There is limited evidence directly comparing different procedures. Given the complexity of current models of depression, there are likely to be multiple sites of therapeutic action. It has been suggested that stereotactic ablation in discrete areas of CLIPST circuitry may alleviate treatment-refractory forms of depression through modification of downstream pathways in the network, in addition to reducing cortical mass and activity within the areas explicitly targeted.

Reductions in volume and function of the reciprocal connections between ACC and several other structures, including OFC, amygdala, hippocampus and PCC, have been observed within 1 year of surgery.[222] Lesions of dorsal ACC might produce disinhibition of rostral ACC, which, in turn, might render patients more responsive to antidepressant pharmacotherapy after surgery. Alternatively, lesions of the cingulum might interrupt ascending influences of the amygdala on the dorsal circuitry.[69] Although neurosurgical treatments have shown some benefit for refractory

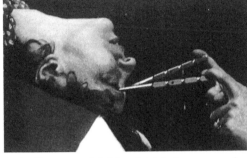

Fig. 7. The transorbital frontal lobotomy procedure, with 2 leucotome orbitoclasts positioned in the orbit. With little or no evidence for extent of lesion or standardized surgical procedures, patients were often given anesthesia in the form of electroconvulsive shock, followed by hammering of sturdy orbitoclasts through the orbital bone and up into neural tissue. (*Courtesy of* Walter Freeman III.)

forms of mood disorders, the current direction of the field is toward electrical, magnetic, and even modulation through focused ultrasound of neural structures for clinical purposes.

DBS

Subgenual anterior cingulate cortex
Following its introduction in the 1990s, high-frequency DBS, a less-invasive, reversible technique, gained popularity as a treatment of intractable forms of MDD.[130,212,214] Based on early circuit models of depression derived primarily from PET scan measures of GLC and CBF, the first region to be targeted was the sgACC (see **Fig. 8**).[130,214] Stimulation of the sgACC or the white matter tracts that lead to it (see **Fig. 8**) has

been shown to induce remission of depression, with poststimulation decreases in cerebral flow to sgACC, and increases to PFC, correlating with clinical improvement.[153,222,224] Studies have further shown reversal and reresponse of effect with off-on-off-on design, lack of response with sham or subthreshold stimulation, and sustained 6- to 12-month improvement, supporting the effectiveness of sgACC DBS for treatment of depression.[212,224] Whether longer-term sustained response (ie, prevention of relapse) correlates with sgACC activity remains to be determined.[224]

Ventral anterior internal capsule/ventral striatum
A second brain region targeted for DBS in refractory depression has been the ventral anterior internal capsule/ventral striatum (VC/VS) (see **Fig. 8**).[132,225] Schlaepfer and colleagues[225] conducted preliminary studies to show that DBS in the nucleus accumbens was associated with clinical improvement when the stimulator was on, and worsening when it was turned off. A case of bilateral DBS of the accumbens for severe anxiety and secondary depression has also been reported.[212] A more recent study reported antidepressant, antianhedonic, and antianxiety effects of DBS to the nucleus accumbens, and associated metabolic decreases in sgACC, OFC, medial thalamus, PCC, and dmPFC.[132]

rTMS

rTMS is another noninvasive method for localized modulation of CLIPST circuitry.[226–232] Since its introduction in 1985, more than 40 randomized controlled trials of rTMS for depression have

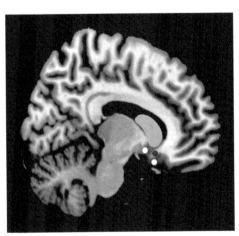
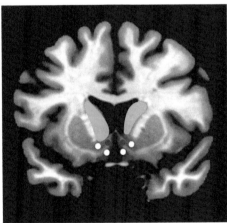

Fig. 8. Targets for stereotactic ablation and DBS treatments of refractory depression (shown in sagittal and coronal sections on a template brain). Red circles indicate targeted sites for subcaudate tractotomy: the substantia innominata (just inferior to the head of the caudate nucleus, in blue) is targeted with the goal of interrupting white matter tracts connecting OFC to subcortical structures. White circles indicate targeted sites (subgenual cingulate, nucleus accumbens) for deep brain stimulation.

been implemented, with mixed results.[232] A subset of these has examined pre- and posttreatment blood flow in rostral ACC. Nadeau and colleagues[229] found that pretreatment rostral ACC blood flow was correlated with reduction in depression severity following 10 days of 20 Hz rTMS over the left DLPFC. Similarly, increased pretreatment activity in rostral ACC was found to predict reduction of depressive symptoms following a 2-week trial of rTMS augmentation, or a 3-week trial of low-frequency stimulation over the right DLPFC.[230] In contrast, other studies have shown that lower pretreatment regional CBF in the rostral ACC was linked to greater rTMS response, whereas some have found no relationship between the 2 variables.[232] A recent meta-analysis concluded that the largest mean effect size for rTMS in treatment-resistant depression has occurred when right DLPFC has been targeted in the absence of pharmacotherapy.[228]

It is likely that ongoing advances in DBS and transcranial magnetic stimulation technologies will improve their clinical efficacy, and that these methods will be supplemented by additional reversible and possibly noninvasive localized treatments, such as focused ultrasound,[233,234] cranial electrotherapy stimulation,[235] or epidural cortical stimulation.[236] Unfolding topics of investigation, such as stem cell–based neuroprotective and neurorestorative strategies[237] and localized protein-based therapies using adeno-associated virus (AAV)–mediated gene transfer,[238] also hold great promise.

SUMMARY

The investigational use of functional neuroimaging has revolutionized understanding of the functional neuroanatomy of psychiatric disorders, giving rise to complex neurocircuitry-based models that provide a foundation for the development of neurosurgical and other targeted biologic treatments for psychiatric disorders. These techniques are also being used to identify biomarkers for risk/resilience factors, to elucidate clinical subtypes and final common pathways, to guide early intervention, and to predict treatment response. Although there is yet to be a standard, scientifically validated role for neuroimaging techniques in the clinical evaluation of individual patients suffering from mental illness, it is our hope that they will ultimately be used to diagnose pathophysiology based subclassifications of psychiatric disease, and to determine corresponding treatment approaches. Interventions requiring neurosurgical expertise are likely to play an important role in targeting specific neuropsychiatric symptom profiles, particularly in refractory cases.

REFERENCES

1. Jackson SW. Melancholia and depression: from Hippocratic times to modern times. New Haven (CT): Yale University Press; 1986.
2. Kutzer M. Tradition, metaphors, anatomy of the brain: the physiology of insanity in the late XVIth and XVIIth centuries, in essays in the history of the physiological sciences: Proceedings of a symposium held at the University Louis Pasteur. Debru C, editor. Atlanta (GA): The Wellcome Institute Series in the History of Medicine; 1993. p. 99–116.
3. Nicolaidis S. Depression and neurosurgery: past, present, and future. Metabolism 2005;54(5 Suppl 1): 28–32.
4. Siegel RE. Galen on psychology, psychopathology and function and diseases of the nervous system. Basel (Switzerland): Karger; 1973.
5. Clarke E, O'Malley CD. The human brain and spinal cord: a historical study illustrated by writings from antiquity to the twentieth century. Norman neurosciences series; no. 2. San Francisco (CA): Norman Publishers; 1996.
6. Gross CG. Brain, vision, memory: tales in the history of neuroscience. Cambridge (MA): MIT Press; 1998.
7. Finger S. Origins of neuroscience: a history of explorations into brain function. New York: Oxford University Press; 1994.
8. Zola-Morgan S. Localization of brain function: the legacy of Franz Joseph Gall (1758–1828). Annu Rev Neurosci 1995;18(1):359–83.
9. Harrington A. Beyond phrenology: localization theory in the modern era. In: Corsi P, editor. The enchanted loom: chapters in the history of neuroscience. New York: Oxford University Press; 1991. p. 207–39.
10. Bouillaud MJ. Traite clinique et physiologique de l'encephalite ou inflammation du cerveau, et de ses suites. Paris: Bailiere; 1825.
11. Finger S. Minds behind the brain: a history of the pioneers and their discoveries. Oxford (UK): Oxford University Press; 2000.
12. Farah MJ, Feinberg TE. Patient-based approaches to cognitive neuroscience. Cambridge (MA): MIT Press; 2000.
13. Finger S, Michael FB, Aminoff J, et al. Chapter 10. The birth of localization theory. In: Finger S, Boller F, Tyler K, editors. History of neurology. New York: Elsevier; 2009. p. 117–28.
14. Damasio H, Grabowski T, Frank R, et al. The return of Phineas Gage: clues about the brain from the skull of a famous patient. Science 1994; 264(5162):1102–5.
15. Ratiu P, Talos IF, Haker S, et al. The tale of Phineas Gage, digitally remastered. J Neurotrauma 2004; 21(5):637–43.
16. McHenry LC Jr. Garrison's history of neurology. Springfield (IL): Charles C Thomas; 1969.

17. Jackson JH. Selected writings of John Hughlings Jackson. London: Hodder and Stoughton; 1931.

18. Maclean PD. The limbic system and its hippocampal formation; studies in animals and their possible application to man. J Neurosurg 1954; 11(1):29–44.

19. Papez JW. A proposed mechanism of emotion. 1937. J Neuropsychiatry Clin Neurosci 1995;7(1): 103–12.

20. Cannon WB. The James-Lange theory of emotions: a critical examination and an alternative theory. Am J Psychol 1927;39:106–24.

21. Alheid GF, Heimer L. New perspectives in basal forebrain organization of special relevance for neuropsychiatric disorders: the striatopallidal, amygdaloid, and corticopetal components of substantia innominata. Neuroscience 1988;27(1):1–39.

22. Ongur D, Price JL. The organization of networks within the orbital and medial prefrontal cortex of rats, monkeys and humans. Cereb Cortex 2000; 10(3):206–19.

23. Amaral DG, Price JL. Amygdalo-cortical projections in the monkey (Macaca fascicularis). J Comp Neurol 1984;230(4):465–96.

24. Krettek JE, Price JL. An audioradiographic study of projections from the amygdaloid complex to the thalamus and cerebral cortex. J Comp Neurol 1977;172:723–52.

25. Nauta WJ. Fibre degeneration following lesions of the amygdaloid complex in the monkey. J Anat 1961;95:515–31.

26. Nauta WJ, Feirtag M. The organization of the brain. Sci Am 1979;241(3):88–111.

27. Heimer L. Pathways in the brain. Sci Am 1971;225: 48–60.

28. Gray TS. Functional and anatomical relationships among the amygdala, basal forebrain, ventral striatum, and cortex: an integrative discussion. In: McGinty JF, editor. Advancing from the ventral striatum to the extended amygdala. New York: The New York Academy of Sciences; 1999. p. 439–45.

29. De Olmos JS, Heimer L. The concepts of the ventral striatopallidal system and extended amygdala. In: McGinty JF, editor. Advancing from the ventral striatum to the extended amygdala. New York: The New York Academy of Sciences; 1999. p. 1–33.

30. Gardner HE. The mind's new science: a history of the cognitive revolution. New York: Basic Books; 1987.

31. Stein DJ. Cognitive science and psychiatry: an overview. Integr Psychiatry 1993;9(1):13–24.

32. Benson DF. Neuropsychiatry and behavioral neurology: past, present, and future. J Neuropsychiatry Clin Neurosci 1996;8(3):351–7.

33. Geschwind N. Disconnexion syndromes in animals and man: Part I. 1965. Neuropsychol Rev 2010; 20(2):128–57.

34. Ross ED. Intellectual origins and theoretical framework of behavioral neurology: a response to Michael R. Trimble. Neuropsychiatry Neuropsychol Behav Neurol 1993;6(1):65–7.

35. LeDoux JE. The emotional brain: the mysterious underpinnings of emotional life. New York: Simon & Schuster; 1996.

36. McGaugh JL, Roozendaal B, Cahill L. Modulation of memory storage by stress hormones and the amygdaloid complex. In: Gazzaniga MS, editor. The new cognitive neurosciences. Cambridge (MA): MIT Press; 2000. p. 1081–98.

37. Ono T, Nishijo H. Neurophysiological basis of emotion in primates: neuronal responses in the monkey amygdala and anterior cingulate cortex. In: Gazzaniga MS, editor. The new cognitive neurosciences. Cambridge (MA): MIT Press; 2000. p. 1099–114.

38. Robbins TW, Everitt BJ. Neurobehavioural mechanisms of reward and motivation. Curr Opin Neurobiol 1996;6(2):228–36.

39. Rolls ET. The orbitofrontal cortex. In: Roberst AC, editor. The prefrontal cortex: executive and cognitive functions. New York: Oxford University Press; 1998. p. 67–86.

40. McEwen BS. Stress and hippocampal plasticity. Annu Rev Neurosci 1999;22(1):105–22.

41. Brothers L. The social brain: a project for integrating primate behavior and neuropsychiatry in a new domain. Concepts Neurosci 1990;1(1):27–51.

42. Cosmides L, Tooby J. The cognitive neurosciences of social reasoning. In: Gazzaniga MS, editor. The new cognitive neurosciences. Cambridge (MA): MIT Press; 2000. p. 1259–70.

43. Jacoby RJ, Levy R, Dawson JM. Computed tomography in the elderly: I. The normal population. Br J Psychiatry 1980;136:249–55.

44. Rangel-Guerra RA, Perez-Payan H, Minkoff L, et al. Nuclear magnetic resonance in bipolar affective disorders. AJNR Am J Neuroradiol 1983;4(3):229–31.

45. Huettel SA, Song AW, McCarthy G. Functional magnetic resonance imaging. 2nd edition. Sunderland (MA): Sinauer Associates ; 2008.

46. Drevets WC, Price JL, Furey ML. Brain structural and functional abnormalities in mood disorders: implications for neurocircuitry models of depression. Brain Struct Funct 2008;213(1/2):93–118.

47. Phillips ML, Drevets WC, Rauch SL, et al. Neurobiology of emotion perception II: implications for major psychiatric disorders. Biol Psychiatry 2003; 54(5):515–28.

48. Price JL, Drevets WC. Neurocircuitry of mood disorders. Neuropsychopharmacology 2010; 35(1):192–216.

49. Dolan RJ, Poynton AM, Bridges PK, et al. Altered magnetic resonance white-matter T1 values in patients with affective disorder. Br J Psychiatr 1990;157:107–10.

50. Soares JC, Mann JJ. The anatomy of mood disorders - review of structural neuroimaging studies. Biol Psychiatry 1997;41(1):86–106.

51. Dougherty D, Rauch SL. Neuroimaging and neurobiological models of depression. Harv Rev Psychiatry 1997;5(3):138–59.

52. Bench CJ, Dolan RJ, Friston KJ, et al. Positron emission tomography in the study of brain metabolism in psychiatric and neuropsychiatric disorders. Br J Psychiatry Suppl 1990;9:82–95.

53. Sheline YI. Neuroimaging studies of mood disorder effects on the brain. Biol Psychiatry 2003;54(3):338–52.

54. Nestler EJ, Carlezon WA Jr. The mesolimbic dopamine reward circuit in depression. Biol Psychiatry 2006;59(12):1151–9.

55. McEwen BS, Magarinos AM. Stress and hippocampal plasticity: implications for the pathophysiology of affective disorders. Hum Psychopharmacol 2001;16(S1):S7–19.

56. Mayberg HS, McGinnis S. Brain mapping: the application, mood and emotions. In: Toga AW, Mazziotta JC, editors. Brain mapping: the systems. San Francisco (CA): Academic Press; 2000. p. 491–521.

57. Liu D, Diorio J, Tannenbaum B, et al. Maternal care, hippocampal glucocorticoid receptors, and hypothalamic-pituitary-adrenal responses to stress. Science 1997;277(5332):1659–62.

58. Sheline YI. Hippocampal atrophy in major depression: a result of depression-induced neurotoxicity? Mol Psychiatry 1996;1(4):298–9.

59. DeCarolis NA, Eisch AJ. Hippocampal neurogenesis as a target for the treatment of mental illness: a critical evaluation. Neuropharmacology 2010;58(6):884–93.

60. Burke HM, Davis MC, Otte C, et al. Depression and cortisol responses to psychological stress: a meta-analysis. Psychoneuroendocrinology 2005;30(9):846–56.

61. Daley SE, Hammen C, Rao U. Predictors of first onset and recurrence of major depression in young women during the 5 years following high school graduation. J Abnorm Psychol 2000;109(3):525–33.

62. Kendler KS, Karkowski LM, Prescott CA. Causal relationship between stressful life events and the onset of major depression. Am J Psychiatr 1999;156(6):837–41.

63. Hammen C, Davila J, Brown G, et al. Psychiatric history and stress: predictors of severity of unipolar depression. J Abnorm Psychol 1992;101(1):45–52.

64. Strakowski SM, Adler CM, DelBello MP. Volumetric MRI studies of mood disorders: do they distinguish unipolar and bipolar disorder? Bipolar Disord 2002;4(2):80–8.

65. Krishnan KR, McDonald WM, Tupler LA. Neuropathology in affective illness. Am J Psychiatr 1993;150(10):1568–9.

66. McDonald WM, Krishnan KR. Magnetic resonance in patients with affective illness. Eur Arch Psychiatry Clin Neurosci 1992;241(5):283–90.

67. Drevets WC, Gadde K, Krishnan KR. Neuroimaging studies of mood disorders. In: Charney DS, Nestler EJ, editors. Neurobiology of mental illness. New York: Oxford University Press; 2004. p. 461–80.

68. Mayberg HS. Defining the neural circuitry of depression: toward a new nosology with therapeutic implications. Biol Psychiatry 2007;61(6):729–30.

69. Rauch SL. Neuroimaging and neurocircuitry models pertaining to the neurosurgical treatment of psychiatric disorders. Neurosurg Clin N Am 2003;14(2):213–23, vii–viii.

70. Lorenzetti V, Allen NB, Fornito A, et al. Structural brain abnormalities in major depressive disorder: a selective review of recent MRI studies. J Affect Disord 2009;117(1–2):1–17.

71. Ongur D, Ferry AT, Price JL. Architectonic subdivision of the human orbital and medial prefrontal cortex. J Comp Neurol 2003;460(3):425–49.

72. Davidson RJ, Irwin W. The functional neuroanatomy of emotion and affective style. Trends Cogn Sci 1999;3(1):11–21.

73. Downhill JE Jr, Robinson RG. Longitudinal assessment of depression and cognitive impairment following stroke. J Nerv Ment Dis 1994;182(8):425–31.

74. Gainotti G. Emotional behavior and hemispheric side of the lesion. Cortex 1972;8(1):41–55.

75. Davidson RJ. Anxiety and affective style: role of prefrontal cortex and amygdala. Biol Psychiatry 2002;51(1):68–80.

76. Davidson RJ, Lewis DA, Alloy LB, et al. Neural and behavioral substrates of mood and mood regulation. Biol Psychiatry 2002;52(6):478–502.

77. Starkstein SE, Mayberg HS, Berthier ML, et al. Mania after brain injury: neuroradiological and metabolic findings. Ann Neurol 1990;27(6):652–9.

78. Robinson RG, Downhill JE. Lateralization of psychopathology in response to focal brain injury. In: Davidson RJ, Hugdahl K, editors. Brain asymmetry. Cambridge (MA): MIT Press; 1995. p. 693–711.

79. Fitzgerald PB, Oxley TJ, Laird AR, et al. An analysis of functional neuroimaging studies of dorsolateral prefrontal cortical activity in depression. Psychiatry Res 2006;148(1):33–45.

80. Davidson RJ, Pizzagalli D, Nitschke JB, et al. Depression: perspectives from affective neuroscience. Annu Rev Psychol 2002;53:545–74.

81. Cerullo MA, Adler CM, Delbello MP, et al. The functional neuroanatomy of bipolar disorder. Int Rev Psychiatry 2009;21(4):314–22.

82. Emsell L, McDonald C. The structural neuroimaging of bipolar disorder. Int Rev Psychiatry 2009;21(4):297–313.

83. Fleck DE, Nandagopal J, Cerullo MA, et al. Morphometric magnetic resonance imaging in psychiatry. Top Magn Reson Imaging 2008;19(2): 131–42.

84. Hallahan B, Newell J, Soares JC, et al. Structural magnetic resonance imaging in bipolar disorder: an international collaborative mega-analysis of individual adult patient data. Biol Psychiatry 2011; 69(4):326–35.

85. Adler CM, DelBello MP, Jarvis K, et al. Voxel-based study of structural changes in first-episode patients with bipolar disorder. Biol Psychiatry 2007;61(6): 776–81.

86. Bremner JD. Structural changes in the brain in depression and relationship to symptom recurrence. CNS Spectr 2002;7(2):129–30, 135–9.

87. Lai T, Payne ME, Byrum CE, et al. Reduction of orbital frontal cortex volume in geriatric depression. Biol Psychiatry 2000;48(10):971–5.

88. Rajkowska G, Miguel-Hidalgo JJ, Wei J, et al. Morphometric evidence for neuronal and glial prefrontal cell pathology in major depression. Biol Psychiatry 1999;45(9):1085–98.

89. Ekman CJ, Lind J, Rydén E, et al. Manic episodes are associated with grey matter volume reduction - a voxel-based morphometry brain analysis. Acta Psychiatr Scand 2010;122:507–15.

90. Li CT, Lin CP, Chou KH, et al. Structural and cognitive deficits in remitting and non-remitting recurrent depression: a voxel-based morphometric study. Neuroimage 2010;50(1):347–56.

91. Critchley HD, Mathias CJ, Josephs O, et al. Human cingulate cortex and autonomic control: converging neuroimaging and clinical evidence. Brain 2003;126(Pt 10):2139–52.

92. Mayberg HS, Brannan SK, Mahurin RK, et al. Cingulate function in depression: a potential predictor of treatment response. Neuroreport 1997;8(4):1057–61.

93. Ressler KJ, Mayberg HS. Targeting abnormal neural circuits in mood and anxiety disorders: from the laboratory to the clinic. Nat Neurosci 2007;10(9):1116–24.

94. Bench CJ, Friston KJ, Brown RG, et al. Regional cerebral blood flow in depression measured by positron emission tomography: the relationship with clinical dimensions. Psychol Med 1993;23(3): 579–90.

95. Botteron KN, Raichle ME, Drevets WC, et al. Volumetric reduction in left subgenual prefrontal cortex in early onset depression. Biol Psychiatry 2002; 51(4):342–4.

96. Coryell W, Nopoulos P, Drevets W, et al. Subgenual prefrontal cortex volumes in major depressive disorder and schizophrenia: diagnostic specificity and prognostic implications. Am J Psychiatr 2005;162(9):1706–12.

97. Drevets WC, Savitz J, Trimble M. The subgenual anterior cingulate cortex in mood disorders. CNS Spectr 2008;13(8):663–81.

98. Ebert D, Ebmeier KP. The role of the cingulate gyrus in depression: from functional anatomy to neurochemistry. Biol Psychiatry 1996;39(12): 1044–50.

99. Hastings RS, Parsey RV, Oquendo MA, et al. Volumetric analysis of the prefrontal cortex, amygdala, and hippocampus in major depression. Neuropsychopharmacology 2004;29(5):952–9.

100. Drevets WC, Price JL, Simpson JR Jr, et al. Subgenual prefrontal cortex abnormalities in mood disorders. Nature 1997;386(6627):824–7.

101. Drevets WC, Ongur D, Price JL. Neuroimaging abnormalities in the subgenual prefrontal cortex: implications for the pathophysiology of familial mood disorders. Mol Psychiatry 1998;3(3):220–6, 190–1.

102. Ongur D, Drevets WC, Price JL. Glial reduction in the subgenual prefrontal cortex in mood disorders. Proc Natl Acad Sci U S A 1998;95(22):13290–5.

103. Rajkowska G. Postmortem studies in mood disorders indicate altered numbers of neurons and glial cells. Biol Psychiatry 2000;48(8):766–77.

104. McKinnon MC, Yucel K, Nazarov A, et al. A meta-analysis examining clinical predictors of hippocampal volume in patients with major depressive disorder. J Psychiatry Neurosci 2009;34(1):41–54.

105. Bremner JD, Narayan M, Anderson ER, et al. Hippocampal volume reduction in major depression. Am J Psychiatr 2000;157(1):115–8.

106. Campbell S, Marriott M, Nahmias C, et al. Lower hippocampal volume in patients suffering from depression: a meta-analysis. Am J Psychiatr 2004;161(4):598–607.

107. Cole J, Toga AW, Hojatkashani C, et al. Subregional hippocampal deformations in major depressive disorder. J Affect Disord 2010;126(1/2):272–7.

108. de Asis JM, Stern E, Alexopoulos GS, et al. Hippocampal and anterior cingulate activation deficits in patients with geriatric depression. Am J Psychiatr 2001;158(8):1321–3.

109. Vakili K, Pillay SS, Lafer B, et al. Hippocampal volume in primary unipolar major depression: a magnetic resonance imaging study. Biol Psychiatry 2000;47(12):1087–90.

110. Neumeister A, Charney DS, Drevets WC. Hippocampus, VI. Depression and the hippocampus. Am J Psychiatr 2005;162(6):1057.

111. Feder A, Nestler EJ, Charney DS. Psychobiology and molecular genetics of resilience. Nat Rev Neurosci 2009;10(6):446–57.

112. Frodl T, Meisenzahl EM, Zetzsche T, et al. Hippocampal changes in patients with a first episode of major depression. Am J Psychiatr 2002;159(7): 1112–8.

113. Drevets W, Gadde K, Krishnan K. Neuroimaging studies of mood disorders. In: Charney DS, Nestler EJ, Bunney BJ, editors. The neurobiological foundation of mental illness. New York: Oxford University Press; 2004. p. 461–90.

114. Drevets WC. Neuroimaging abnormalities in the amygdala in mood disorders. Ann N Y Acad Sci 2003;985:420–44.

115. Sheline YI, Gado MH, Price JL. Amygdala core nuclei volumes are decreased in recurrent major depression. Neuroreport 1998;9(9):2023–8.

116. Bowley MP, Drevets WC, Ongür D, et al. Low glial numbers in the amygdala in major depressive disorder. Biol Psychiatry 2002;52(5):404–12.

117. Krishnan KR, McDonald WM, Escalona PR, et al. Magnetic resonance imaging of the caudate nuclei in depression. Preliminary observations. Arch Gen Psychiatry 1992;49(7):553–7.

118. Baumann B, Danos P, Krell D, et al. Reduced volume of limbic system-affiliated basal ganglia in mood disorders: preliminary data from a post-mortem study. J Neuropsychiatry Clin Neurosci 1999;11(1):71–8.

119. Carlson PJ, Singh JB, Zarate CA Jr, et al. Neural circuitry and neuroplasticity in mood disorders: insights for novel therapeutic targets. NeuroRx 2006;3(1):22–41.

120. Krishnan KR, McDonald WM, Doraiswamy PM, et al. Neuroanatomical substrates of depression in the elderly. Eur Arch Psychiatry Clin Neurosci 1993;243(1):41–6.

121. Aylward EH, Roberts-Twillie JV, Barta PE, et al. Basal ganglia volumes and white matter hyperintensities in patients with bipolar disorder. Am J Psychiatr 1994;151(5):687–93.

122. Bonelli RM, Kapfhammer HP, Pillay SS, et al. Basal ganglia volumetric studies in affective disorder: what did we learn in the last 15 years? J Neural Transm 2006;113(2):255–68.

123. Bhatia KP, Daniel SE, Marsden CD. Familial parkinsonism with depression: a clinicopathological study. Ann Neurol 1993;34(6):842–7.

124. Martinelli P, Giuliani S, Ippoliti M, et al. Familial idiopathic strio-pallido-dentate calcifications with late onset extrapyramidal syndrome. Mov Disord 1993;8(2):220–2.

125. Drevets WC. Functional neuroimaging studies of depression: the anatomy of melancholia. Annu Rev Med 1998;49:341–61.

126. Baxter LR Jr, Phelps ME, Mazziotta JC, et al. Cerebral metabolic rates for glucose in mood disorders. Studies with positron emission tomography and flu-orodeoxyglucose F 18. Arch Gen Psychiatry 1985; 42(5):441–7.

127. Buchsbaum MS. Brain imaging in the search for biological markers in affective disorder. J Clin Psychiatr 1986;47(Suppl):7–12.

128. Ketter TA, George MS, Kimbrell TA, et al. Functional brain imaging, limbic function, and affective disorders. Neuroscientist 1996;2(1):55–65.

129. Bench CJ, Friston KJ, Brown RG, et al. The anatomy of melancholia–focal abnormalities of cerebral blood flow in major depression. Psychol Med 1992;22(3):607–15.

130. Mayberg HS. Limbic-cortical dysregulation: a proposed model of depression. J Neuropsychiatry Clin Neurosci 1997;9(3):471–81.

131. Goldapple K, Segal Z, Garson C, et al. Modulation of cortical-limbic pathways in major depression: treatment-specific effects of cognitive behavior therapy. Arch Gen Psychiatry 2004;61(1):34–41.

132. Bewernick BH, Hurlemann R, Matusch A, et al. Nucleus accumbens deep brain stimulation decreases ratings of depression and anxiety in treatment-resistant depression. Biol Psychiatry 2010;67(2):110–6.

133. Blumberg HP, Stern E, Martinez D, et al. Increased anterior cingulate and caudate activity in bipolar mania. Biol Psychiatry 2000;48(11):1045–52.

134. Blumberg HP, Stern E, Ricketts S, et al. Rostral and orbital prefrontal cortex dysfunction in the manic state of bipolar disorder. Am J Psychiatr 1999; 156(12):1986–8.

135. Thayer JF, Lane RD. A model of neurovisceral integration in emotion regulation and dysregulation. J Affect Disord 2000;61(3):201–16.

136. Bush G, Luu P, Posner MI. Cognitive and emotional influences in anterior cingulate cortex. Trends Cogn Sci 2000;4(6):215–22.

137. George MS, Ketter TA, Parekh PI, et al. Blunted left cingulate activation in mood disorder subjects during a response interference task (the Stroop). J Neuropsychiatry Clin Neurosci 1997;9(1):55–63.

138. Pizzagalli DA, Oakes TR, Fox AS, et al. Functional but not structural subgenual prefrontal cortex abnormalities in melancholia. Mol Psychiatry 2004;9(4):393–405.

139. Mayberg HS. Clinical correlates of PET- and SPECT-identified defects in dementia. J Clin Psychiatr 1994;55(Suppl):12–21.

140. Kumar A, Newberg A, Alavi A, et al. Regional cerebral glucose metabolism in late-life depression and Alzheimer disease: a preliminary positron emission tomography study. Proc Natl Acad Sci U S A 1993; 90(15):7019–23.

141. Liotti M, Mayberg HS. The role of functional neuroimaging in the neuropsychology of depression. J Clin Exp Neuropsychol 2001;23(1):121–36.

142. Anand A, Li Y, Wang Y, et al. Activity and connectivity of brain mood regulating circuit in depression: a functional magnetic resonance study. Biol Psychiatry 2005;57(10):1079–88.

143. Kumano H, Ida I, Oshima A, et al. Brain metabolic changes associated with predisposition to onset of

major depressive disorder and adjustment disorder in cancer patients–a preliminary PET study. J Psychiatr Res 2007;41(7):591–9.

144. Siegle GJ, Carter CS, Thase ME. Use of FMRI to predict recovery from unipolar depression with cognitive behavior therapy. Am J Psychiatr 2006; 163(4):735–8.

145. Kennedy SH, Evans KR, Krüger S, et al. Changes in regional brain glucose metabolism measured with positron emission tomography after paroxetine treatment of major depression. Am J Psychiatr 2001;158(6):899–905.

146. Beauregard M, Leroux JM, Bergman S, et al. The functional neuroanatomy of major depression: an fMRI study using an emotional activation paradigm. Neuroreport 1998;9(14):3253–8.

147. George MS, Ketter TA, Parekh PI, et al. Regional blood-flow correlates of transient self-induced sadness or happiness. Biol Psychiatry 1994;35(9):647.

148. Fu CH, Williams SC, Cleare AJ, et al. Neural responses to sad facial expressions in major depression following cognitive behavioral therapy. Biol Psychiatry 2008;64(6):505–12.

149. Damasio AR. Descartes' error: emotion, reason, and the human brain. New York: Avon Books; 1994.

150. Osuch EA, Ketter TA, Kimbrell TA, et al. Regional cerebral metabolism associated with anxiety symptoms in affective disorder patients. Biol Psychiatry 2000;48(10):1020–3.

151. Drevets WC, Bogers W, Raichle ME. Functional anatomical correlates of antidepressant drug treatment assessed using PET measures of regional glucose metabolism. Eur Neuropsychopharmacol 2002;12(6):527–44.

152. Nobler MS, Oquendo MA, Kegeles LS, et al. Decreased regional brain metabolism after ECT. Am J Psychiatr 2001;158(2):305–8.

153. Mayberg HS, Lozano AM, Voon V, et al. Deep brain stimulation for treatment-resistant depression. Neuron 2005;45(5):651–60.

154. Mayberg HS. Modulating dysfunctional limbic-cortical circuits in depression: towards development of brain-based algorithms for diagnosis and optimised treatment. Br Med Bull 2003;65:193–207.

155. Thomas KM, Drevets WC, Dahl RE, et al. Amygdala response to fearful faces in anxious and depressed children. Arch Gen Psychiatry 2001; 58(11):1057–63.

156. Siegle GJ, Thompson W, Carter CS, et al. Increased amygdala and decreased dorsolateral prefrontal BOLD responses in unipolar depression: related and independent features. Biol Psychiatry 2007;61(2):198–209.

157. Malberg JE, Eisch AJ, Nestler EJ, et al. Chronic antidepressant treatment increases neurogenesis in adult rat hippocampus. J Neurosci 2000; 20(24):9104–10.

158. Price JL, Carmichael ST, Drevets WC. Networks related to the orbital and medial prefrontal cortex; a substrate for emotional behavior? Prog Brain Res 1996;107:523–36.

159. Baxter LR Jr, Schwartz JM, Phelps ME, et al. Reduction of prefrontal cortex glucose metabolism common to three types of depression. Arch Gen Psychiatry 1989;46(3):243–50.

160. Strakowski SM, Delbello MP, Adler CM. The functional neuroanatomy of bipolar disorder: a review of neuroimaging findings. Mol Psychiatry 2005; 10(1):105–16.

161. Epstein J, Pan H, Kocsis JH, et al. Lack of ventral striatal response to positive stimuli in depressed versus normal subjects. Am J Psychiatr 2006; 163(10):1784–90.

162. McCabe C, Cowen PJ, Harmer CJ. Neural representation of reward in recovered depressed patients. Psychopharmacology (Berl) 2009;205(4): 667–77.

163. Forbes EE, Dahl RE. Neural systems of positive affect: relevance to understanding child and adolescent depression? Dev Psychopathol 2005; 17(3):827–50.

164. Harvey PO, Pruessner J, Czechowska Y, et al. Individual differences in trait anhedonia: a structural and functional magnetic resonance imaging study in non-clinical subjects. Mol Psychiatry 2007; 12(8):703, 767–75.

165. Beck AT. The evolution of the cognitive model of depression and its neurobiological correlates. Am J Psychiatr 2008;165(8):969–77.

166. Dichter GS, Felder JN, Petty C, et al. The effects of psychotherapy on neural responses to rewards in major depression. Biol Psychiatry 2009;66:886–97.

167. Paulus MP, Stein MB. Interoception in anxiety and depression. Brain Struct Funct 2010;214(5/6): 451–63.

168. Craig AD. Interoception: the sense of the physiological condition of the body. Curr Opin Neurobiol 2003;13(4):500–5.

169. Craig AD. Emotional moments across time: a possible neural basis for time perception in the anterior insula. Philos Trans R Soc Lond B Biol Sci 2009;364(1525):1933–42.

170. Craig AD. Interoception and emotion. In: Lewis M, Haviland-Jones JM, Feldman Barrett L, editors. Handbook of emotions. New York: Guilford Press; 2008. p. 272–88.

171. Critchley HD, Wiens S, Rotshtein P, et al. Neural systems supporting interoceptive awareness. Nat Neurosci 2004;7(2):189–95.

172. Wiebking C, Bauer A, de Greck M, et al. Abnormal body perception and neural activity in the insula in depression: an fMRI study of the depressed "material me". World J Biol Psychiatry 2010;11(3): 538–49.

173. Lee KH, Siegle GJ. Common and distinct brain networks underlying explicit emotional evaluation: a meta-analytic study. Soc Cogn Affect Neurosci 2009. [Epub ahead of print].

174. Phillips ML, Drevets WC, Rauch SL, et al. Neurobiology of emotion perception. I: The neural basis of normal emotion perception. Biol Psychiatry 2003; 54(5):504–14.

175. Davidson RJ, Irwin W, Anderle MJ, et al. The neural substrates of affective processing in depressed patients treated with venlafaxine. Am J Psychiatr 2003;160(1):64–75.

176. Buckner RL, Andrews-Hanna JR, Schacter DL. The brain's default network: anatomy, function, and relevance to disease. Ann N Y Acad Sci 2008; 1124:1–38.

177. Raichle ME, Snyder AZ. A default mode of brain function. Proc Natl Acad Sci U S A 2001;98(2): 676–82.

178. Biswal B, Yetkin FZ, Haughton VM, et al. Functional connectivity in the motor cortex of resting human brain using echo-planar MRI. Magn Reson Med 1995;34(4):537–41.

179. Greicius MD, Supekar K, Menon V, et al. Resting-state functional connectivity reflects structural connectivity in the default mode network. Cereb Cortex 2009;19(1):72–8.

180. Shehzad Z, Kelly AM, Reiss PT, et al. The resting brain: unconstrained yet reliable. Cereb Cortex 2009;19(10):2209–29.

181. Andrews-Hanna JR, Reidler JS, Huang C, et al. Evidence for the default network's role in spontaneous cognition. J Neurophysiol 2010;104(1): 322–35.

182. Gusnard DA, Akbudak E, Shulman GL, et al. Medial prefrontal cortex and self-referential mental activity: relation to a default mode of brain function. Proc Natl Acad Sci U S A 2001;98(7):4259–64.

183. Mason MF, Norton MI, Van Horn JD, et al. Wandering minds: the default network and stimulus-independent thought. Science 2007;315(5810): 393–5.

184. Fox MD, Raichle ME. Spontaneous fluctuations in brain activity observed with functional magnetic resonance imaging. Nat Rev Neurosci 2007;8(9): 700–11.

185. Northoff G, Heinzel A, de Greck M, et al. Self-referential processing in our brain–a meta-analysis of imaging studies on the self. Neuroimage 2006; 31(1):440–57.

186. Greicius MD, Flores BH, Menon V, et al. Resting-state functional connectivity in major depression: abnormally increased contributions from subgenual cingulate cortex and thalamus. Biol Psychiatry 2007;62(5):429–37.

187. Grimm S, Boesiger P, Beck J, et al. Altered negative BOLD responses in the default-mode network during emotion processing in depressed subjects. Neuropsychopharmacology 2009;34(4):932–843.

188. Sheline YI, Price JL, Yan Z, et al. Resting-state functional MRI in depression unmasks increased connectivity between networks via the dorsal nexus. Proc Natl Acad Sci U S A 2010;107(24):11020–5.

189. Broyd SJ, Demanuele C, Debener S, et al. Default-mode brain dysfunction in mental disorders: a systematic review. Neurosci Biobehav Rev 2009;33(3):279–96.

190. Berman MG, Peltier S, Nee DE, et al. Depression, rumination and the default network. Soc Cogn Affect Neurosci 2010. [Epub ahead of print].

191. Chepenik LG, Raffo M, Hampson M, et al. Functional connectivity between ventral prefrontal cortex and amygdala at low frequency in the resting state in bipolar disorder. Psychiatry Res 2010;182(3):207–10.

192. Hasler G, van der Veen JW, Tumonis T, et al. Reduced prefrontal glutamate/glutamine and gamma-aminobutyric acid levels in major depression determined using proton magnetic resonance spectroscopy. Arch Gen Psychiatry 2007;64(2): 193–200.

193. Horn DI, Yu C, Steiner J, et al. Glutamatergic and resting-state functional connectivity correlates of severity in major depression - the role of pregenual anterior cingulate cortex and anterior insula. Front Syst Neurosci 2010;4:33.

194. Ende G, Demirakca T, Tost H. The biochemistry of dysfunctional emotions: proton MR spectroscopic findings in major depressive disorder. Prog Brain Res 2006;156:481–501.

195. Moore CM, Breeze JL, Gruber SA, et al. Choline, myo-inositol and mood in bipolar disorder: a proton magnetic resonance spectroscopic imaging study of the anterior cingulate cortex. Bipolar Disord 2000;2(3 Pt 2):207–16.

196. Koenigs M, Grafman J. The functional neuroanatomy of depression: distinct roles for ventromedial and dorsolateral prefrontal cortex. Behav Brain Res 2009;201(2):239–43.

197. Drevets WC. Functional anatomical abnormalities in limbic and prefrontal cortical structures in major depression. Prog Brain Res 2000;126:413–31.

198. Mayberg HS. Modulating limbic-cortical circuits in depression: targets of antidepressant treatments. Semin Clin Neuropsychiatry 2002;7(4):255–68.

199. Price JL. Prefrontal cortical networks related to visceral function and mood. Ann N Y Acad Sci 1999;877:383–96.

200. Mashour GA, Walker EE, Martuza RL. Psychosurgery: past, present, and future. Brain Res Rev 2005;48(3):409–19.

201. Delgado MR, Olsson A, Phelps EA. Extending animal models of fear conditioning to humans. Biol Psychol 2006;73(1):39–48.

202. Vallenstein ES. History of psychosurgery. In: Greenblatt SH, editor. The history of neurosurgery. Park Ridge (IL): AANS; 1997. p. 499–516.

203. Bechara A, Damasio H, Damasio AR. Emotion, decision making and the orbitofrontal cortex. Cereb Cortex 2000;10(3):295–307.

204. Andersen SL, Teicher MH. Stress, sensitive periods and maturational events in adolescent depression. Trends Neurosci 2008;31(4):183–91.

205. Hare TA, Tottenham N, Galvan A, et al. Biological substrates of emotional reactivity and regulation in adolescence during an emotional go-nogo task. Biol Psychiatry 2008;63(10):927–34.

206. Maller JJ, Thomson RH, Lewis PM, et al. Traumatic brain injury, major depression, and diffusion tensor imaging: making connections. Brain Res Rev 2010; 64(1):213–40.

207. Charney DS. Psychobiological mechanisms of resilience and vulnerability: implications for successful adaptation to extreme stress. Am J Psychiatr 2004;161(2):195–216.

208. Goldman-Rakic PS. The prefrontal landscape: implications of functional architecture for understanding human mentation and the central executive. Philos Trans R Soc Lond B Biol Sci 1996;351(1346):1445–53.

209. Drevets WC. Neuroimaging and neuropathological studies of depression: implications for the cognitive-emotional features of mood disorders. Curr Opin Neurobiol 2001;11(2):240–9.

210. Seminowicz DA, Mayberg HS, McIntosh AR, et al. Limbic-frontal circuitry in major depression: a path modeling metanalysis. Neuroimage 2004; 22(1):409–18.

211. Ochsner KN, Gross JJ. The cognitive control of emotion. Trends Cogn Sci 2005;9(5):242–9.

212. Larson PS. Deep brain stimulation for psychiatric disorders. Neurotherapeutics 2008;5(1):50–8.

213. Nitsche MA, Boggio PS, Fregni F, et al. Treatment of depression with transcranial direct current stimulation (tDCS): a review. Exp Neurol 2009;219(1): 14–9.

214. Mayberg HS. Targeted electrode-based modulation of neural circuits for depression. J Clin Invest 2009;119(4):717–25.

215. Anderson CA, Arciniegas DB. Neurosurgical interventions for neuropsychiatric syndromes. Curr Psychiatry Rep 2004;6(5):355–63.

216. Feldman RP, Goodrich JT. Psychosurgery: a historical overview. Neurosurgery 2001;48(3):647–57 [discussion: 657–9].

217. Pressman JD. Last resort: psychosurgery and the limits of medicine. New York: Cambridge University Press; 1998.

218. Vallenstein ES. Great and desperate cures. The rise and decline of psychosurgery and other radical treatments for mental illness. New York: Basic Books; 1986.

219. Malhi GS, Bartlett JR. Depression: a role for neurosurgery? Br J Neurosurg 2000;14(5):415–22 [discussion: 423].

220. Bridges PK. Investigating psychosurgery. Br J Psychiatr 1990;157:619.

221. Hodgkiss AD, Malizia AL, Bartlett JR, et al. Outcome after the psychosurgical operation of stereotactic subcaudate tractotomy, 1979–1991. J Neuropsychiatry Clin Neurosci 1995;7(2): 230–4.

222. Feldman RP, Alterman RL, Goodrich JT. Contemporary psychosurgery and a look to the future. J Neurosurg 2001;95(6):944–56.

223. Marino Junior R, Cosgrove GR. Neurosurgical treatment of neuropsychiatric illness. Psychiatr Clin North Am 1997;20(4):933–43.

224. Tye SJ, Frye MA, Lee KH. Disrupting disordered neurocircuitry: treating refractory psychiatric illness with neuromodulation. Mayo Clin Proc 2009;84(6): 522–32.

225. Schlaepfer TE, Cohen MX, Frick C, et al. Deep brain stimulation to reward circuitry alleviates anhedonia in refractory major depression. Neuropsychopharmacology 2008;33(2):368–77.

226. Levkovitz Y, Harel EV, Roth Y, et al. Deep transcranial magnetic stimulation over the prefrontal cortex: evaluation of antidepressant and cognitive effects in depressive patients. Brain Stimul 2009;2(4): 188–200.

227. Rosenberg O, Zangen A, Stryjer R, et al. Response to deep TMS in depressive patients with previous electroconvulsive treatment. Brain Stimul 2010; 3(4):211–7.

228. Slotema CW, Blom JD, Hoek HW, et al. Should we expand the toolbox of psychiatric treatment methods to include repetitive transcranial magnetic stimulation (rTMS)? A meta-analysis of the efficacy of rTMS in psychiatric disorders. J Clin Psychiatr 2010;71(7):873–84.

229. Nadeau SE, McCoy KJ, Crucian GP, et al. Cerebral blood flow changes in depressed patients after treatment with repetitive transcranial magnetic stimulation: evidence of individual variability. Neuropsychiatry Neuropsychol Behav Neurol 2002;15(3):159–75.

230. Gershon AA, Dannon PN, Grunhaus L. Transcranial magnetic stimulation in the treatment of depression. Am J Psychiatr 2003;160(5):835–45.

231. Pascual-Leone A, Rubio B, Pallardó F, et al. Rapid-rate transcranial magnetic stimulation of left dorsolateral prefrontal cortex in drug-resistant depression. Lancet 1996;348(9022):233–7.

232. D'Agati D, Bloch Y, Levkovitz Y, et al. rTMS for adolescents: safety and efficacy considerations. Psychiatry Res 2010;177(3):280–5.

233. Gavrilov LR, Tsirulnikov EM, Davies IA. Application of focused ultrasound for the stimulation of

neural structures. Ultrasound Med Biol 1996; 22(2):179–92.

234. Martin E, Jeanmonod D, Morel A, et al. High-intensity focused ultrasound for noninvasive functional neurosurgery. Ann Neurol 2009;66(6): 858–61.

235. Gunther M, Phillips KD. Cranial electrotherapy stimulation for the treatment of depression. J Psychosoc Nurs Ment Health Serv 2010;48(11):37–42.

236. Lefaucheur JP. Principles of therapeutic use of transcranial and epidural cortical stimulation. Clin Neurophysiol 2008;119(10):2179–84.

237. Hung CW, Liou YJ, Lu SW, et al. Stem cell-based neuroprotective and neurorestorative strategies. Int J Mol Sci 2010;11(5):2039–55.

238. Alexander B, Warner-Schmidt J, Eriksson T, et al. Reversal of depressed behaviors in mice by p11 gene therapy in the nucleus accumbens. Sci Transl Med 2010;2(54):54ra76.

239. Fu CH, Williams SC, Cleare AJ, et al. Attenuation of the neural response to sad faces in major depression by antidepressant treatment: a prospective, event-related functional magnetic resonance imaging study. Arch Gen Psychiatry 2004;61(9):877–89.

Development of a Clinical Functional Magnetic Resonance Imaging Service

Laura Rigolo, MA[a,b], Emily Stern, MD[c],
Pamela Deaver, MD[b], Alexandra J. Golby, MD[a,b],
Srinivasan Mukundan Jr, PhD, MD[b,*]

KEYWORDS

- fMRI • BOLD imaging • Stimulus delivery • CPT

From the discovery of the Roentgen Ray more than a century ago, the primary focus of radiology has been the noninvasive demonstration of structural anatomy of the human body. Through the demonstration of alterations of normal anatomy, the identification of pathologic conditions was elicited. The wide availability of cross-sectional imaging modalities, first with computed tomography (CT) followed by magnetic resonance imaging (MRI), resulted in marked improvements in the quality of the depiction of anatomic structures in 3-dimensional (3D) space. The anatomic region most affected by these techniques was the neuraxis, which had been previously hidden by the calvarium and vertebral column.

As this issue of the *Clinics* demonstrates, a new focus on physiologic imaging has developed over the past 2 decades. Through these methods, the imaging aim has shifted from the demonstration of anatomy to the evaluation of physiology. Many of these so-called functional imaging approaches are being refined, including the imaging of blood flow (perfusion), specific metabolites (spectroscopy), and regional blood oxygenation (blood oxygen level–dependent, or BOLD imaging). Taken as a whole, each of these methods can be considered as functional imaging, although the aim of this article is to describe approaches involving BOLD imaging.

As more completely described elsewhere in this issue, BOLD imaging is based on a phenomenon first described by Roy and Sherrington[1] in Cambridge in 1890, demonstrating that neural activation induces increased blood flow in the blood vessels supplying and draining that area of cerebral cortex. This phenomenon remained unexploited for nearly a century until the development of positron emission tomography (PET) imaging in the 1980s. The phenomenon was further leveraged with the development of BOLD functional MRI (fMRI) in 1990.[2] The power of the BOLD method was made evident in early studies when regions of brain activation associated with various motor, sensory, visual, and language tasks were mapped in normal subjects.[3] These early demonstrations of feasibility were followed by the development of paradigms used to evaluate pathologic states, including brain tumors, multiple sclerosis, strokes, epilepsy, and Alzheimer disease.

The fMRI technique remained largely a research modality until 2007, when the Centers for Medicare and Medicaid Services (CMS) issued 3 separate current procedural terminology (CPT) codes for its clinical use (**Table 1**). The recommendation

[a] Department of Neurosurgery, Brigham and Women's Hospital, Harvard Medical School, 75 Francis Street, Boston, MA 02115, USA
[b] Department of Radiology, Brigham and Women's Hospital, Harvard Medical School, 75 Francis Street, Boston, MA 02115, USA
[c] Department of Radiology, fMRI Service, Functional and Molecular Neuroimaging, Brigham & Women's Hospital/Harvard Medical School, 824 Boylston Street, Chestnut Hill, MA 02143, USA
* Corresponding author.
E-mail address: smukundan@partners.org

Neurosurg Clin N Am 22 (2011) 307–314
doi:10.1016/j.nec.2011.01.001

Table 1
Summary of the CPT codes for fMRI

CPT Code	Description
70554	Functional MRI selected and performed by a technologist. Do not report with CPT 96020 or CPT 70555.
70555	Complex paradigms for fMRI selected and performed by a physician or psychologist, involving neurofunctional testing. Report with CPT 96020.
96020	Neurofunctional testing by physician or psychologist, with review of results and report. Report with CPT 70555.

for the development of CPT codes was based largely on experience at major academic medical centers that had begun to use fMRI as a presurgical technique for mapping eloquent regions of the brain, typically under the auspices of a protocol approved by the institutional review board. Using this approach, the typical study consisted of developing fMRI paradigms for the identification of motor areas, speech centers, and sensory regions that should be avoided by the surgeon during a craniotomy. This development of clinical CPT codes has led to significantly increased interest in the use of fMRI by clinicians and consequent increases in the number of studies ordered in many institutions. The aim of this short article is to describe both the rationale for establishing a clinical fMRI service and the basic requirements for hardware and software. In addition, there is a short discussion on the implementation of the CPT codes.

RATIONALE FOR ESTABLISHING AN FMRI CENTER IN SUPPORT OF BRAIN TUMOR CENTERS

According to the Brain Tumor Society, there are in excess of 200,000 newly diagnosed brain tumors (primary or metastatic) each year within the United States. Despite significant advances in both chemotherapy and radiation treatments, neurosurgery remains the preeminent treatment modality in most cases. Numerous outcomes of gross-total resection of a brain tumor include relief of mass effect, decreased risk of epilepsy, increased time to tumor progression, and increased survival.[4–6] However, the preoperative goal of gross-total resection can be thwarted intraoperatively by the difficulty in determining tumor boundaries. This is

particularly true for infiltrating gliomas, which may be difficult to distinguish from healthy brain due to indistinct infiltrative margins with healthy brain parenchyma. Moreover, the proximity of tumor to eloquent brain carries the risk of functional loss after surgery, if those regions are violated. By mapping the boundaries of eloquent brain in the context of tumor-distorted anatomy, neurofunctional testing approaches have been used over the past 25 years to improve surgical outcomes.

Functional Imaging

fMRI is a noninvasive MR-based brain mapping technique that requires no exogenous contrast agents. Through the investment in a minimal amount of hardware and software that can be obtained at incremental cost, fMRI can be added to most existing MR scanners. Evaluation of multiple functions is feasible in patients with cerebral tumors using fMRI,[7] and preoperative maps depicting brain areas activated during motor, sensory, and language tasks can be obtained using task paradigms specific to the function or functions of interest. Typical paradigms include motor mapping (eg, hand clenching, finger tapping, toe movement), language (word generation, sentence completion, and similar tasks), and visual stimulation (typically a flashing checkerboard or annulus). The resulting maps are useful for presurgical planning and can be integrated into neuronavigation systems to guide intraoperative decision making (**Fig. 1**).[8–17] Strong evidence that a more radical tumor resection may be

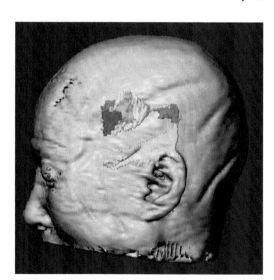

Fig. 1. An example of intraoperative display of BOLD data. The tumor volume (*green*), language task BOLD activations (*pink*), and DTI-based fiber tractography (*yellow*) are displayed as 3D renderings.

achieved by using fMRI information during neuro-surgery has been demonstrated by Krishnan and colleagues[11] and Haberg and colleagues.[18] Diffusion tensor imaging (DTI)–based tractography has recently emerged as another potentially valuable tool to visualize white matter anatomy for preoperative planning[19–25] and postoperative follow-up[26] of surgically treated brain tumors and vascular malformations (**Fig. 2**). In addition, the use of fMRI has been shown to significantly reduce operative time and facilitate preoperative decision making as to whether to perform surgeries awake or under general anesthesia.[27]

SOFTWARE AND HARDWARE REQUIREMENTS

Although most mid-field and high-field MRI scanners in clinical use are capable of performing fMRI, most require upgrades of scanner software and hardware to perform the imaging. In addition, software "keys" for specialized pulse sequences required for performing fMRI on the MRI scanner, such as BOLD or DTI echo planar sequences, may be required. Specialized software is required for both administering the test and interpreting the test results properly. These results are discussed separately later. There is also a specific need for specially trained individuals to administer and interpret the test.

Stimulus Delivery Software and Hardware

The specialized software required for performing the study is known as stimulus delivery software. This software handles several tasks that are not part of standard MRI studies. Specifically, the software must perform 3 tasks: (1) synchronize with the MRI scanner software to initiate the proper pulse sequences to be performed by the scanner at the appropriate time, (2) provide the appropriate stimulus to the subject to activate the brain area of interest at the proper time, and (3) record any

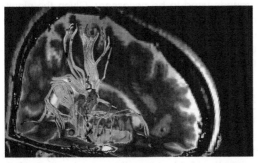

Fig. 2. DTI tractography (tubes) with tract seed point (*red sphere*), the segmented tumor volume (*transparent green*), and a proximal fMRI activation.

associated data, such as feedback from response devices, at the appropriate times. To perform these tasks, there are many solutions offered by both the original equipment manufacturers (OEMs) and third parties.

The ability to synchronize with the native scanner software to perform the appropriate pulse sequence is central to the fMRI experiment. The synchronization is critical because precise knowledge of the task timing relative to image acquisition is required to tease out the small signal differences between task and control conditions. When using OEM stimulus software, it may reside on the scanner console itself. In contrast, when using third-party stimulus software, it typically resides on another computer that is linked to the scanner computer, usually through a specialized hardware synchronization device (**Fig. 3**).

There are several different stimulus devices that are available that may need to be powered by the stimulus software. In many instances, visual stimuli are provided to the subject, as such, several different kinds of visual display devices may potentially be used. Typically a video projector or special MRI-compatible eye goggles are used to display a visual stimulus at appropriate times to the subject (see **Fig. 3**). More recently, several vendors have developed MRI-compatible high-definition liquid crystal display (HD-LCD) monitors. In fact, the development of the HD-LCD monitors has necessitated computer hardware upgrades because older systems do not have the high-definition video output that is capable of supporting the HD-LCD monitors. Alternatively, auditory stimuli are commonly used and delivered through nonmagnetic headsets or ear buds, and high-quality audio systems are also available for auditory stimulus presentation. The third component of the stimulus delivery software is the ability to record behavioral data and subject response data at the proper time point. The types of data recorded can be from a variety of devices, such as button boxes and eye tracking cameras (see **Fig. 3**).

Analysis Software

The analysis software generates the work product of the entire process. To be useful, it must be able to accept both BOLD datasets and high-resolution anatomic datasets. At present, analysis software typically accepts other types of data, including perfusion, DTI, and angiographic datasets. In almost all instances, the analysis software packages are run on a postprocessing workstation, whether the software has been provided by the OEM or not. The analysis software performs two

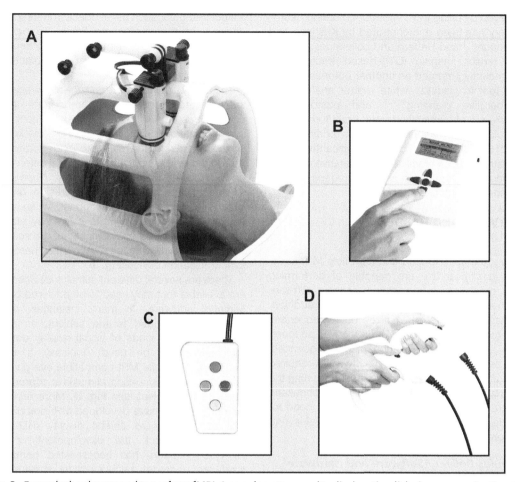

Fig. 3. Examples hardware used to perform fMRI. A goggle system used to display stimuli during an examination. (*A*) A synchronization box used to synch the paradigm and scanner. (*B*) Input devices for response recording (*C*) and (*D*).

main tasks: data reduction and data display. Software subroutines that are useful for the analysis of each of these datasets frequently include BOLD data, DTI data, and high-resolution anatomic data. It should be noted that the typical fMRI experiment generates thousands of images and that a separate data transfer protocol from the scanner to the post processing station is usually required. The images then need to be appropriately grouped according to the analytic module and statistically analyzed. Activations are then identified based on a user-defined threshold and displayed as a 3D map that is superimposed on the anatomic images. Typically, it possible to both modify the data in real time and cut planes and rotate projections viewed in the 3D and orthogonal view displays. More advanced systems allow the operator to display activations from multiple task paradigms simultaneously and toggle them on and off (**Fig. 4**).

For archival purposes, a threshold level is chosen by the user and then orthogonal views are output in digital imaging and communications in medicine format (DICOM) for loading into institutional picture archiving and communication systems (PACS). Surgeons also appreciate the ability to export the processed fMRI data to neuro-navigation systems for use intraoperatively, and this function is now frequently offered in commercial packages, although data transfer work arounds used to be necessary. Given the significant effect that these software packages have in clinical decision making, many vendors have obtained approval by US Food and Drug Administration for their clinical software packages.

Scanner Hardware Requirements

The main hardware requirement obviously is a mid-field or high-field MRI scanner (1.5–3.0 T). There is improved signal observed at higher magnetic field strengths, such that fMRI performed at 3 T MRI is of significantly higher quality than at 1.5 T.[28,29] Echo planar imaging is

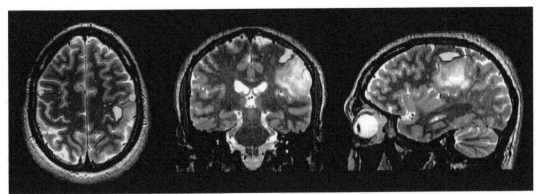

Fig. 4. An example of thresholded data used for presurgical planning from both a hand-clenching task (*red*, t = 5.31) and a finger-tapping task (*green*, t = 7.35).

typically used for fMRI, and as such, the scanner gradient coils must be capable of rapidly switching gradients. A multichannel head coil also provides improved signal acquisition over a single-channel coil. The scanner should be approved for fMRI use before implementing a program, and the pulse sequences should then be assessed according to routine quality control guidelines by the institutional MRI physicist.

Retrofitting of an existing MRI scanner to perform fMRI requires physical modifications to the scanner room. The specific hardware required for fMRI stimulus delivery should be installed. Devices for visual display include goggles, projectors, or MRI-compatible LCD panels; audio devices include headphones or ear buds, as described earlier. Frequently, optical cables are used to transfer the signals from the control room to the scanner room through a device known as a wave guide. Access to the scanning room via a penetration panel may also be necessary for other instrumentation, such as physiologic recording equipment. In addition, appropriate mounts for cameras and LCD panels may need to be installed. Once the system is set up, several test runs with control subjects should be performed to test all components and train personnel.

Personnel and Training

Personnel administering the fMRI examination need specific training to use the fMRI hardware and software, as well as training regarding methodological issues related to the functional tasks. In many cases the examinations are performed by technologists, and often, the equipment/software manufacturer provides on site training. The visual display devices must be set up to demonstrate clear images to the subject that are observed by both eyes and can stimulate all of the visual fields. Therefore, goggles are often

adjustable for the interophthalmic distance and requisite visual corrections as needed for each subject. Similarly, projectors or LCD monitors must be positioned such that the subjects can properly see them. When setting up the audio system, care must be taken to ensure that the subjects can adequately hear the presented content independently in each ear while the scanner is running.

In addition, before scanning, the technologist should instruct the patient and assist with practicing the behavioral task paradigms that will be run. This step is crucial to ensure that the tasks are performed correctly, so that the functions of interest can be assessed. Patients who are aphasic or have motor deficits may require additional coaching. Ensuring patient comfort and reducing head motion with appropriate padding are paramount because both factors can affect task performance. Task performance should also be monitored during the scanning session to ensure the task paradigms are followed. After the scan, the data need to be analyzed by the technologist or additional trained personnel.

The American College of Radiology (ACR) in collaboration with the American Society of Neuroradiology published guidelines for performing fMRI studies in 2007. In these guidelines, the physician supervising and interpreting fMRI is tasked with being clinically informed about the patient and understanding the "specific questions to be answered before the procedure to plan and perform it safely and effectively." The physician should also have experience or formal training in the performance of fMRI.

As with any MRI study, the supervising physician must understand indications, risks, and benefits of the examination, as well as the alternative imaging procedures, such as a Wada test. Risk assessment involves knowledge of patient factors, including the presence of a pacemaker or other medical device that is potentially hazardous in the MR environment. An understanding of the hazards of MRI contrast encompassing both allergies and the potential of nephrogenic systemic fibrosis in the setting of significant renal impairment is critical if contrast administration is being considered.

The physician interpreting the study should be familiar with the patient's clinical presentation, relevant prior history, and imaging studies. Obviously, the physician performing the fMRI interpretation must also have appropriate knowledge and understanding of the anatomy and pathophysiology to render a meaningful interpretation. Experience with fMRI paradigm design, selection, administration, and validation is also critical to rendering a quality interpretation. Rigorous quality assessment of every study should take into account factors such as patient compliance with the protocol and patient motion. Confounding issues such as magnetic susceptibility artifact at the skullbase or the presence of blood products or metal is essential to performing high-quality interpretation. Also, the interpreting physician must understand the BOLD effect and potential sources of neurovascular uncoupling that could cause false-negative activations.

CPT CODES

In the CPT code book in 2007, 3 new CPT codes were added for fMRI (see **Table 1**). The codes can be separated into 2 main categories: (1) simple paradigms that are performed by a technologist (70554) and (2) complex paradigms that are administered by a physician or neuropsychologist (70555 + 96020). One example of the 70554 code would be simple motor paradigms performed by a technologist without input from a physician to map motor activations. When using the second code, there are many specific criteria that must be met including the need to perform at least two fMRI paradigms, with one of the tests being designed to identify higher cognitive function running the gamut from memory and attention tasks to language to executive functioning. Moreover, the physician or psychologist is expected to select the test, demonstrate the test to the subject, administer the test, interpret the results, and consult with the referring physician. After this test is performed, the 70555 code is billed to report the fMRI portion of the study and 96020 is used to report on the neurocognitive testing. It should be noted that standard neurocognitive testing should not be performed on the same day as functional MRI. Similarly, it is the practice of the American Medical Association, which manages the CPT coding system, that standard MRI is usually not performed on the same day as the fMRI study. If such a study is to be performed on the same day as the fMRI, a separate order is required for each study and a special modifier code is used to demonstrate that MRI brain evaluation beyond the fMRI was also performed.

As with most MRI examinations, many third-party payers require that the site performing the fMRI be accredited. The main accrediting bodies in the United States include the ACR, Joint Commission on Accreditation of Health Care Organizations, Accreditation Association for Ambulatory Health Care (Accreditation Association) and the Intersocietal Commission for the Accreditation of Magnetic Resonance Laboratories. Although varying by agency, the accreditation process is comprehensive. For example, the ACR requires that sites submit deidentified images obtained from actual patient studies for quality evaluation by central readers. In addition, there are specified phantom studies that also need to be submitted.

POSITION OF PROFESSIONAL SOCIETIES

Several imaging-based professional societies have adopted positions in support of the development of clinical fMRI programs. These positions are summarized below. At present, the American Association of Neurological Surgeons and the Congress of Neurological Surgeons do not have any official policy, whereas the American Academy of Neurology and the American Society of Functional Neuroradiology are at present conducting systematic reviews of the literature and developing clinical fMRI guidelines.

Radiological Society of North America Position

According to the Radiological Society of North America (2007), fMRI is becoming the diagnostic method of choice for learning how a normal, diseased, or injured brain is working, as well as for assessing the potential risks of surgery or other invasive treatments of the brain. Physicians perform fMRI to:

- Examine the anatomy of the brain.
- Determine precisely which part of the brain is handling critical functions such as thought, speech, movement, and sensation, which is called brain mapping.
- Help assess the effects of stroke, trauma, or degenerative disease (such as Alzheimer disease) on brain function.
- Monitor the growth and function of brain tumors.

- Guide the planning of surgery, radiation therapy, or other surgical treatments for the brain.

ACR Position

In October 2007, ACR published a new practice guideline "for the Performance of Functional Magnetic Resonance Imaging of the Brain (fMRI)." The ACR states that BOLD fMRI is an appropriate method for evaluation of eloquent cortex in relation to focal brain lesions. Typically, either neoplasm or vascular malformation is the suspected lesion.

Primary indications for fMRI include:

A. Assessment of Intracranial Tumoral Disease
1. Presurgical planning, assessment of eloquent cortex (eg, language, sensory motor, visual) in relation to a tumor.
2. Surgical planning (biopsy or resection), use of fMRI data for surgical guidance or resection procedure.
3. Therapeutic follow-up, evaluation of preserved eloquent cortex.
B. Assessment of Language Functions for Epilepsy Surgery

In fact, this support by professional organizations combined with the wealth of developing literature led to CMS approving CPT codes for fMRI based on clinical indications summarized earlier.

SUMMARY

The growing body of evidence demonstrating the utility of fMRI as a means for presurgical evaluation led to the development of CPT codes for performing clinical fMRI examinations. This development has been followed by an increased demand in the number of studies ordered. Structurally, a clinical fMRI service can be established by adding additional hardware and software components to most existing mid-field and high-field MRI scanners. There is also a need for specific training for the personnel who will be performing and interpreting the examinations.

ACKNOWLEDGMENTS

This work was supported by NIH P41 RR019703, NIH P01 CA067165, The Brain Science Foundation, and the Klarman Family Foundation.

REFERENCES

1. Roy CS, Sherrington CS. On the regulation of the blood-supply of the brain. J Physiol 1890;11: 85–158 17.

2. Ogawa S, Lee TM, Kay AR, et al. Brain magnetic resonance imaging with contrast dependent on blood oxygenation. Proc Natl Acad Sci U S A 1990;87:9868–72.

3. Kwong KK, Belliveau JW, Chesler DA, et al. Dynamic magnetic resonance imaging of human brain activity during primary sensory stimulation. Proc Natl Acad Sci U S A 1992;89:5675–9.

4. Berger MS. Lesions in functional ("eloquent") cortex and subcortical white matter. Clin Neurosurg 1994; 41:444–63.

5. Claus EB, Horlacher A, Hsu L, et al. Survival rates in patients with low-grade glioma after intraoperative magnetic resonance image guidance. Cancer 2005;103:1227–33.

6. Piepmeier J, Christopher S, Spencer D, et al. Variations in the natural history and survival of patients with supratentorial low-grade astrocytomas. Neurosurgery 1996;38:872–8 [discussion: 878–9].

7. Mueller WM, Yetkin FZ, Hammeke TA, et al. Functional magnetic resonance imaging mapping of the motor cortex in patients with cerebral tumors. Neurosurgery 1996;39:515–20 [discussion: 520–1].

8. Ganslandt O, Fahlbusch R, Nimsky C, et al. Functional neuronavigation with magnetoencephalography: outcome in 50 patients with lesions around the motor cortex. J Neurosurg 1999;91:73–9.

9. Gralla J, Ganslandt O, Kober H, et al. Image-guided removal of supratentorial cavernomas in critical brain areas: application of neuronavigation and intraoperative magnetic resonance imaging. Minim Invasive Neurosurg 2003;46:72–7.

10. Jannin P, Morandi X, Fleig OJ, et al. Integration of sulcal and functional information for multimodal neuronavigation. J Neurosurg 2002;96:713–23.

11. Krishnan R, Raabe A, Hattingen E, et al. Functional magnetic resonance imaging-integrated neuronavigation: correlation between lesion-to-motor cortex distance and outcome. Neurosurgery 2004;55: 904–14 [discusssion: 914–5].

12. Lehericy S, Duffau H, Cornu P, et al. Correspondence between functional magnetic resonance imaging somatotopy and individual brain anatomy of the central region: comparison with intraoperative stimulation in patients with brain tumors. J Neurosurg 2000;92:589–98.

13. Maldjian JA, Schulder M, Liu WC, et al. Intraoperative functional MRI using a real-time neurosurgical navigation system. J Comput Assist Tomogr 1997; 21:910–2.

14. Nimsky C, Ganslandt O, Kober H, et al. Integration of functional magnetic resonance imaging supported by magnetoencephalography in functional neuronavigation. Neurosurgery 1999;44:1249–55 [discussion: 1255–6].

15. O'Shea JP, Whalen S, Branco DM, et al. Integrated image- and function-guided surgery in eloquent

cortex: a technique report. Int J Med Robot 2006;2: 75–83.

16. Reithmeier T, Krammer M, Gumprecht H, et al. Neuronavigation combined with electrophysiological monitoring for surgery of lesions in eloquent brain areas in 42 cases: a retrospective comparison of the neurological outcome and the quality of resection with a control group with similar lesions. Minim Invasive Neurosurg 2003;46:65–71.

17. Roessler K, Donat M, Lanzenberger R, et al. Evaluation of preoperative high magnetic field motor functional MRI (3 Tesla) in glioma patients by navigated electrocortical stimulation and postoperative outcome. J Neurol Neurosurg Psychiatry 2005;76: 1152–7.

18. Haberg A, Kvistad KA, Unsgard G, et al. Preoperative blood oxygen level-dependent functional magnetic resonance imaging in patients with primary brain tumors: clinical application and outcome. Neurosurgery 2004;54:902–14 [discussion: 914–5].

19. Coenen VA, Krings T, Axer H, et al. Intraoperative three-dimensional visualization of the pyramidal tract in a neuronavigation system (PTV) reliably predicts true position of principal motor pathways. Surg Neurol 2003;60:381–90 [discussion: 390].

20. Field AS, Alexander AL, Wu YC, et al. Diffusion tensor eigenvector directional color imaging patterns in the evaluation of cerebral white matter tracts altered by tumor. J Magn Reson Imaging 2004;20:555–62.

21. Holodny AI, Schwartz TH, Ollenschleger M, et al. Tumor involvement of the corticospinal tract: diffusion magnetic resonance tractography with intraoperative correlation. J Neurosurg 2001;95:1082.

22. Mori S, Frederiksen K, van Zijl PC, et al. Brain white matter anatomy of tumor patients evaluated with diffusion tensor imaging. Ann Neurol 2002;51:377–80.

23. Tummala RP, Chu RM, Liu H, et al. Application of diffusion tensor imaging to magnetic-resonance-guided brain tumor resection. Pediatr Neurosurg 2003;39: 39–43.

24. Wieshmann UC, Symms MR, Parker GJ, et al. Diffusion tensor imaging demonstrates deviation of fibres in normal appearing white matter adjacent to a brain tumour. J Neurol Neurosurg Psychiatry 2000;68: 501–3.

25. Witwer BP, Moftakhar R, Hasan KM, et al. Diffusion-tensor imaging of white matter tracts in patients with cerebral neoplasm. J Neurosurg 2002;97:568–75.

26. Field AS, Alexander AL. Diffusion tensor imaging in cerebral tumor diagnosis and therapy. Top Magn Reson Imaging 2004;15:315–24.

27. Petrella JR, Shah LM, Harris KM, et al. Preoperative functional MR imaging localization of language and motor areas: effect on therapeutic decision making in patients with potentially resectable brain tumors. Radiology 2006;240:793–802.

28. Soher BJ, Dale BM, Merkle EM. A review of MR physics: 3T versus 1.5T. Magn Reson Imaging Clin N Am 2007;15:277–90, v.

29. Tieleman A, Vandemaele P, Seurinck R, et al. Comparison between functional magnetic resonance imaging at 1.5 and 3 Tesla: effect of increased field strength on 4 paradigms used during presurgical work-up. Invest Radiol 2007;42:130–8.

Index

Neurosurg Clin N Am 22 (2011) 315–320
doi:10.1016/S1042-3680(11)00014-3
1042-3680/11/$ – see front matter © 2011 Elsevier Inc. All rights reserved.

Printed and bound by CPI Group (UK) Ltd, Croydon, CR0 4YY

03/10/2024

01040352-0001